Observing Behavior

Volume I

Theory and Applications in Mental Retardation

Proceedings of the conference, Application of Observational/Ethological Methods to the Study of Mental Retardation, held at Lake Wilderness, Washington in June 1976.

Jointly sponsored by the National Institute of Child Health and Human Development of the United States Public Health Services, and by the Child Development and Mental Retardation Center of the University of Washington.

NICHD—Mental Retardation Research Centers Series

OBSERVING BEHAVIOR

Volume I
Theory and Applications in Mental Retardation

Edited by
Gene P. Sackett, Ph.D.
Professor of Psychology
Associate Director for Behavioral Research
Child Development and Mental Retardation Center
University of Washington

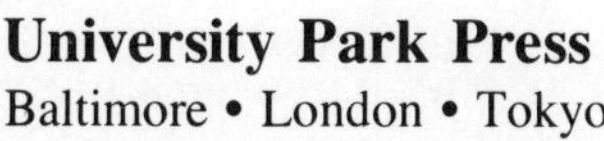
University Park Press
Baltimore • London • Tokyo
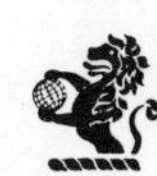

UNIVERSITY PARK PRESS
International Publishers in Science and Medicine
233 East Redwood Street
Baltimore, Maryland 21202

Typeset by The Composing Room of Michigan, Inc.
Manufactured in the United States of America by
Universal Lithographers, Inc.,
and The Optic Bindery Incorporated.

Library of Congress Cataloging in Publication Data

Main entry under title:

Observing behavior.

Bibliography: v. 2, p.
CONTENTS: v. 1. Theory and applications in mental retardation.—v. 2. Data collection and analysis methods.
1. Mental deficiency research—Congresses.
I. Sackett, Gene P. II. United States. National Institute of Child Health and Human Development. III. Washington (State). University. Child Development and Mental Retardation Center.
RC569.9.027 618.9′28′588 77-25276

ISBN 0-8391-1167-3 (v. 1)
ISBN 0-8391-1168-1 (v. 2)

Contents

Contributors

Steven R. Abernathy, M.A.
Demonstration and Research Center for Early Education (DARCEE)
The John F. Kennedy Center for Research on Education and Human Development
George Peabody College for Teachers
Nashville, Tennessee 37203

Mary Lou Ashe
Demonstration and Research Center for Early Education (DARCEE)
The John F. Kennedy Center for Research on Education and Human Development
George Peabody College for Teachers
Nashville, Tennessee 37203

Kathryn Barnard, Ph.D.
Professor of Nursing
Child Development and Mental Retardation Center
University of Washington
Seattle, Washington 98195

Patricia T. Becker
Department of Biobehavioral Sciences
The University of Connecticut
Storrs, Conneticut 06268

Gershon Berkson, Ph.D.
Illinois Institute for Developmental Disabilities
University of Illinois at Chicago Circle
Chicago, Illinois 60608

Arne T. Bjaanes, Ph.D.
Program Director
Client Centered Evaluation Model Project
Center for the Study of Community Perspectives
2831 University Avenue
Riverside, California 92502

Patricia Black-Cleworth, Ph.D.
Neuropsychiatric Institute
The Center for the Health Sciences
University of California at Los Angeles
760 Westwood Plaza
Los Angeles, California 90024

Lois Bloom, Ph.D.
Teachers College
Columbia University
New York, New York 10027

Edgar W. Butler, Ph.D.
Professor of Sociology
University of California
Riverside, California 92502

Earl C. Butterfield, Ph.D.
Professor of Pediatrics
Ralph L. Smith Center for Research in Mental Retardation
University of Kansas Medical Center
Kansas City, Kansas 66103

Joseph K. Carrier, Jr., Ph.D.
136 Linden
Fort Collins, Colorado 80521

William R. Charlesworth, Ph.D.
Institute of Child Development and Research, Development and Demonstration Center
University of Minnesota
Minneapolis, Minnesota 55455

Thomas J. Ciborowski, Ph.D.
Department of Psychology
University of Hawaii
Honolulu, Hawaii 95822

Susan Crawley
Department of Psychology
George Peabody College for Teachers
Nashville, Tennessee 37203

Philip S. Dale, Ph.D.
Department of Psychology, and Child Development and Mental Retardation Center WJ-10
University of Washington
Seattle, Washington 98195

Robert B. Edgerton, Ph.D.
The Center for the Health Sciences
University of California
760 Westwood Plaza
Los Angeles, California 90024

Gretchen Faulstich
Demonstration and Research Center for Early Education (DARCEE)
The John F. Kennedy Center for Research on Education and Human Development
George Peabody College for Teachers
Nashville, Tennessee 37203

Margaret P. Freese
Psychology Department
Indiana University
Bloomington, Indiana 47401

Jay Gottlieb, Ph.D.
Nero & Associates
1901 North Moore Street
Arlington, Virginia 22209

Bruce A. Grellong, Ph.D.
Child Development Project
Albert Einstein College of Medicine
Yeshiva University
Bronx, New York 10461

Lois Hood, Ph.D.
Department of Psychology
Program in Developmental Psychology
Teachers College
Columbia University
New York, New York 10027

Maria Iaccobo
Department of Psychology
George Peabody College for Teachers
Nashville, Tennessee 37203

Margaret Lahey, Ph.D.
Teachers College
Columbia University
New York, New York 10027

Sharon Landesman-Dwyer, Ph.D.
Department of Psychiatry and Behavioral Sciences, and Child Development and Mental Retardation Center WJ-10
University of Washington
Seattle, Washington 98195 and Office of Research
Department of Social and Health Services

Lewis L. Langness, Ph.D.
Department of Psychiatry
School of Medicine
Neuropsychiatric Institute
The Center for the Health Sciences
University of California
Los Angeles, California 90024

Karin Lifter, Ph.D.
Teachers College
Columbia University
New York, New York 10027

Thomas C. Lucas
Psychology Department
Clark University
Worcester, Massachusetts 01610

Ross D. Parke, Ph.D.
Professor of Psychology
Chairman, Division of Developmental Psychology
University of Illinois at Urbana-Champaign
Champaign, Illinois 61820

Martha Perry, Ph.D.
Department of Psychology
University of Washington
Seattle, Washington 98195

Richard H. Porter, Ph.D.
Department of Psychology, and the
John F. Kennedy Center for Research on Education and Human Development
Post Office Box 154
George Peabody College
Nashville, Tennessee 37203

Douglass R. Price-Williams, Ph.D.
Department of Psychiatry
School of Medicine The Center for the Health Sciences
University of California
Los Angeles, California 90024

Barbara Ramsey
Department of Psychology
George Peabody College for Teachers
Nashville, Tennessee 37203

Nancy M. Robinson, Ph.D.
Psychiatry and Behavioral Sciences
Child Development and Mental Retardation Center
University of Washington
Seattle, Washington 98195

Gene P. Sackett, Ph.D.
Professor of Psychology
Associate Director for Behavior Research
Child Development and Mental Retardation Center WJ-10
University of Washington
Seattle, Washington 98195

Phil Schoggen, Ph.D.
Department of Human Development
and Family Studies
New York State College of Human Ecology
Martha van Rensselear
Cornell University
Ithaca, New York 14850

Jody G. Stein
Psychiatry and Behavioral Sciences Research
Program
Behavioral Research Unit
Child Development and Mental Retardation
Center
University of Washington
Seattle, Washington 98195

Evelyn B. Thoman, Ph.D.
Department of Biobehavioral Sciences
The College of Liberal Arts and Sciences
The University of Connecticut
Storrs, Connecticut 06268

Ann Tremblay
Department of Psychology
George Peabody College for Teachers
Nashville, Tennessee 37203

Ina C. Uzgiris, Ph.D.
Department of Psychology
Clark University
Worcester, Massachusetts 01610

Peter M. Vietze, Ph.D.
Social and Behavioral Sciences Branch
National Institute of Child Health and Human
Development
Auburn Building 220
Bethesda, Maryland 22014

Foreword
Michael J. Begab, Ph.D.
Mental Retardation Program
National Institute of Child Health
and Human Development
Bethesda, Maryland 20014

Foreword

Mental retardation, whatever its etiology or the degree of its severity, is defined by manifestations in intellectual and behavioral impairment. Unfortunately, standardized instruments for measuring intelligence, although fairly predictive of school success or failure, are less useful in assessing daily problem-solving behavior. The measurement of adaptive behavior is even more complex, for adaptation is dependent, in part at least, on the demands and expectations of the environment. Environments, in turn, vary markedly from culture to subculture, between communities, and among families. Thus, an individual may adapt satisfactorily in specific behavior settings at one point in his development and not in another place at another time.

The importance of behavioral observation extends well beyond matters of classification and diagnosis, into issues of etiology and development. It is becoming increasingly apparent that biological factors associated with neonatal and perinatal distress, such as prematurity and anoxia, may be necessary but not sufficient causes of later learning deficits. These conditions, and others subsumed under the "continuum of reproductive casualty" concept, are more likely to result in developmental disorders in the presence of environmental risk factors than in healthy child-rearing conditions. Biologic stress, except in cases of severe and extensive trauma, *predisposes* to learning and behavior problems, but it is the caregiving environment that usually determines the ultimate outcome. Careful specification of living environments, especially mother-child interaction during infancy and early childhood, is vital in this regard.

The biosocial approach to behavior has great potential for identifying the origins of deviancy in the constitutional or experiential history of the individual, and for directing preventive and treatment efforts. To achieve this goal, we have yet to reconcile differential views and theories among developmental psychologists regarding continuities of functioning throughout the life span, and the relation of cognitive development to changes in structural organization at different stages of growth. Progress in this area is being made, however, and we stand today on the threshhold of new advances in the understanding of human behavior, in general, and mental retardation in particular.

Recent advances in sophisticated computer technology, statistical analysis, and techniques for observing behavior are contributing significantly to this objective. These techniques have been applied to humans and animals under natural and structured conditions in a wide range of field and laboratory settings, including homes, classrooms, hospital nurseries, institutions, day care centers, sheltered workshops, and a variety of other behavior settings. The emergence of ethology as one approach to the systematic study of the formation of human character and the growing application of ecological methods toward understanding the relationship of the human organism to its environment have markedly facilitated this process.

These conceptual and technological developments come at a most opportune time for behavioral scientists engaged in the study of retarded or potentially retarded individuals. Much of the past and current research in mental retardation has relied on standard psychometric instruments, task performance tests, questionnaires, interviews, adaptive behavior measures, and clinical judgements. Although of unquestionable value for certain purposes, these approaches tell us little about the process of adaptation or how the retarded individual applies his learning, communicative, and interpersonal skills to real life situations. Furthermore, they do not assess the setting-specific nature of most behavior nor specify the environmental context in which behavior is shaped. In addition, these data-generating strategies may not be the most feasible approach to retarded persons who lack verbal skills and cannot articulate their needs, wants, or motives.

This book represents the proceedings of a conference cosponsored by The National Institute for Child Health and Human Development and The Child Development and Mental Retardation Center at the University of Washington. It is part of an ongoing series of seminars devoted to varied topics in mental retardation and developmental disabilities that are of interest to research scientists and professional practitioners in a wide range of disciplines, to students, and to lay citizens.

Through this publication and in those preceding, the NICHD presents the most current thinking of experts in the field. It is hoped that, through this medium, the dissemination of scientific knowledge will be advanced, services will be improved, and new and promising directions for future inquiry will be stimulated.

Michael J. Begab

Preface

These two volumes were sponsored jointly by the Mental Retardation Program of the National Institute of Child Health and Human Development and the Child Development and Mental Retardation Center at the University of Washington. The books are part of a conference series organized each year by one of the 12 Mental Retardation Research Centers funded by the Mental Retardation Program. The Mental Retardation Program staff has provided administrative support and scientific expertise to these Center's Research Series volumes. This staff is headed by Dr. Theodore Tjossem, Director of the Mental Retardation Program. Our volumes owe much to the leadership of Dr. Michael J. Begab, Head, Mental Retardation Research Centers. Dr. Begab provided us with sound advice, coordination, and his professional input, from inception of the idea for the conference, through publication.

The Mental Retardation Center Program was established by an act of congress in 1963. A major goal is to solve problems of retarded people in our society through multidisciplinary research. To accomplish this goal, the Mental Retardation Research Centers were located at major universities across the United States. The Child Development and Mental Retardation Center at the University of Washington is one of these multidisciplinary facilities. Our center is an integral part of the Health Sciences Center at the University. As such, we receive administrative support from the Vice President for Health Affairs, Dr. J. Thomas Grayston, and his associate, Dr. Maureen Henderson.

We are organized in four overlapping units. A Medical and a Behavioral Research Unit consist of faculty from the health science and medical school departments, as well as the behavioral and social science faculty from the College of Arts and Sciences and the School of Social Work. Our Experimental Education Unit contains a school for retarded and similarly handicapped children who come from school districts in and around the Seattle area. This unit obtains faculty from the College of Education, trains students in special education and related fields, and conducts basic and applied research. Our Clinical Training Unit provides services to clients throughout the state of Washington. This unit trains health scientists and clinicians in areas related to mental retardation and also conducts basic and applied research. A major goal of this unit is to put into practice relevant findings from medical, behavioral, and educational investigations. Portions of the Experimental Education and Clinical Training Units form a University Affiliated Facility (UAF), which is a part of the overall Child Development and Mental Retardation Center program.

The center staff includes over 150 faculty members who receive salaries from academic departments of the University, 25 other professionals holding advanced degrees who are salaried through the center or other grants, and 350 supervisory and technical personnel who support the center research and training activities. This large staff working in the four buildings which house center programs make our facility the largest of the 12 Mental Retardation Research Centers.

The center director, Dr. Irvin Emanuel, is a pediatrician and epidemiologist who assumed his duties in 1973. His background in medical and social aspects of mental retardation has provided expert leadership in defining center goals and instituting programs for attaining these goals. Our mission is to conduct a coordinated and broad-based program of research and training in mental retardation and related aspects of human development. The goals underlying this mission are to facilitate the prevention of mental retardation and related problems of human development; to enhance the quality of life for mentally retarded and similarly handicapped persons; to help ensure that adequate numbers of specialists are available for research, training, and delivery of services necessary to prevent mental retardation and to enhance the quality of life for affected persons; and to develop exemplary professional services for retarded persons so that they may be demonstrated for the purposes of training, research, and application. Dr. Emanuel's considerable support of behavioral observation research in our center was one of the instrumental factors leading to the conference that produced these books.

The conference, Application of Observational-Ethological Methods to the Study of Mental Retardation, was held at the University of Washington Lake Wilderness Conference Center in June, 1976. The general topic concerned theoretical and methodological issues involved in using direct observation of behavior as a basic research tool. Our overall goal was to see how this tool could be used a) to enlarge the descriptive base of facts about the behavior of retarded people, and b) to test specific hypotheses under laboratory conditions and in the everyday environments of retarded people.

One motive underlying the conference came from my belief that in studying mental retardation the basic scientific phase of systematic description and fact gathering had been largely bypassed. In reviewing the rather sparse literature on *quantitative* observation of retarded people, I found that most investigations gathered data to solve a specific, immediate problem. This approach seemed incompatible with generating useful and valid descriptive facts from which general problems of individual and social behavior could be defined, studied under varied conditions, and perhaps even understood. Given these assumptions, my hope was to bring together a group or scientists interested in developing a systematic ''science of behavioral observation,'' which might have an immediate impact on the study of mental retardation.

To initiate this perhaps overly ambitious task, we invited Dr. William Charlesworth and Dr. Phil Schoggen to set the major theoretical tone for the conference. Their chapters in volume I describe ethological and ecological approaches to the study of behavior. Both theories utilize direct observation as their primary methodological tool. They also illustrate how a systematic viewpoint can be used to define the problems under study and the types of behavioral dimensions that need to be measured. These theories were also selected because their assumptions and concepts for explaining behavior seem directly applicable to many problems in mental retardation. Thus, I believed that these views might provide a focus for designing experiments to describe and understand the variations in behavioral adaptation used by retarded people living under various ecological-social conditions.

Other scientists attending the conference had either conducted observational studies on retarded people, or had developed observational techniques for testing hypotheses in areas relevant to mental retardation. Thus, the remainder of volume I consists of examples from a variety of research areas involving a wide range of observational methods. These examples serve as models illustrating research strategies to a) form testable questions, amenable to answering by direct observation of behavior, b) design behavioral coding and sampling systems for measuring the phenomena of interest, and c) choose appropriate environmental settings that might actually yield data relevant to the problem at hand. These papers were discussed in terms of their specific content area, with emphasis placed on the potential relevance of each contribution for understanding problems of mental retardation. A rapporteur was assigned to summarize the discussion of each model research area. Their comments form the basis for the introductory chapters in each section of both books.

A final set of conference participants had expertise in the major technical areas involved in collecting or analyzing observational data. With the exception of Dr. Rosenblum's presentation on "behavioral taxonomy," their papers were not formally presented at the conference. These individuals contributed by offering criticisms of methodological issues raised in the formal presentations and suggestions for improving the research methodologies. Their formal papers are presented in volume II. Although a great deal has been written concerning methodological and statistical problems in observational research, most of this material is scattered in a number of books and journals. Many of these are either not easily accessible or are presented in highly technical or mathematical form. Our goal in volume II was to describe the basics of observational methodology. The areas covered span problems of definition and category design, measurement and sampling techniques, statistical analysis, within and between observer reliabilitiy, and equipment used to collect the data. The volume is meant to be an exposition of methodology and a "laboratory" manual to aid researchers in conducting observational investigations.

Success for the conference was almost assured by typical Pacific Northwest June weather. The first day had bright sun and extremely blue skies. This was followed by 3 days of pouring rain; a major factor in actually achieving the 12-hr daily conference schedule. The sun shone again on the fifth day, allowing us to visit "nearby" Mount Rainier, one of the northwest's major tourist attractions. The conference ended with the general feeling that it is actually possible to gather an extremely heterogeneous collection of scientists together for an intensive week of productive interaction. Many of us came away with at least an understanding of the problems tackled by different disciplines if not actual agreement on the best way to approach these problems.

Conference organization and manuscript preparation relied almost exclusively on the organizational talents, foresight, and cheery goodwill of Ms. Tali Ott, Administrative Assistant to the Associate Directors at our center. Without her efforts our days or rain might have been terminally oppressive. Ms. Ott was aided in manuscript preparation by Ms. Kathleen Schmidt, Research Publications Editor at the Regional Primate Research Center, University of Washington. I am also indebted to Dr. H. Carl Haywood, Dr. Peter Vietze, and Dr. Richard Porter of the Kennedy Center for Research on Education and Human Development, George Peabody College. They provided expert assistance in selecting conference participants and planning the conference format. Finally, I must mention my wife, Barbara. With patience and understanding she looked after *all* arrangements for our wedding, which took place the day after the week-long conference ended.

Gene P. Sackett

Dedication

This book is dedicated to those past, present, and future investigators of humanity who hope to find order observing the streams of behavior emitted by people going about their everyday activities. Their greatest research pitfall—observer bias—is nicely illustrated by a story passed on by my friend, Leonard Rosenblum.

> Three umpires were asked to explain their methods for making decisions during baseball games. The first umpire, an empiricist, said, "I calls 'em the way I sees 'em." The second umpire, an optimist, insisted that, "I calls 'em the way they are." The third umpire, obviously a typical observational theorist, sagely stated "they ain't nothing 'til I calls 'em."

Ethological and Ecological Theories and their Implications for the Study of Mental Retardation

Introduction

Gene P. Sackett

During the past 10 years major advances have been made in developing quantitative methods for observing behavior. This methodology has produced data concerning the daily activities of people and animals related to social group structure and ecology. Research problems using observational procedures include social and individual behavior of human and nonhuman primates measured in laboratory and field settings; behavior of developing children in home, school, and institutional settings; pupil-teacher interactions; and interactions among family members in home, hospital, and laboratory environments. The purpose of the two volumes constituting this book is to describe theoretical issues, research problems, and methodological techniques involved in making quantitative behavioral observations that can be applied to understanding mental retardation and related behavioral handicapping conditions.

In this volume we describe two major theories—one ethological and the other ecological—which explain behavior on the basis of data collected using observational methods. These theories specify important behavioral and environmental variables that might be measured in conducting observational research on retarded subjects. We also present examples of specific observational studies designed to describe behavior and to test hypotheses in research areas relevant to mental retardation. When possible, the examples are taken from studies of mentally retarded people. However, much data in this book deal with nonretarded subjects because few investigators of mental retardation have used quantitative observational methods in their studies.

The measures reported in most of the published literature on mental retardation include scores on standard psychological tests, performance on tasks designed to measure specific intellectual or motor abilities, questionnaires, rating scales, and nonquantitative subjective evaluations. Many of these information sources have been valuable in identifying and defining skills and abilities of particular individuals and of etiological groups. However, these data do not answer questions about what mentally retarded people actually do with their motor, perceptual, learning, communicative, and social skills. Furthermore, questionnaires, rating scales, and subjective evaluations tend to have limited possibilities for identifying specific variables that do and do not support adaptive behavior in real life situations. Our major premise in this book is that quantitative observational methods can be used to address both basic research questions concerning mental retardation and to help solve practical problems of retarded people. These practical problems involve economic, political, ecological, social, and ethical decisions concerning the life styles of retarded people living in a complex society.

A major misunderstanding about quantitative observation methods concerns the distinction between laboratory and naturalistic research. Observational research is not synonymous with naturalistic investigation. The distinguishing feature of quantitative observation is that human perceptual abilities and judgments are used to identify particular responses occurring in the ongoing flow of behaviors. The particular type of environment in which observations are made does not determine whether observational or some other measurement technique will be most appropriate for solving a research question. Direct observation will be useful in natural *or* laboratory settings when either 1) there are no machines or standardized instruments that can make the required measurements, or 2) the research problem deals with behavior in situations that place few or no constraints on the responses that can be omitted by the subjects.

There is, however, one principal difference between controlled laboratory experiments and natural observation research that seems especially important for studying mental retardation. This concerns the question of what people *can do* under ideal conditions versus what they *actually do* when given the opportunity to respond freely. Laboratory experiments identify variables that might be important outside of the specific measurement setting. But these experiments cannot determine the actual importance of such variables outside the laboratory. In discussing this issue, Patterson (1977) suggests that powerful variables such as reinforcement contingencies which definitely control behavior in the laboratory may not even be attended to in real life situations. "That being the case, even the most compelling laboratory evidence attesting to the significance of [a variable] is of little moment. For final status within a theory, a variable, like a successful debutante, must put in an appearance in the real world of [everyday behavior]."

Patterson's ideas seem especially important for the study of handicapped populations. For example, until recently, severely retarded people were thought to be incapable of living independently and earning their own living. Most such individuals resided in institutions or other settings that provided 24 hr care and surveillance. A large number of experimental studies suggested that these people were untrainable in many basic adaptive skills (e.g., studies reviewed in Cleland and Talkington, 1975, 1976). However, work by Gold (1972) and by Bellamy et al. (1975) refutes many of these ideas. Gold and Bellamy successfully trained profoundly retarded people to earn a living doing assembly line work tasks while living independently in noninstitutional residences. Thus, conclusions about many of these people derived from experiments and standardized tests did not accurately predict the possible range of their actual attainments.

A major focus in this book is on such adaptive behavior involving retarded people interacting in a complex social and nonsocial world. This world provides the physical and psychological supports by which the person "makes a living." According to both ethological and ecological viewpoints, making a living consists of adjusting adaptive behavioral functions to the demands placed on a person's behavioral repertoire. Such demands may be met by simply performing behaviors that have been made a number of times in the past. However, demands made by changes in the environment or by maturation of anatomical or physiological systems may require a new set of behaviors for adaptive responding. The variables leading to successfully meeting such demands form the complex subject matter of theories dealing with the concept of adaptive behavior.

Adaptiveness has been a major concept in studies of mental retardation and forms one of the bases for classifying levels of retardation (Nihara et al., 1974). However, descriptions of adaptive behavior, and exactly what attributes constitute such behavior, seem singularly missing from the retardation literature. For example, one test purportedly measuring adaptive behavior was to drop a sheaf of papers and note whether the retarded testee picked them up. How this represents adaptive responding is unclear. There could be a number of perfectly adaptive reasons why the subject would choose not to pick up the papers.

A primary purpose of quantitative observational research is to generate information relevant to describing and identifying adaptive functions in the course of everyday person-environment transactions. Our hope is that this book and its companion volume may lead to theoretical progress in defining adaptive functions of retarded people and to an understanding of how the social and nonsocial environment allows these functions to operate successfully. We believe that this can best be done by measuring the behavior of mentally retarded people while they attempt to make a living during their daily activities.

REFERENCES

Bellamy, G. T., Peterson, L., and Close, D. W. 1975. Habilitation of the Severely and Profoundly Retarded: Illustrations of Competence. Monograph of Center on Human Development, University of Oregon, Eugene, Oregon.

Cleland, C. C., and Talkington, L. W. (eds.). 1975. Research with Profoundly Retarded: A Conference Proceedings. The Brown Schools, Austin, Texas.

Cleland, C. C., and Talkington, L. W. (eds.). 1976. Second Western Research Conference on Mental Retardation. The Brown Schools, Austin, Texas.

Gold, M. W. 1972. Stimulus factors in skill training of retarded adolescents on a complex assembly task: Acquisition, transfer, and retention. Am. J. Ment. Defic. 76:517–526.

Nihara, K., Foster, R., Shellhaas, M., and Leland, H. 1974. AAMD Adaptive Behavior Scale. American Association on Mental Deficiency, Washington, D.C.

Patterson, G. R. 1977. A performance theory for coercive family interaction. In: R. Cairns (ed.), Social Interaction: Methods, Analysis, and Illustration. Monogr. Soc. Res. Child Dev.

chapter 1

Ethology: Its Relevance for Observational Studies of Human Adaptation

William R. Charlesworth

The ethological approach to the study of behavior is discussed along with the concept of adaptation and its relevance for behavioral research in humans. The importance of studying individuals longitudinally as they interact with their environment is stressed and contrasted with more convenient and usually less expensive ways of obtaining information on adaptation, such as tests, questionnaires, and laboratory experiments. An application of the ethological approach is made in the form of studying *intelligent behavior* (cognitively guided behavior that mediates between the individual and his or her environment) rather than *intelligence,* which is a disposition measured by tests that reveal little or nothing about the role of environment in eliciting and influencing intelligent behavior, and allow only partial predictions about future adaptation. The rationale and procedure for observing intelligent behavior (defined specifically as problem-solving) in individuals as they go about their everyday activities is presented along with a pilot study of a young Down's syndrome child and a normal child. A brief summary of some of the main results is presented along with a general discussion.

As a behavioral science within biology, ethology investigates a wide range of topics and uses a wide range of methodologies shared by other sciences. Hence it is not possible to set ethology off from other disciplines in terms of a specific subject matter or approach. It is much too variegated for that. However, it is possible to view ethology as a distinct discipline engaged in an aggregate of related research activities which are guided primarily by a particular conceptual orientation, namely the synthetic theory of evolution. For a definition of ethology in these and other terms, see Eibl-Eibesfeldt, 1970; Hess, 1970; Blurton-Jones, 1972; and Freedman, 1974.

Most ethologists would probably not object if one simply defined their discipline as the complete study of behavior as it occurs in the natural habitat. What is meant by "complete" is, of course, the big question. It seems an ethological study, at minimum, has to include a detailed and comprehensive description of the nature and frequency of the animal's total behavior repertoire (or some major part of it), show an understanding of the adaptive function of the behavior and its relationship to the animal's environment, and aim for some idea of its underlying neurophysiological mechanisms. Ideally, along with all this there should also be a demonstrated awareness of the comparative status of the behavior, hence its possible evolutionary significance, as well as knowledge of its current ecological value for the individual and the species. Finally, there should be good descriptive knowledge of the development of the behavior within the individual over ontogenesis. To achieve all this, ethologists have to do many things: 1) observe and record the behavior of animals in their natural habitats, 2) analyze behavior in terms of immediate stimulus conditions and consequences, 3) investigate behavior in terms of wider social/ecological conditions, especially those bearing upon the animals' ability to survive, 4) view behavior in terms of its possible evolutionary significance and thereby its connections with the behaviors of other species, living or dead; 5) search for underlying neurophysiologic/endocrinologic mechanisms that control the behavior; and 6) view the total behavioral repertoire of the animal in terms of individual reproductive fitness and its significance for the population to which the individual belongs.

This is a big order, to say the least, but most ethologists would probably not find their curiosity about a particular animal and its behavior exhausted until these factors were satisfactorily explored. If we look closely at an animal and learn something about its phylogenetic origins, its place in the local ecology, and its physical makeup, we cannot help but be drawn further into the vast complexity of interacting factors that surround its behavior. If a "final" picture of the behavior is ever to correspond to what is directly observed and what is deduced from other observations, it must be a comprehensive, logically consistent, and empirically valid construction of everything known about the animal and its origins. The picture must be as complete as possible, and every part of it connected in some manner to every other part. In short, it must be holistic and integrative in nature, and it is this requirement that gives ethology its distinctive place in the behavioral sciences.

This ideal picture does not disclose itself after just observing a particular animal for hundreds of hours. Although observation is the bedrock requirement, the complete picture of the animal's behavior must have its conceptual basis in the synthetic theory of evolution (see Mayr, 1970). This theory, which has as its key concept *adaptation,* is based on a multitude of facts concerning dead and living animals, some related to the particular animal under study, some totally unrelated.

Furthermore, the theory is based on knowledge of the molecular nature of the chemicals of life and reproduction that constitute the genetic foundations of living things, as well as knowledge of past and present ecological conditions that affect the behavior of animals in general. In short, an ethologist studying any particular animal does so in full view of a tremendous network of ideas and data held together by the synthetic theory of evolution. This network makes it virtually impossible to study any behavior in isolation, or to study it without statements about some aspect of it being potentially vulnerable to falsification at one level or another. The plenitude of hypotheses and data about the same or similar behavior in other animals makes any single study only a small part of a total picture (whether the investigator likes it or not), which means it is exposed to a great range of potentially damaging (or supporting) data and arguments.

Being part of such a great picture creates the occasion for many comparisons between man and animals, which in turn can set the stage for great scientific debate and public discord. The political and social implications of evolutionary theory for man have been immense over the past century, and still continue to arouse strong passions. The reaction to E. O. Wilson's book, *Sociobiology: A New Synthesis* (1975), is a good example of their power (see Wade, 1976). Such reactions are understandable, but they might not be so strong if certain basic points were clarified by those who generate hypotheses linking man to other animals.

First, most behavioral links between man and animals are based on analogy, i.e., on evidence of overt similarity that is usually most parsimoniously traceable to common environments, rather than on homology which attributes similarity to common ancestry. This distinction does not necessarily eliminate the issue of biological or phylogenetic determination of behavior, but it does give strong impetus toward seeking environmental/cultural explanations of behavioral origins. Second, human culture as a product of symbolic and linguistic functioning is indeed an infrequent (if not unique) form of adaptation in the animal kingdom. Such functioning hardly seems totally reducible in a meaningful way to any existing biological laws. Finally, those who apply evolution to human behavior are, by the logic of their own methodology, committed to studying their subject matter as it is, not as they think it should be. Hence, they cannot neglect man's symbolic/linguistic behavior and the phenomenal cultural achievements connected with it. Such neglect would violate the holistic/integrative nature of the ethologist's picture of behavior.

There is no reason for psychologists to panic at the thought of ethology invading the domain of human behavior. Nor should ethologists feel that studying humans merely means extrapolating their successful approach with animals to the study of humans without any special accommodations. The issue in establishing a human ethology is not straightforward, but it is not an impossibility. Applying ethology to human behavior may well reveal that some aspects of the latter are refractory to standard ethological analysis and hence require great assistance from psychologists, anthropologists, and sociologists.

In my opinion, ethology's potential offering to the study of human behavior is many faceted, and actually reflects some of the profound aspects of human behavior not totally reflected by other disciplines. Its offering can be very great because of the intrinsic strength of ethology's methodology, its underlying theory, and perhaps more importantly, its well established connections with other disciplines such as genetics, ecology, and neurophysiology, which already play an important role in unraveling the secrets of human nature. For these reasons it is probably incorrect to consider ethology a passing fancy of biological determinists, or a ploy by reactionaries to shape social policy, as some of the opponents of human ethology argue. There is a great difference between a scientific discipline that aims to understand a phenomenon and is therefore committed to being totally objective about it, and a quasiscientific discipline that aims to influence phenomena for ideological purposes. Ethology is clearly the former and those who argue otherwise are misleading themselves and others.

Ethology's offering can be described more specifically as coming in three forms: *factual, conceptual,* and *methodological*. This chapter does not discuss the factual, by which is meant the vast amount of data on animal adaptation that serve the ethologist as a necessary background for viewing human adaptation. These data, much of which have been collected by comparative psychologists and naturalists as well as ethologists, form an indispensable body of knowledge for any student of human behavior. As for the conceptual, primarily the concept of adaptation and, briefly, what it takes to achieve adaptation as a member of *Homo sapiens* are mentioned. Regarding the methodological, this chapter deals exclusively with naturalistic observation, the hallmark of the Darwinian approach and much of ethology. In concrete terms, the use of this method in studying one form of human adaptation, namely, intelligence or problem solving is discussed.

ADAPTATION

The concept of adaptation is imprecise, but useful. It can be found in biology, psychology, psychiatry, anthropology, and other disciplines sensitive to the fact that every living being has an environment with which it has to cope at one time or another. The word ''adapt'' is derived from the Latin prefix *ad* meaning to, toward, at, about, and *aptus* meaning fitted, fitting, appropriate. Thus, the verb ''to adapt'' means to fit or adjust to. In the biological context, adaptation usually refers to two separate things: a condition or the process that brings about the condition. Ernst Mayr (1970), for example, defines adaptation as ''the condition of showing fitness for a particular environment, as applied to characteristics of a structure, function, or entire organism'' (p. 413), and Wilson (1975) defines it as the ''evolutionary process leading to the formation of such a trait'' (p. 577). In both definitions adaptation can refer to physical traits (or the processes involved in bringing them into existence)—the fur of the polar bear is an adaptation to Arctic conditions—or adaptation can refer to behavioral traits, a somewhat more recent notion. As Darwin long intimated, behavior could represent an adaptation extremely crucial for evolution. Mayr (1970) considers behavior an important factor in initiating the process of adaptation to new ecological niches. Only after some members of a species make the appropriate behavioral adaptations to a new niche do the structural or physical adaptations associated with them begin to appear with greater frequency in subsequent generations. It should be clear that evolutionary changes, which by definition are intergenerational, operate through genetic programs that control the ontogenesis of each individual. Behavior contributes to evolution only to the extent that it has genetic determination. There is no convincing evidence for the Lamarckian hypothesis that behavior characteristics acquired as a result of experience are transmitted through some nongenetic mechanisms to the next generation. Transmission is either genetic or traditional, that is, by means of one generation learning from an older generation.

The special value of adaptation as a concept for studying behavior, as general or imprecise as it is, lies in its being a relational term connecting two elements: a living organism and an environment which requires something of the organism. Unfortunately, in psychological research this relational aspect is frequently neglected in at least two ways. First, the subject's environment is usually not studied in much detail, if at all; the subject attracts nearly all the attention—is tested, interviewed, and trained—without any attention paid to the subject's environment. Second, the actual process of subject/environment interaction is scarcely looked at; when looked at it is usually in laboratory conditions which have only partial ecological validity, if any. The larger, more important job of observing subject-environment interaction over subject-relevant (not research-relevant) time periods has been done by only a small, intrepid minority of researchers (see Willems and Raush, 1969).

The study of adaptation in humans seems to have origins quite different from those of ethology. The impetus to define human adaptive behavior and to develop behavioral taxonomies of adaptation (and maladaptation) seems to have come primarily from researchers and practitioners working in mental retardation and psychiatry, both areas dealing with individuals who are by definition maladapted to major aspects of their environments (Heber, 1961; Leland et al. 1966; Phillips, 1968; Robinson and Robinson, 1976). In ethology the emphasis is mostly reversed. Attention is paid to varying degrees of adaptation present in *all* animals, usually within a prescribed geographic area. Although sick and injured animals are not ignored, the main focus is on normal animals which vary in their ability to attract mates, reproduce, and maintain the viability of their offspring, etc. There are usually no clear-cut definitions of what is normal and what is not where behavior is concerned, at least not in the beginning phases of research. Biologists frequently use a dichotomous criterion such as whether or not the animal is reproductively successful.

Psychology and the other human sciences have great difficulty in defining what is normal, and somewhat less difficulty in defining what is abnormal, although this has changed somewhat recently. Trying to pin down what is normal and abnormal in a pluralistic open society deeply concerned with individual freedom and social tolerance is frequently viewed as a dangerous authoritarian move to label individuals in order to put them in groups, and ultimately to suppress them. In addition, intrinsic to many ideas about what is normal is the concept of an established plan prescribing the pathways of individual development (within varying limits), thereby limiting the options open to individual choice. For many this suggests a biological determinism which, regardless of whether or not it has a basis in reality, can lead to fatalistic attitudes having disastrous individual and social consequences. In spite of these problems, the practical if not theoretical or methodological question of what is normal still remains. There are many unhappy and socially disruptive individuals who need assistance, and setting a standard, even if loosely defined, is necessary if the goals of this assistance are to be in any way defined.

ADAPTATION FOR WHAT?

Whereas the concept of adaptation includes two principal components—a living organism and an environment, of which both can be observed individually as well as in interaction with each other—it also includes the vague and tacit notion of a prearranged goal or design that designates what the adaptation is for, or what its aim really is. Without this prearranged goal, even if it is prescriptive in only a very rough sense, the organism would not "know" when to start or stop adapting, or even "know" what had to be adapted to.

This notion creates a difficult problem for biologists because of its inherent teleological nature (Williams, 1966). The problem becomes more complex when humans are studied. Despite their notorious unpredictability and conscious control over much of what they do, humans display some predictable organization in their behavior (e.g., reactions to frustrations, novel objects, and threatening situations) and in their development (e.g., major aspects of physical, cognitive, moral, and social development). This organization is shared in some rough form by the majority of any individual's age and sex group despite cultural or historical differences. Ethologists and other biologists view this commonality as no coincidence. There is an underlying reason for it just as there is for the many cross cultural similarities between widely separated humans, and for the chemical, anatomical, embryological, and neurophysiological similarities between man and nonhuman primates.

To complicate matters, the organization of human behavior, especially over the life span, gives the strong impression that there is a rough but inexorable purposiveness to it in the sense that such organization seems appropriately adapted to life conditions. This impression may be incorrect, but it is difficult to overlook that many adaptations during the various phases of ontogenesis correspond to patterns of changes in the individual's surrounding environment. For example, it seems hardly fortuitous that the onset of walking, curiosity, and personal autonomy coincide with the decline in care and nurturance on the part of parents and, in many species, is related to the appearance of a newborn sib. Strong infant attachment gives way to detachment at the time when there is growing sensitivity to peers along with growing peer pressure. An ethologist with an overview of the animal kingdom can see that a human progresses in a manner that is roughly analogous to that of many other species: from a dependent, nonreproductive, parasitic relationship with an older generation to an independent, reproductive relationship with its own generation. It would be surprising if a developmental potential for such similarities were not represented by some form of genetically transmitted blueprint as a result of eons of ancestral adaptations.

All this relates to the question of what is normal human behavior. Any definition of normal behavior must include at least three criteria: 1) it must be typical for most same-age and same-sex members of the species, 2) it must lead to self-maintenance or preservation, and 3) it must result in the production or care of succeeding generations of the species. Maslow's (1954, 1972) formulations of need hierarchies can be used to expand on these, and studies of developmental norms can provide empirically established definitions to expand or verify Maslow's. However, all such definitions are incomplete if the environmental dimension is left out. One cannot ignore defining what constitutes a normal environment for humans (regardless of the great number and variety of such environments) if one wants a meaningful picture of normal behavior.

As diffuse and circular as definitions of normality are, they are hardly useless or fictional. For example, Harlow (1971) has shown that functioning as a normal rhesus monkey in adulthood does not occur if infancy and early childhood are characterized by wide deviations from some unspecified but nevertheless very real norm of rhesus early environment. Such research works on the assumption of some probably very loose definition of normality and abnormality in both behavior and environment. Assumptions must underlie most human deprivation/enrichment research, but the nature and degree of variation characterizing behavior and the environment in which it takes place have not been defined and spelled out in sufficient detail, and maybe never will be, given man's great ability and nouveaumaniacal compulsion to change things at an astounding rate.

In all of this one should not overlook two distinctive and major attributes of human behavior: 1) nearly all of it is learned and hence more directly connected to tradition and culture than to genetic dispositions (although there may be genetic predispositions to learn certain behaviors and not others); and 2) there is great individual variation in behavior. These attributes have not traditionally been the focus of ethological research, but times have changed. Leading ethologists such as Lorenz (1969) and Wilson (1975) are very aware of these attributes and are attempting to find a place for them in their overall formulations.

Man's ability to learn and create novelty in whatever he touches is recognized at least tacitly by most ethologists as limiting their methodology and certain working concepts. However, learning ability is not viewed as falling outside the realm of an evolutionary framework; it is viewed as another adaptation, just as morphological features are. According to Lorenz (1969, 1971), man's adaptive speciality is in being unspecialized, and he can afford to be unspecialized because he inherits general learning abilities to help him learn the specific behaviors that the environment requires of him. These abilities are not viewed as just "there at birth." They have phylogenetic origins and hence are biological, not cultural. Most ethologists do not totally reject Locke's *tabula rasa* theory: they know humans are written upon by experience. But they want to know more about the tabula itself and feel that a good theory will try to account for it, rather than ignore it as many environmentalists have purportedly done. Simply evoking man's great malleability, his great ability to learn and adapt, does not explain much when one does comparative studies and gets the overwhelming suspicion that a chimp's tabula is radically different from a turtle's and somewhat less different from a human's.

INDIVIDUAL DIFFERENCES

One of the misconceptions shared by many who view ethology with dissatisfaction is that ethologists tend to look for behavioral universals (e.g., Eibl-Eibesfeldt, 1970; Ekman and Friesen, 1971) and thereby play down or totally disregard variations in behavior. This may not seem to be a serious tendency at first, but for those who have misconceptions it carries with it strong arguments for biological determinism. The argument is that if man behaves essentially the same independently of culture, such behavior must be genetically determined and hence out of man's control. Although such a misconception may have social or political value for those opposed to viewing man as predestined to play out biological roles or for those opposed to attempting to reduce the great variety of human groups to one or a few superbly adapted prototypes, it does not have much scientific value. Those who share this misconception overlook the most basic fact of all biology and evolutionary theory, namely that there would be no species if there were no variation between species, and no evolution of species if there were no variation between individuals within a species. In short, variation is one of the most overwhelming distinctive features of living organisms. It is true that some ethologists may overlook variations in their search for universal behavior patterns, general laws, and trends, but they are constantly faced with the raw empirical fact of individual differences (whether they like them or not), and are forced to realize that without these differences there would be no variation to work on. Without individual differences evolutionary arguments for the appearance of behavior patterns as adaptations would simply be invalid. As a group, ethologists search for both similarities and differences and try to account for both in the most plausible way possible; they differ from most psychologists in that they emphasize their biological basis more than psychologists do.

Awareness of individual differences involves more than the recognition of its role in evolution: it has methodological significance as well. It is impossible to obtain a complete ethogram of behavior without knowing the nature of its ontogenesis, and there is no way of knowing its ontogenesis without studying the individual animal over time as it interacts with its environment. In human research, retrospective, psychometric, and laboratory studies of different age groups are valuable in generating hypotheses about age differences (as well as explicating to some extent the nature of short term behavioral mechanisms), but they shed little or no light on how age changes occur. Currently it is extremely difficult, if not impossible, to account for age changes in behavior in terms of underlying neurophysiological mechanisms. Thirty-minute learning experiments with well measured physiological concomitants cannot explain in any adequate way what happens during development. The only method that will disclose something about the nature of ontogenesis of behavior and its determinants is longitudinal/observational studies of individuals, and even they have limitations.

As is well known, it is with these limitations that the trouble begins. The cost, time, and effort of doing such studies are very great. But no other alternative is evident, especially for those disciplines in which intervention in the lives of individuals is the ultimate goal. There is much talk today of doing meaningful research and although much of this talk seems to be based upon an emotional reaction to what is perceived as a cold, impersonal, fragmentary and therefore artificial experimental approach of most behavioral sciences, it has an important and perhaps inadvertent scientific truth to it. This truth is that the most satisfactory account of behavior will have to include all major contributing factors; individual as well as group, sociological as well as psychological and biological, everyday as well as laboratory. Recall what was said earlier about the complete picture of behavior, the integrative holistic nature of the ethologist's goal.

What all this adds up to in practical terms is that ''research of convenience,'' a term that aptly describes much of what psychologists have been engaging in, has to give way to ''research of relevance'' (not ideological, but epistemic relevance, i.e., relevance for scientific knowledge). This has to be achieved without losing rigor in the process. Research of relevance will probably be carried out initially by those doing observational/longitudinal research. Such research is inconvenient and time consuming, but is absolutely necessary to establish the foundation of primary descriptive data which the field, as Tinbergen (1972) and others have pointed out, is so blatantly lacking. For the most part, interviewing and testing will be given minor emphasis until the primary data indicate what is worth collecting by such approaches. Interviews and tests are not constructed to provide reliable information on the nature of the individual's environment (they have other functions), but this information is desperately needed to complete the picture of the individual and to aid one in making better and more relevant predictions about his or her future adaptation. It will no longer do to take the short cut of labeling environments as middle class, enriched, ghetto, authoritarian, democratic, or culturally deprived. These labels are far too abstract and imprecise to have any scientific or practical significance.

More accurate and precise descriptions are necessary for general scientific reasons and especially for planning future intervention.

AN APPLICATION

The following is more explicit about ways in which the ethological orientation can allow a relevant approach to human behavior. The core concept is individual adaptation to the environment, and researchers view it in many different ways. There are those who suscribe to the AAMD definitions of mental retardation, the Leland et al. (1966, 1967) definition, the more operationally rigorous working definition used by behavior modifiers, the more traditional maladaptation view of mental illness, and the sociocultural view (e.g., Mercer, 1973). The ethological view does not seem to conflict in any fundamental way with any of these, primarily because of its wide generality. What the ethologist's view could offer to implement such definitions is the following. 1) a greater emphasis upon obtaining hard observational data on subject/environment interaction; 2) greater attention to the immediately functional as well as long term adaptive value of behavior as it relates to short and long term goals of the individual; 3) greater awareness of similarities of man's problems of adaptation to those of other animals, and hence greater awareness of the mutual descriptive and possibly explanatory benefits of such comparisons; and 4) a sense of the historical as well as contemporary significance of the synthetic theory of evolution for understanding human behavior.

As noted earlier, ethologists view any behavior that mediates between the animal and its environment as having immediate or potential adaptive value. Traditionally, they have concentrated heavily on social behaviors, behaviors directed toward conspecifics or predators and prey. Behaviors that could be defined as epistemic (that is, based on cumulated information, hence cognitive) and directed primarily toward the physical world, such as problem solving and tool using, have been studied more by comparative psychologists in the laboratory or seminatural settings than by ethologists. Only recently in the work of Jane van Lawick-Goodall has the field study approach been more than casually focused upon tool-using behavior in nonhuman primates. This does not mean that ethologists have been unaware of the clever, cognitive things animals do to survive; it means that ethologists have not developed a coherent and systematic method and theory to deal with epistemic behavior. The kind of in-depth work they have done with social behavior has, apparently, not been done with the epistemic. Developing an ethological approach to epistemic behavior is one of our current tasks. What follows is an attempt to concretize this approach in field studies of what is generally called intelligent behavior.

INTELLIGENT BEHAVIOR

The empirical portion of this paper deals with intelligent behavior as observed in two children, one normal and one retarded. The concept of intelligence has recently been evaluated (see Resnick, 1976), and once again reveals itself to be a very complex, unwieldly concept that many would like to do without but cannot. This chapter avoids many of the present issues associated with it and concentrates instead upon one specific behavioral aspect, namely, problem solving.

The behavioral aspect of intelligence is emphasized for a number of reasons. First, the term *intelligence* is used to account for a particular dispositional characteristic of an individual as measured by tests. Consequently, it does not include environmental measures to interpret the behavioral aspect. Second, from an evolutionary perspective, selection operates directly on behavior, not on tendencies to behave (tendencies may be very numerous and varied and yet never occur). Whereas test measures of intelligence may be correlated with actual behaviors upon which selection acts, it is too premature to assume this without a more thorough study of intelligent behavior in the natural habitat and the extent to which factors of the habitat release and reinforce such behavior. A more extensive discussion of these points can be found in Charlesworth (1976). A final reason for concentrating on behavior rather than test scores is simply that behavior is more amenable to modification than test scores and hence is more relevant.

Intelligent behavior is here defined as behavior that generally aids the individual in the attempt to adapt to problematic situations causing imbalances in interactions with the environment. Such behavior is distinguished from reflexes, taxis, tropisms, and fixed action patterns in that it is organized and controlled by cognitive processes, processes that are inferred from the nature of the behavior itself or from what is known of the individual's past experience. This definition has a number of problems. For one, there is no way to qualitatively evaluate such behaviors in terms of long term adaptiveness. They are evaluated simply in terms of whether they are successful in removing barriers or satisfying needs, and hence in re-establishing a short term balance with the environment. For another, the definition overemphasizes the problem-solving aspect of intelligent behavior. That is, intelligent behavior by this definition occurs only in reaction to a problem, disruption, or blocking of behavior; it is not considered a problem-avoiding behavior (as one would have no way of knowing this from observation), or behavior one could observe when the individual is in relaxed, problem-free play conditions. Finally, this emphasis upon behavior may seem contradictory in light of the definition that intelligent behavior is controlled by nonbehavioral processes.

The first weakness can probably be remedied with the aid of long term longitudinal studies, although it is too soon to attempt to link intelligent behaviors to more global measures of adaptation. As for the second weakness, a rigorous way to observe or identify intelligent behavior outside of specific and reliably identifiable stimulus/response conditions has not been found. What is observed fairly reliably is a disruption in the subject-environment relationship that interrupts ongoing behavior and requires some coping response. Without this disruption one would not know when and where to look for a response or how to define it. As for the third weakness, it is possible to infer (with varying degrees of certainty) whether or not a response has cognitive mediation behind it. Verbal individuals can be asked to report on their behavior, although verbal reports are not necessary. A behavioral response is the crucial response, not a verbal one, which may be superfluous or misleading. If verbalizations and cognitions make no behavioral difference, they will have no impact on the environment and hence have no potential survival value for the individual. Let us now look at intelligent behavior in terms of its purported value.

Intelligent behavior (no matter how defined) must have played some role in the evolution of man in terms of its survival value (Mayr, 1970; Jerison, 1973; Klein, 1973). Although one has no direct knowledge of how such behavior actually made a difference to survival, some inferences can be made from artifacts, geological data, etc. and from what we see today among various cultures, such as the hunters and gatherers of Kalahari, whose living conditions resemble those of early man. One thing seems fairly certain: wherever man can be found he has made a more or less successful adaptation to his environment, and some of this adaptation was achieved by more than physical strength, endurance, and locomotor speed; cognitive skills were also involved. The ingenuity of preindustrial peoples in solving various everyday problems requiring forethought, planning, and the shrewd weighing of alternatives is impressive from any standpoint. To get an idea of this, one need only read Mason's (1966) account of the origins of invention in primitive peoples, or Gladwin's (1970) more up-to-date account of the navigational and logical skills used by the inhabitants of the Puluwat Atoll in the South Pacific. Such accounts also give a good idea of how intelligent behavior, even though its nature may vary considerably, is equally distributed across various human populations inhabiting geographically different environments, and of how intelligent behavior is triggered by problems encountered in the physical as well as the social environment.

Early man's intelligent behavior can be inferred from fossil remains as well as current comparisons with other higher primates. Reed (1965) speculates that the ancestors of early man probably had intellectual capacities not much higher than today's apes, and that intelligence of early man himself was most probably much lower than today's average. Assuming that primitive man's IQ was around 30 points, Reed calculates that over 35,000 generations it would take a 0.002-point increase per generation to reach today's average of 100. Such a gradual increase could be compatible with existing genetic models of change. How correct his estimate is or whether it overlooks qualitative changes between nonhuman primate intelligence and human intelligence which do not correspond to a model of gradual change is immaterial for the present discussion. The point of interest is whether a phylogenetic change in intelligence was related to forces of natural selection, and if such changes were in any way similar to changes in mental age as we define them today.

If selection did occur it may have operated, as Williams (1966) argues, on basic cognitive skills such as comprehension, memory, and simple problem-solving skills rather than much higher intellectual functioning. As Williams points out, there is no reason to believe that geniuses have more children than the rest of us. However, it is true that the retarded tend to have fewer offspring than the normal population (Higgins, Reed, and Reed, 1962), and this may account for any gradual increases in intelligence over human evolution. Also, it is possible that in addition to lower reproductive rates, retarded adults throughout history may have suffered a higher rate of prereproductive mortality. They may have had higher accident rates, been the first to be deprived during food shortages, and been more vulnerable to parasites and predators as well as hostile humans. If this was the case, such selection must have become more relaxed with increases in food supplies through farming, greater control over environmental dangers, more humane attitudes, and the like. Today, the retarded probably suffer no greater rate of prereproductive mortality than the general population. What will happen in the future is anyone's guess. Maybe some traits other than intelligence, such as sociability or expressivity, will play a more important role in survival.

In discussing the phylogenesis of intelligence, reference is usually made to environmental factors that for some reason exerted powerful selective pressures upon early man. The Pleistocene with its long periods of intense cold, excessive snow, and diminished food sources is thought to have put the greatest strain on emerging man's cognitive powers, and fossil remains support such a hypothesis. What the effects of the Pleistocene climate were on single individuals and how each one of them dealt with it is virtually impossible to reconstruct. But such information is necessary if one wants an adequate test of the hypothesis. A weaker test can be carried out theoretically at least by long term studies of individuals today. This is partly what the empirical work to be presented here is about.

If one takes the individual as the unit for study and looks at the question of intelligence, it is found that the great bulk of information is made up of samples of the individual's ability to respond to test items. This information is obtained most frequently by paper and pencil tests, which last minutes or at most no more than 2 hr, and less frequently by the individual's performance in problem-solving situations. Although this information is important, it says next to nothing about the individual's everyday behavior. It also gives no clue about how the individual acquired such abilities, and no indication about what role environmental factors played in the acquisition. In short, although there are excellent measures of intelligence as a disposition to act intelligently on future tests and in school situations, these measures give only an approximate idea of what the individual actually does in real life and what other factors are involved when he or she acts intelligently in everyday situations. Furthermore, although knowing what the individual can do allows one to make some predictions about the future (such as how well the child will do in school on verbal assignments), such predictions are highly dependent upon the nature of the environmental conditions the individual is in at the time. Without foreknowledge of these conditions, there is no way of predicting an individual's future chances of adaptive success. The report by Jencks et al. (1972) showing that many factors other than measured intelligence play important roles in determining how well an individual will adapt is evidence of how much information must be amplified before a reasonable prediction about anyone's future can be made.

For these reasons it is concluded that a way to study intelligent behavior in everyday situations must be developed if we ever want to know how it relates to environmental conditions. In the process, we will find out what these conditions really are, both during early ontogenesis and later in life, and these findings ought to improve our intervention procedures and predictions.

OBSERVING INTELLIGENT BEHAVIOR

Our first attempt to observe intelligent behavior was in a study of tool using. About 200 children between 1 and 4 years of age were given eight to fifteen problems that involved obtaining desired objects that were not immediately available without using a tool. We focused on instrumental behaviors, such as reaching, grasping, picking up a stick, using a stick to rake in an object, etc. Whenever the child could go no further a standard set of graded prompts were given until a solution was achieved. It was soon discovered that obtaining reliable observational records of seemingly simple instrumental behaviors was not as easy as first thought. The observer-training period was lengthened and the behavior of the 1-year-olds was videotaped because they were disorganized and did a lot of unexpected, ambiguous things.

Meanwhile, informal observations showed almost no tool-using behavior in preschool children in the home. Parents were then instructed to record all instances of problem situations that required their child to use a tool. The parents did this for 4 weeks and the number of problems that were reported turned out to be extremely small. This was intriguing. If children had relatively few experiences of solving problems with tools, how were they able to solve the problems on the tests, especially those that were novel and hence had no representation in their experience?

By this time I began to conceptualize the problems in terms of adaptation, and to distinguish between measuring intelligence as a disposition, and observing intelligent behavior as an adaptive response to an environmentally imposed problem. This approach was compatible with my interests in ethology. However, as mentioned earlier, ethologists historically have not looked at problem-solving behavior in animals in any concentrated, systematic way. Neither have there been studies of human problem-solving behavior as it occurs "spontaneously" in the natural habitat; at home, on the job, at play, etc.

What is known about children's problem-solving abilities comes mostly from tests, and what is known about their performance at home comes almost exclusively from baby biographies and other anecdotal sources.

The first task was to define, in general terms, a problem and its behavioral solution so that they could be observed and applied to all humans as well as to animals, if necessary. Whether this was successful remains to be seen. For now we have settled on the following working definition, which represents a composite of conventional ideas about the nature of a problem and of ideas we gathered inductively after recording large numbers of subject/environment interactions.

A *problem* is defined as a situation in which an individual's ongoing behavior is interrupted or blocked by certain external or internal stimulus conditions. This is a term applied to the relationship between two separate entities: an individual and a particular stimulus condition. A problem is not a statement solely about a particular aspect of an environment which blocks behavior, since what is a blocking condition for one individual may not be for another. Nor is a problem a statement solely about a particular individual since the same individual may be blocked by one stimulus condition and not by another. It is the particular nature of the interaction between the individual and the stimulus that defines a problem. This may seem obvious, but one commonly talks about problems independently of individuals, even though one knows that what is a problem for a 4-year-old child is usually not for a 10-year-old. It is only when an individual has difficulty with a stimulus condition that we label the situation as problematic. Conversely, it is frequently assumed that an individual who fails problem-solving tasks will fail to solve other problems he or she encounters. But this is obviously incorrect, because it depends on the nature of those other problems. An individual labeled retarded on the basis of an intelligence test score may solve problems of social relations in a way superior to a gifted child.

Blocking conditions are problematic in the sense that they halt or slow down ongoing behavior and require that the individual change his or her behavior to deal with their particular demand properties. Such conditions can be social, physical, or cognitive in nature; another person can demand that the individual stop what he is doing and do something else, a door can resist being opened immediately, or the individual can fail to remember where he or she put something.

The behavior elicited in response to the blocking condition is defined as problem-solving behavior (whether it removes the blocking condition or not). Many types of responses can be elicited by a blocking condition. For example, a particular blocking condition can elicit a single, well learned response of a short latency, or a complicated chain of familiar as well as novel responses occurring in what may be described as a trial-and-error fashion, or a single ingenious or creative response for which one has to wait many minutes. In all instances it is assumed that such responses are mediated by cognitive (symbolic or linguistic) processes or, in the case of well learned, habitual responses, have been mediated by such processes earlier in the individual's history when cognitive mediation was necessary. In this respect, problem-solving behavior is learned behavior (a point discussed by Gagne, 1965) and therefore distinguished from reflexes, taxis, fixed action patterns, and other behaviors for which there is no reason to believe that cognitive mediation is necessary.

The immediate effects of problem-solving behavior range from successfully removing the blocking condition and allowing the individual to resume the ongoing behavior, to completely failing to remove the conditions and thereby requiring that the individual engage in something else. Doing something else usually has the consequence of having to relinquish the ongoing behavior more or less permanently. The long term effects of problem-solving behavior range from strengthening already established responses to adding completely novel responses to the individual's repertoire.

In some respects the present definition of a problem is similar to conventional definitions. Problems have been defined as obstacles, perceived difficulties, or predicaments that halt or interfere with ongoing or goal-directed behavior and require that the individual do something about them (see Kohler, 1925; Dewey, 1933; Maier, 1940; Wertheimer, 1945; Duncker, 1945; Berlyne, 1965; Resnick and Glaser, 1976). Most of these authors generally assume that what the individual does in response to a problem is novel, otherwise there would be no problem. However, I feel that assumption is too restrictive. Many situations outside the laboratory or test situation disrupt behavior and require that the individual cope with them, and in most cases it is impossible to determine whether or not the coping responses or their organization are novel. Our feeling is that most disruptions elicit familiar, well learned coping responses rather than novel or clever response, but this could be wrong. The present definition relieves us of this uncertainty by going beyond the definition of a problem as being a condition that requires a novel response and including as problems all conditions that block or interrupt behavior and require that the individual deal with them. Expanding the definition in this manner makes it possible to include a wide range of everyday conditions that compel adaptation.

Expanding the definition to include commonplace problematic conditions also makes it possible to assess the extent to which the individual has dealt with similar conditions earlier in development. We assume that problem-solving behavior, as in-novel and non-cognitive as it may seem, was novel and cognitive at an earlier period of the individual's life. In this respect the definition has utility for a developmental analysis of adaptive capacities. An individual can either solve or fail a problem immediately, or after a lot of difficulty. After sufficient normative data have been collected at different age levels and under different environmental conditions, a subject's performance can be evaluated in terms of individuals of a similar age and in similar environmental conditions. Only in this way is it possible to get a representative sample of the range and level of the individual's adaptive capacities.

Another way in which the present definition differs from most of the conventional definitions is its emphasis on observable behavior as an indication that a particular stimulus condition is problematic. Unlike the experimenter or tester who creates novel problematic situations and presents them to subjects, the observer of problem-solving behavior in natural situations has no control over the stimulus situation and hence (with one exception) cannot *a priori* designate them as problematic. The observer must rely solely upon changes in the individual's behavior to determine whether a condition is creating a problem for the individual. The exception is when a social stimulus condition is observed which is "clearly" intended as a blocking condition to the individual's behavior; for example, when the mother demands that the child stop playing. In most such cases a behavioral change follows: the child stops playing, or the child momentarily stops playing and says "No." Sometimes, though, the child continues playing and says "No," or the child stops playing and starts to cry, etc. (We also record instances when the child does not respond; this does not qualify as a problem in the strict sense, but gives us an idea of how potentially problematic the child's environment is.) In short, the present definition focuses much more on actual behavior than on conventional definitions and makes an attempt to identify the exact environmental conditions involved. The only requirement made on the observer (whose task is to identify problems when they occur) is that he or she make the inference that cognitive processes are implicated in dealing with the blocking condition.

The blocking conditions that disrupt the individual's ongoing behavior can be divided into two major categories: 1) those that are immediately visible in the sense that one can observe them to be impositions on the individual or as sources of resistance to the individual's behavior (for example, another person physically restrains the individual from doing something, or a chair is clearly too high for the child to climb upon); and 2) those that are not visible, but have to be inferred (as a need or want) because the individual's behavior indicates that he or she cannot continue as intended until certain conditions are met (for example, the individual cannot start or continue to eat until he or she solves the problem of getting the mother to bring food). The latter involves the lack of needed object or person. This constitutes a barrier condition since it interrupts or blocks the individual's behavior and forces him or her to engage in other behaviors to make the object or person available.

Both categories of blocking conditions, the observed and the inferred, can be classified three ways in terms of content: social, physical, or cognitive. Table 1 contains

Table 1. Six classes and examples of blocking conditions (BC's) and responses (R's) to them observed in problem situations

Blocking conditions	Social	Physical	Cognitive
	(Someone imposes on child)	(Object or aspect of physical environment resists child)	(Someone imposes demand for cognitive response upon child)
Observed (imposition; resistance)	Mother tells child to stay seated (BC); child complies (R)	Child tries to open jar, but fails (BC); child persists in trying to turn cap, cries, then calls mother (R)	Mother asks child where she put the crayons (BC); child tells her (R)
	Father holds child back from TV set (BC); child squirms free, reaches TV and starts turning knobs (R)	Child cannot ride tricycle up slight incline (BC); tricycle rolls back, child gets off, and pulling tricycle, walks up incline (R)	Sister asks child to repeat a long word after her (BC); child does not answer (R)
	(Child wants someone or someone's behavior)	(Child wants object)	(Child wants information)
Inferred (need; want)	Mother leaves room (BC); child begins crying (R)	Child in high chair, juice on counter out of reach (BC); child stand in high chair, leans way over to reach bottle, fails, crawls out of chair and picks up bottle of juice (R)	Mother leaves room (BC); child asks father where mother is going (R)
	Child and mother looking at book (BC); child asks mother to turn pages (R)	Toy train in box in closet (BC); child asks mother to get box down for him (R)	Child and mother looking at picture book (BC); child asks mother name of animal pictured in book (R)

the six resulting classes of blocking conditions and the responses to them along with representative examples.

The examples of blocking conditions and responses in Table 1 are relatively simple. However, there is a fairly large number of others (observed in the field) that consist of complicated blends of the six classes.

Initially we expected that blocking conditions, as unplanned disruptions of the child's behavior, would range from those requiring relatively complicated cognitive operations (e.g., recalling information and finding ways to apply it to the problem, or analyzing the problem into components) to those requiring overlearned responses (e.g., pushing an obstructing object until it moves away, or saying "no" to someone making a demand). In Piagetian terms, the problems would range from those requiring much accommodation and little assimilation (that is, struggle for a solution through trial-and-error, a search for new information or new insights, etc.) to those simply requiring little accommodation and much assimilation (that is, a relatively automatic application of already learned responses). It was expected that a fairly large number of the former would be detected in the developing child, who presumably is faced frequently throughout the day with challenges requiring some form of coping behavior. That our results have not confirmed this expectation is an interesting finding, which is discussed later. The point is that it was decided originally to focus as much as possible upon that part of the child's interaction with his or her environment that is disruptive and problematic and hence compels the child to respond to it. Other aspects of adaptation could have been focused on, but it was found that theoretically and methodologically, as far as observation is concerned, a disruption model makes the best sense. We recognize that it may be too narrow a definition to warrant the use of intelligent behavior, but it is a practical way to identify problematic situations requiring that the individual react to them.

The child's *response* to the blocking conditions constitutes the problem-solving behavior (whether it is successful is discussed below). Some examples are: *social responses*—tries to get the other to do something, ignores the other, refuses, yields, or complies; *physical responses*—uses force, a tool, or manipulation; *cognitive responses*—asks for information, answers a question, or searches overtly for a missing object.

The response is followed by one of two *results*: the blocking condition is removed, or it is not removed. Sometimes the observer checks off "neither" because it was impossible to determine which occurred.

The result of the response, in return, is followed by one of two *outcomes*: the ongoing behavior before the blocking condition is resumed, or it is not resumed and the individual engages in another behavior. Here, too, as in the case of the response, the observer may record "neither."

This is an oversimplified version of the schema developed, but it must do for now. It should be pointed out that the final schema for defining and describing what went on during a problem episode involved analyzing more than a thousand problems, took over a year to develop, and went through 29 revisions.

A sample problem is as follows:

> S is playing with a ballpoint pen while sitting in the playpen (*Ongoing behavior, playing*). S's pen gets stuck in the railings of the playpen (*Physical blocking condition*). S cries (*Negative emotional response*). Father comes over to S. S gets the pen out from the railings (*Response*

unknown; probably manipulating pen) (*Result, barrier removed*). S begins to write on her arms with pen (*Outcome, continues playing*).

Our first study involved 30 observation hours of stratified sampling during all waking hours of the day over a 7-week period (excluding weekends) during June and July. Subjects were two girls and two boys ranging in age from 1 year 2 months to 2 years 7 months; all children were normal, white, "middle class" with at least one sib in the family. A follow-up study conducted a year later consisted of 15 observation hours per child. We chose children of this age for a number of reasons: their behavior and demands are relatively simple; they are capable of relatively unambiguous instrumental behavior, and the younger the child, the better are the chances for implementing an intervention program based on these methods.

The second study involved observing a Down's syndrome girl, 1 year 10 months, with a Bayley Score of 75, and a normal girl of the same age, with a Bayley Score of 132. Both girls came from white, "middle class" families with no siblings, and each was observed for 16 hr distributed over 4½ weeks.

The third study (Spiker, 1976) involved observing six nursery school children, three girls and three boys ranging in age from 3 years 8 months to 4 years 4 months, all white and all attending the same nursery school. Each child was observed for a total of 450 min at different times on five separate mornings distributed over a 6-week period.

All three studies involved the same basic observational methodology: 1) on-the-minute time sampling of nonproblem behavior using 12 to 14 predetermined categories, which for our purposes accounted for all nonproblem-solving behaviors, and 2) a narrative recording of the problem episodes. The purpose of the studies was to obtain several pieces of information: 1) the number, kinds, and lengths of problems the children faced during the day in their normal environment, 2) the kinds and number of responses the children made to the problems, 3) the results of their responses, 4) the outcomes of the results, 5) how successful their responses were, 6) to what extent other persons intervened, helped, etc., and 7) within what contexts the problems occurred (i.e., physical and social settings, ongoing behavior as measured by the categories, time of day, and anything else that seemed relevant to the observer, such as whether the child was not feeling well, was tired, etc.).

The predetermined categories of nonproblem behavior included: playing, interacting socially, locomoting toward a goal, looking intently (excludes casual, "normal" looking), caring for body, dressing, attempting to acquire an object, self-stimulating, toileting, eating, doing nothing (includes aimless activity), and unknown (used to fill in empty cells).

In the next section a portion of the results are presented (namely, gross frequencies and percentages of problems and their components) from the study of the Down's syndrome and normal children.

PROBLEM SOLVING IN A DOWN'S SYNDROME CHILD AND A NORMAL CHILD

The parents of both children were contacted through friends and, after being told in general terms what the study was about, were very willing to have female observers in the home for approximately 20 hr. While the observers trained for 4 hr over a 3-day period, observers, parents, and child became acquainted. During this time each child apparently learned that when the observer had her clipboard, she was not to be interrupted. After about 3 hr the observers noticed no substantial disruption of anyone's behavior and began ''feeling like furniture.'' All observations subsequently were made with no interruptions.

To obtain a measure of interobserver agreement, simultaneous observations were carried out on 38% of the 16 hr of observations for each child. These observations were spread across the total observation period to monitor and prevent ''drifting.'' The principal observer for this study trained for 7 hr under two observers who had already completed 82 observation hours. Interobserver agreement (number of agreements divided by number of agreements plus disagreements) was obtained separately for problem narratives and for categories. To qualify as an agreement both problem narratives had to specify the same blocking condition in the same time period, and the same response to the block. Observer pairs agreed on 274 of 331 problems observed (83% agreement). Observer agreement on categories was also calculated on 38% of the total number of observations. Various procedures were used to calculate agreements, but are not discussed here. The most conservative procedure revealed that the two observers agreed between 84% and 89% of the time.

As noted earlier, it took over a year to develop a schema for reliably defining and describing in standard fashion what went on during a problem episode. The resulting schema makes it possible to reduce narratives to essential information that can be fed into a computer. For the present study three persons ''schematized'' the narrative information on 42 problem cards selected randomly from both children. Agreements ranged from 74% to 84%, with an overall mean of 81% agreement. The results of this study are presented in Tables 2 to 4.

Table 2. Frequencies of problems and blocking conditions and time spent on problems for the Down's Syndrome (DS) child and normal control (N)

Observations	DS	N
Problems and blocking conditoins (BC)		
Frequency of problems	328	535
Frequency of BC's (one problem can include one or more BC's)	814	1350
Time spent on problems		
Total time spent on problems	77 min	155 min
% total observation time (960 min.) spent on problems	8%	16%
Mean time spent on single problem	14 sec	18 sec
Range of time spent on problems	2 sec to 6.5 min	2 sec to 4.1 min
One problem occurs on the average every:	2.9 min	1.8 min
One block occurs on the average every:	1.2 min	0.7 min

Table 3. Frequency (f) and percentages of blocking conditions

Blocking conditions	Down's f	Down's %	Normal f	Normal %
Three classes of blocking conditions (BC's)				
Social	702	86	1208	89
Physical	13	2	80	6
Cognitive	89	11	51	4
Unknown (S cries, screams for unknown reason)	10	1	11	1
Sum =	814		1350	
Subclasses of social blocking conditions				
Observed (imposition)				
Other makes prohibitive demands	176	25	355	29
Other demands S to do something	220	31	345	28
Other asks S to do something	18	2	41	3
Other nonverbally blocks S (physical threat, force, takes away object, disrupts S's activity)	210	30	245	20
Other makes an ambiguous statement which could be considered as a blocking condition (''You should play outside.'' ''Wait just a minute.'')	71	10	173	14
Other asks S rhetorical question (''Why did you do that?'')	4	<1	16	1
Other scolds or spanks S	2	<1	4	<1
Other refuses to do something for S	0	0	18	1
Inferred (need)				
S wants other to do something	1	<1	11	1
Sum =	702		1208	
Subclasses of physical blocking conditions				
Observed (imposition)				
Object blocks gross movement	1		5	6
Object cannot be manipulated, handled, etc.	4		6	7
Inferred (need)				
Object unavailable or prohibited	5		55	69
Instances of S slipping, falling, dropping objects etc.	3		14	18
Sum =	13		80	
Subclasses of cognitive blocking conditions				
Observed (imposition)				
Other demands S to say something	14	16	13	25
Other asks S to say something	8	9	3	6
Other asks S to identify something	48	54	1	2
Other seeks information from S	19	21	31	60
Inferred (need)				
S asks information	0	0	3	6
Sum =	89		51	

Table 4. Frequency (f) and percentages of responses to blocking conditions, blocking conditions removed, and resumption of ongoing behaviors

	Down's		Normal	
Observations	f	%	f	%
Frequency and percentage of responses to blocking conditions				
Response to all blocking conditions	643		1258	
Social responses	556	87	1024	81
Physical responses	15	2	42	3
Cognitive responses	8	1	32	3
Unclassified, ambiguous responses	64	10	160	13
Avoids prohibition, shifts to new behavior, engages in irrelevant behavior	11		74	
Whines, crys, frowns	46		71	
Smiles, laughs	4		2	
Stares, stands, walks "aimlessly"	0		3	
Stops crying	3		10	
Percentage of blocking conditions removed by responses (close-to-accurate estimates)		36		41
Percentage of ongoing behavior resumed after problems (close-to-accurate estimates)		31		28
Other-intervention: approximate percentage of problem episodes in which another person intervened in the problem-solving process		6		11

DISCUSSION OF FINDINGS

Because of the small N and the exploratory nature of this study, the findings reported here only illustrate what our method can produce. Although one cannot generalize from these findings, it should be pointed out that preliminary analyses of data from the other studies reveal many similar results.

The everyday problems of the two children in this sample consisted of a wide range of different interruptions; most were social in nature, and relatively few were physical or cognitive. On the average, the Down's syndrome child encountered one problem every 2.9 min and the normal child one problem every 1.8 min. When viewed in terms of blocks, the Down's child experienced one blocking condition every 1.2 min on the average and the normal child one every 0.70 minute. Most of the blocks consisted of demands or requests to do or stop doing something. Physical blocks occurred very infrequently; the most frequent occurred for the normal child in the form of objects the child wanted and could not immediately acquire. Cognitive blocks were also relatively infrequent: the highest percentage occurred in the Down's child while her mother was engaged in teaching her how to identify objects. Neither child engaged in any clever problem-solving behavior, but there did not seem to be any blocking conditions that required clever behavior or tools to remove the block. In short, the problematic nature of the child's environment was overwhelmingly social and consisted heavily of the parents telling the child what to do and not do. The physical environment was only slightly problematic and usually involved the lack of objects rather than the presence of objects or physical conditions that restricted behavior. Both social and physical problems may have reflected the parent's level of control over the environment, which in turn may have reflected their perception of the child's age and developmental level. It could be argued that the parents structured the physical environment to make it safe and nonproblematic for the child and structured the social environment to enhance its effectiveness as a socializing and educating agent in the child's life. Perhaps the very low level of cognitive problems reflected a developmental factor (both children were at an age when rudimentary symbolic and linguistic skills were only beginning to develop). The low level of cognitive problems may also be an artifact of the method in that it may be very difficult at this age to observe valid behavioral correlates of cognitive processes involved in problem solving.

Differences between the two children were evident in both the quantity of problems the child experienced and the quality. As the frequencies indicate, the normal child experienced many more problems than the Down's syndrome child (and consequently spent much more time with them), had longer problems on the average than the Down's child, and (from the data not presented here) was involved in more complicated problems that had multiple blocking conditions and required many responses. For example, 30% of the normal child's problems involved three or more blocks as contrasted with 19% for the Down's child. Qualitative differences between the problems for both children have not been determined systematically as yet; however, it is apparent from a cursory examination of problem content that the Down's child's problems were relatively more elementary than those for the normal child. For example, the Down's child was frequently asked to eat, bite, chew, talk to someone, say words such as "Moo" or "Bye-bye," put her feet or butt down, play patty-cake or itsy-bitsy spider, etc. In contrast, the normal child was asked to eat with a fork, drink from a cup, stop playing with food, say "Thank you," call Daddy to come from the other room, throw the ball, turn the light on, empty the tub, put the guitar back, etc. Physical problems were also different for the two children: the Down's child could not reach a pillow, toy, jar, or climb a rocking horse; the normal child could not get out of the crib, get shampoo from her eyes, look over the window sill, open the door, get the earphones of the stereo untangled, or reach many desired objects. Cognitive problems, although relatively infrequent, occurred more frequently for the Down's child as a result of the mother's training exercises. However, the normal child was asked more frequently than the Down's child for information (60% versus 21% of all cognitive problems).

The two children did not differ in the relative proportion of various problems and problem subclasses. They both had approximately the same number of social problems (86% of total problems for the Down's child, 89% for the normal), physical problems (2% and 6%, respectively), and cognitive problems (11% and 4%, respectively). Subclasses also showed similar proportions in distribution, especially social problems, although what may be significant differences did occur as in the case of some subclasses of cognitive problems. The same can be said of the distribution of various classes of responses made by each child; the two children varied slightly if at all. It is also interesting that success in problem solving, as measured by the percentage of blocking conditions removed by the child's responses, did not differ between the children (the Down's child removed blocks 36% of the time, the normal child 41%). Furthermore, neither differed significantly in the extent to which her ongoing behavior before the blocking condition occurred was resumed after the block was dealt with (31% of ongoing behavior resumed for the Down's child, 28% for the normal).

What is interesting to note is that in quite a few instances, the parents (usually the mother) intervened in the problem-solving process in one way or another. In the case of the Down's child, the mother intervened in 6% of all problems; in the case of the normal child she (sometimes the father as well) intervened in 11% of the problems. Whether interventions of this sort are conducive or detrimental to the development of effective problem solving skill is a question well worth further investigation.

In addition to obtaining a preliminary idea of the problematic nature of the young child's environment and how a normal and retarded child go about dealing with it, the present study also sheds some light on the nature of problems that occur in natural everyday settings. By beginning with some preconceived notions about problems, applying these notions to the development of a provisional observational schema, and carrying out the observations, it became possible to collect a large number of subject-environment interactions which in various degrees fit the preconceived notions. Where a fit did not occur either the schema was changed (as noted earlier, our problem schema underwent 29 revisions), or the observations dispensed with, if they were totally refractory to analysis (this usually happened because the observations in turn resulted in seemingly sounder conceptions). By proceeding more or less inductively in this manner it gradually became possible to expand and come up with a more differentiated picture of problems and problem-solving behavior. This method has added three things to our knowledge of problems. 1) It is now methodologically and theoretically feasible, as indicated earlier, to analyze a problem into five basic elements: ongoing behavior, a blocking condition, a response to the blocking condition, a result of the response (block removed or not), and the outcome of this process (ongoing behavior resumed or not). 2) Problems can be defined and classified in an empirically observable and theoretically meaningful manner: the six classes of problems illustrated in Table 1. 3) The nature of problems and their distribution in everyday settings is much more complicated than ever anticipated. There is not space to discuss this in detail, so let it suffice to mention that problems or blocking conditions can occur singly or in multiples. They can be grouped in terms of a general theme and better understood than when left as isolated units. Blocking conditions can occur so quickly that the individual cannot respond to them and becomes confused because some of the blocks are removed before he can react. Some blocks cease to act as blocks but the individual still responds to them. Another person may intervene and remove the block that is contributing to the problem or ignore the block and carry the problem into a new direction. Or problems can occur within problems as a new block appears on the scene interrupting the individual's ongoing problem-solving behavior. In short, what happens in everyday reality is, as most of us would expect, vastly more complex and confusing than what happens when an individual is presented with problems in a test or laboratory situation. As far as we can tell, the young children we have studied manage to survive in the midst of this complexity. To some extent they have already come to adapt to it, and seem to be in the process of adapting to it during the moments we observe them.

CONCLUSION

What is presented here is a glimpse of what goes on in the lives of a few preschool children as they face everyday problems that require some form of adaptive response. Many of these problems are brief and uncomplicated, some are fairly complex and drawn out, all provide information about the child's environment and his or her way of dealing intelligently with it. It is our argument that the reactions to these problems are the basic stuff of adaptation. Each individual encounter with a problematic portion of the environment probably contributes very little to later success and happiness of the individual as an adult. However, the cumulative effect of all encounters must certainly make a difference to later adaptation, especially when these encounters occur during the early periods of development. For it is during this period that the individual is acquiring the cognitive skills to cope with the myriad of physical and social problems that he or she will eventually have to face as an adult.

Individuals whose capacity to acquire these skills is impaired or less developed than the average are especially vulnerable to adaptational failure as adults. Hence it is important to know firsthand in as much detail as possible how these individuals and their environments interact. It is also important to know exactly what the various adaptational requirements for adults are. One likes to think that this knowledge can be obtained by applying the general methodological principles and basic orientation used in the present study to older children and adults. If this is done there will have to be major alterations in the method to cope with the increasingly dominant role that verbal and symbolic behaviors play in the growing child and especially the adolescent and the adult. By knowing exactly what environmental adaptations are required of adults we will be in a much better position to predict future outcomes for individual children. The present method allows us to draw a better picture of these demands.

The method described here is clearly an eclectic one. It involves basic concepts from cognitive and test psychology, the findings and theories of developmental psychology, the axioms and major concepts of the synthetic theory of evolution, and the methodological and conceptual orientation of ethology. It is the latter that seems to have made the most crucial contribution to this approach. The ethologist's insistence on the importance of naturalistic observation for understanding behavior has been very convincing. As time consuming and painfully tedious as such observation is, it is the only way of really knowing what is going on during the complex interactions between the individual and his environment. By collecting longitudinal information (which adds to the difficulty of this approach, but is nevertheless indispensable), constructing a relevant observational schema, and obtaining representative samples of behavior/environment interactions through naturalistic observations, it will eventually be possible to get a clearer picture of the problematic nature of the child's environment and how the child responds to it. Only then will it be possible to understand the individual. And with such understanding, it will be possible to make better predictions about future adaptation as well as develop a more rational program of intervention for children who need it.

REFERENCES

Berlyne, D. E. 1965. Structure and Direction in Thinking. John Wiley & Sons Inc., New York.

Blurton-Jones, N. G. (ed.). 1972. Ethological Studies of Child Behavior. Cambridge University Press, Cambridge, England.

Charlesworth, W. R. 1976. Human intelligence as adaptation: an ethological approach. In: L. B. Resnick (ed.), The Nature of Intelligence. Lawrence Erlbaum Associates, Publishers, Hillsdale, New Jersey.

Dewey, J. 1933. How We Think. D. C. Heath and Company, New York.

Duncker, K. 1945. On problem solving. Psychol. Monogr. 58, Whole No. 270.

Eibl-Eibesfeldt, I. 1970. Ethology: The Biology of Behavior. Holt, Rinehart & Winston, New York.

Ekman, P., and Friesen, W. V. 1971. Constants across cultures in the face and emotion. J. Pers. Soc. Psychol. 17(2):124–129.

Freedman, D. G. 1974. Human Infancy: An Evolutionary Perspective. Holshear Press (Wiley), New York.

Gagne, R. M. 1965. The Conditions of Learning. Holt, Rinehart & Winston, New York.

Gladwin, T. 1970. East is a Big Bird: Navigation and Logic on Puluwat Atoll. Harvard University Press, Cambridge, Massachusetts.

Harlow, H. F. 1971. Learning to Love. Albion Publishing Company, San Francisco.

Heber, R. F. (ed.). 1961. A manual on terminology and classification in mental retardation. Am. J. Ment. Defic., monogr. suppl.

Hess, E. 1970. Ethological and developmental psychology. In: P. H. Mussen (ed.), Manual of Child Psychology, Vol. 1. pp. 1–38. John Wiley & Sons, Inc., New York.

Higgins, J. V., Reed, E. W., and Reed, S. C. 1962. Intelligence and family size: a paradox resolved. Eugenics Q. 9:84–90.

Jencks, C., Smith, M., Acland, H., Bane, H., Cohen, D., Gintis, H., Heyns, B., and Michelson, S. 1972. Inequality: A Reassessment of the Effect of Family and Schooling in America. The Macmillan Company, New York.

Jerison, H. J. 1973. Evolution of the Brain and Intelligence. Academic Press, New York.

Klein, R. G. 1973. Ice-age Hunters of the Ukraine. The University of Chicago Press, Chicago.

Kohler, W. 1925. The Mentality of Apes. Harcourt, Brace & Co., New York.

Leland, H., Nihara, K., Foster, R., Shellhaas, M., and Kagin, E. 1966. Conference on Measurement of Adaptive Behavior, II. Parsons State Hospital and Training Center, Parsons, Kansas.

Leland, H., Shellhaas, M., Nihara, K., and Foster, R. 1967. Adaptive behavior: a new dimension in the classification of the mentally retarded. Ment. Retard. Abstr. 4:359–387.

Lorenz, K. 1969. Innate bases of learning. In: K. Pribram (ed.), On the Biology of Learning. Harcourt, Brace & World Inc., New York.

Lorenz, K. 1971. Psychology and phylogeny. In: K. Lorenz (ed.), Studies in Animal and Human Behavior, Vol. 2. Harvard University Press, Cambridge, Massachusetts.

Maier, N. R. 1940. The behavior mechanisms concerned with problem solving. Psychol. Rev. 47:43–58.

Maslow, A. H. 1954. Motivation and Personality. Harper & Brothers, New York.

Maslow, A. H. 1972. The Farther Reaches of Human Nature. Viking Press, New York.

Mason, O. T. 1966. The Origins of Invention. M.I.T. Press, Cambridge, Massachusetts (originally published in 1895).

Mayr, E. 1970. Populations, Species, and Evolution. Harvard University Press, Cambridge, Massachusetts.

Mercer, J. R. 1973. Labelling the Mentally Retarded. University of California Press, Berkeley.

Phillips, L. 1968. Human Adaptation and Its Failures. Academic Press, New York.

Reed, S. C. 1965. The evolution of human intelligence. Am. Sci. 53:317–326.

Resnick, L. B. 1976. The Nature of Intelligence. Lawrence Erlbaum Associates, Publishers, Hillsdale, New Jersey.

Resnick, L. B., and Glaser, R. 1976. Problem solving and intelligence. In: L. B. Resnick (ed.), The Nature of Intelligence. Lawrence Erlbaum Associates, Publishers, Hillsdale, New Jersey.

Robinson, N. M., and Robinson, H. B. 1976. The Mentally Retarded: A Psychological Approach. 2nd Ed., The McGraw-Hill Book Company, New York.

Spiker, D. 1976. An observational study of problem-solving behavior in six preschoolers. Unpublished manuscript, University of Minnesota.

Tinbergen, N. 1972. Forward. In: N. Blurton-Jones (ed.), Ethological Studies of Child Behaviour. Cambridge University Press, Cambridge.

Wade, N. 1976. Sociobiology: troubled birth for new discipline. Science 191:1151–1155.

Wertheimer, M. 1945. Productive Thinking. Harper & Brothers, New York.

Willems, E. P., and Raush, H. L. (eds.). 1969. Naturalistic Viewpoints in Psychological Research. Holt, Rinehart & Winston, Inc., New York.

Williams, G. C. 1966. Adaptation and Natural Selection. Princeton University Press, Princeton, New Jersey.

Wilson, E. O. 1975. Sociobiology: The New Synthesis. The Belknap Press of Harvard University Press, Cambridge, Massachusetts.

chapter 2

Ecological Psychology and Mental Retardation

Phil Schoggen

It is the purpose of this paper to present an overview of the main features of theory and method of ecological psychology as developed primarily at the University of Kansas by Roger G. Barker, Herbert F. Wright, and their colleagues and students (e.g., Barker and Wright, 1955; Barker, 1963b; Barker and Gump, 1964; Wright, 1967; Barker, 1968; Barker and Schoggen, 1973) and to suggest some implications this line of research may have for the field of mental retardation. The paper is divided into three major sections: the first gives an orientation by identifying the main historical roots of the field, sketching features of the ecological perspective, and comparing ecology with ethology; the second section presents the basic tenets of ecological psychology and summarizes the two major research strategies used by the ecologists—the specimen record and the behavior setting survey; and the final section discusses the possible relevance of this work to mental retardation.

BACKGROUND

In dedicating her recent book (1972) on the evolution of primate behavior to G. S. Hutchinson, Alison Jolly says that Hutchinson once defined ecology as "the study of the universe." Although there may be an important message here, most writers in the animal and plant sciences seem to work within a less ambitious formulation of the domain of ecology as the study of the relations between living entities (plant or animal) and their natural, real life environments.

In the social sciences, human ecology now has a history of some 50 years as a recognized area of theory and research within sociology. The pioneer work of Robert Ezra Park, R. D. McKenzie, and Ernest W. Burgess opened the way for a long series of fruitful studies that attempted to apply the ecological approach to human communities. The work in human ecology has been concerned primarily with variables at the demographic level, e.g., spatial distribution, crime rates, incidence of delinquency, and mental illness in relation to environmental characteristics such as areas of the city. Hawley (1944) described the concept of human ecology thus:

> Human ecology, like plant and animal ecology, represents a special application of the general viewpoint to a particular class of living things. It involves both a recognition of the fundamental unity of animate nature and an awareness that there is differentiation within that unity. Man

> is an organism and as such he is dependent on the same resources, confronted with the same elementary problems, and displays in essential outline the same mode of response to life conditions as is observed in other forms of life. Thus the extension of patterns of thought and techniques of investigation developed in the study of the collective life of lower organisms to the study of man is a logical consummation of the ecological point of view. One important qualification is necessary, however; the extraordinary degree of flexibility of human behaviour makes for a complexity and a dynamics in the human community without counterpart elsewhere in the organic world. It is this that sets man apart as an object of special inquiry and gives rise to a human as distinct from a general ecology (p. 464).

In psychology, an ecological approach to the study of individual behavior was early attempted by Brunswik (1952) and Lewin (1951d). Although their conceptions were markedly different, they shared a concern for the relation between the psychological functioning of the person and the properties of the environment in which the behavior occurred.

Brunswik was the first to argue for the careful sampling of environmental situations on a basis fully equal to the recognized importance of the sampling of individual subjects. Brunswik believed that the research psychologist was obligated to obtain representative sampling of both concrete environmental situations and research subjects in order to achieve acceptable design of psychological experiments, and that psychological research should maintain a certain degree of naturalness or situational representativeness:

> According to the much-stressed requirement of "representative sampling" in differential psychology, individuals must be randomly drawn from a well-defined population; in the same manner, the study of functional organism-environment relationships would seem to require that not only mediation but especially also focal events and other situational circumstances should be made to represent, by sampling or related devices, the general or specific conditions under which the organism studied has to function. This leads to what the writer has suggested to call representative design of experiments (1952, pp. 29, 30).

Although Brunswik recognized objective regularity and lawfulness in nature as revealed in the laws of physics, he believed that the environment as experienced by the individual is semierratic at best and often chaotic, so that only probabilistic laws linking behavior with the environment are possible:

> . . . his environment remains for all practical purposes a semierratic medium; it is no more than partially controlled and no more than probabilistically predictable. The functional approach in psychology must take cognizance of this basic limitation of the adjustive apparatus; it must link behavior and environment statistically in bivariate or multivariate correlation rather than with the predominant emphasis on strict law, which we have inherited from physics (Brunswik, 1956, p. 157).

In his critique of Brunswik's work, Leeper (1966) summarizes these points with characteristic simplicity and clarity:

> The situation faced by psychology is basically the same as the situation faced by an individual with reference to the life situations to which he must learn how to respond as well as possible. He has to learn that the behavior that is effective in one type of situation is not effective in another, and that the factors that are very highly correlated with success in one type of situation have only a much lower correlation with success in a different type of situation. In each type of situation, there will be variations that will go beyond what he can anticipate; but the individual nevertheless could well express the lessons from his learning by saying, "I have learned that, at different points, I am in such and such different ecologies, and I've had to learn different

laws about how to proceed and what to expect in those different ecologies. My knowledge still is probabilistic, but it is a darn sight better when I recognize these different settings in which I'm operating than when I disregard them or do not know about them." In the same way, although it is true that psychology wants to describe ecologies in more abstract terms than the individual person would be likely to do, the attainment of good explanations by psychology depends on the recognition of a great host of ecologies, separated out by some understanding of the key factors operating in various life situations, even for a given individual (p. 434).

In contrast to Brunswik's probabilistic functionalism, the topological and vector psychology of Kurt Lewin (1935, 1936, 1938) was concerned almost exclusively with the environment as it exists psychologically for the person at a particular time. Whereas Brunswik believed that psychology's task was to study the probabilistic, statistical relations between behavior and the objective, concrete situations of the ecological or preperceptual environment, Lewin was convinced that psychology is an autonomous science, the constructs and theories of which cannot be reduced to those of any other science. He argued, therefore, that psychologists should limit themselves to work with purely psychological variables. His goal was the development of exceptionless scientific laws of behavior, which he saw as possible only by staying strictly within the psychological domain. At the heart of Lewin's system is his concept of the *life space,* which he defined as the totality of psychological facts that determine the behavior of the individual at a particular time. It includes the person and the psychological environment, the environment as seen by the person. Lewin wrote:

> . . . to understand or to predict behavior, the person and his environment have to be considered as *one* constellation of interdependent factors. We call the totality of these factors the life space (LSp) of that individual, and write B = F (P,E) = F (LSp). The life space, therefore, includes both the person and his psychological environment. The task of explaining behavior thus becomes identical with (1) finding representation of the life space (LSp) and (2) determining the function (F) which links the behavior to the life space. This function (F) is what one usually calls a law (1951a, pp. 239, 240).

In another paper, Lewin commented on his preference for seeking strict, psychological laws in contrast to Brunswik's interest in establishing probabilistic rules or correlations.

> To my mind, the main issue is what the term "probability" refers to. Does Brunswik want to study the ideas of the driver of a car about the probability of being killed or does he want to study the accident statistics which tell the "objective probability" of such an event. If an individual sits in a room trusting that the ceiling will not come down, should only his "subjective probability" be taken into account for predicting behavior or should we also consider the "objective probability" of the ceiling's coming down as determined by the engineers. To my mind, only the first has to be taken into account (1951b, p. 58).

Although nothing is more central to Lewin's psychology than this concept of the environment only in terms of its psychological significance to the person, Lewin recognized explicitly the role of nonpsychological factors in addressing certain kinds of problems.

> I can see why psychology should be interested even in those areas of the physical and social world which are not part of the life space or which do not affect its boundary zone at present. If one wishes to safeguard a child's education during the next years, if one wishes to predict in what situation an individual will find himself as a result of a certain action, one will have to

> calculate this future. Obviously, such forecast has to be based partly on statistical considerations about nonpsychological data.
>
> Theoretically, we can characterize this task as discovering what part of the physical or social world will determine during a given period the "boundary zone" of the life space. I would suggest calling it "psychological ecology" (1951b, pp. 58, 59).

Barker, whose own work owes more to Lewin than to any other, describes Lewin as in serious conflict between his view of psychology as a conceptually autonomous science, an encapsulated system of purely psychological constructs, on the one hand, and his recognition that nonpsychological events often have profound importance for people on the other. Lewin saw no way to incorporate such nonpsychological phenomena into a science of psychology.

> So Lewin led an uneasy life with this dilemma. He saw very clearly that an adequate applied behavioral science requires conceptual bridges between psychology and ecology, and even though his conception of science told him that this is impossible, much of his effort from the Iowa period onward was preoccupied with it. Sometimes he approached the psychological-ecological breach directly and explicitly, as in his gatekeeper theory of the link between food habits and food technology and economics [1951d]; sometimes he approached it obliquely and implicitly, as in his attempt to treat the social field as a psychological construct [1951c]. He seemed unable to avoid the interface between ecology and psychology and to work within his own system, as he had done in the earlier studies of tension systems, psychological satiation, and level of aspiration. I think the reason is clear: Lewin's total life experience and his conception of psychology as a science were in irreconcilable conflict. He could not ignore his life experiences, and he could not give up his conception of psychology. It was a painful conflict (Barker, 1963a, pp. 18, 19).

Although the theoretical explorations of Brunswik and Lewin are seen as the primary intellectual antecedents in the development of ecological psychology, other work in psychology that has had a clearly identifiable influence includes that of Fritz Heider (1959), E. C. Tolman (1932), Henry Murray (1938), William McDougall (1923), and Karl Muenzinger (1942).

The problems addressed in ecological psychology have much in common with time-honored concerns of social anthropology (e.g., Mead, 1928; Kluckhohn, 1940; Whiting and Child, 1953). Although they acknowledged their incursion into anthropological territory without so much as a "by your leave" (Barker and Wright, 1955, pp. 5, 6), the ecologists asserted their interest in taking a more strictly psychological approach and they saw promise in the attempt to develop new, more systematic, and readily quantifiable techniques of field research. Whether this promise has been realized during the intervening 20 years might be judged differently by different observers.

An Ecological Perspective

It may be useful to identify next some of the main features that distinguish the ecological from other approaches to the study of behavior. Over the past 10 years, Edwin P. Willems has addressed himself to this task in at least three different papers (1965, 1969, 1977). His most recent and comprehensive statement discusses a number of emphases, assumptions, and programmatic implications of what he calls "behavioral ecology." What follows in this section is a brief summary of Willems' points that seem most directly relevant to ecological psychology.

Behavior and Environment The ecological perspective stresses the mutual interdependence between organism, behavior, and environment. Brunswik put it this way:

> Both organism and environment will have to be seen as systems, each with properties of its own, yet both hewn from basically the same block. Each has surface and depth, or overt and covert regions . . . the interrelationship between the two systems has the essential characteristic of a "coming-to-terms." And this coming to terms is not merely a matter of the mutual boundary or surface areas. It concerns equally as much, or perhaps even more, the rapport between the central, covert layers of the two systems. It follows that, much as psychology must be concerned with the texture of the organism or of its nervous processes and must investigate them in depth, it also must be concerned with the texture of the environment as it extends in depth away from the common boundary (1957, p. 5).

Site Specificity: The Importance of Place For the ecological psychologist, it is important to specify with precision the location of the organism in time and space. Bruner (1965) commented "I am still struck by Roger Barker's ironic truism that the best way to predict the behavior of a human being is to know where he is: in a post office he behaves post office, at church he behaves church" (p. 1016). In other words, place-behavior systems have such strong principles of organization and constraint that their standing patterns of behavior remain essentially the same although individuals come and go. Wicker (1972) has discussed this process which he calls "behavior-environment congruence."

Molar Phenomena and Nonreductionism The ecological perspective tends, generally, to emphasize molar as opposed to molecular phenomena. There is a related emphasis upon environmental, behavioral, and organismic holism and simultaneous, complex relationships. This reflects ecology's persistent concern, at various levels of analysis, with the organism's and the population's behavioral commerce with the environmental packages they inhabit.

Systems Concepts The ecologist's emphasis upon holism and the study of complex, simultaneous, and sequentially interdependent phenomena sends him searching for new ways of thinking about such problems. Increasingly, systems theory and concepts seem to be helpful. Willems says:

> Psychology is emerging from a period in which the definition and selection of problems, the procedures of research, the processes of inference, and the formulation and testing of models have been closely intertwined with, if not dominated by, the available tools of probability statistics and sampling distributions of statistics. *Independence* of events, variables, and data points is the bedrock of such procedures and of experimental analysis. We are beginning to sense the inappropriateness of the assumption of independence for many important phenomena. Just the opposite of independence characterizes many of the phenomena whose understanding is being sought and the interdependency must be reflected in appropriate models, terms, and procedures. Systems theory and its various derivatives offer the tools for representing *interdependence* and simultaneous, time-related complexity (1977).

Ecological Diagnosis One of the most memorable parts of Willems' paper tells the story of an ornithologist with a European zoo who wished to add a small bird called the bearded tit to the zoo's collection. Willems describes the story as a central parable of behavioral ecology and credits Robert B. Lockard as the source.

> Armed with all the relevant information he could find about the tit, the ornithologist went to great pains to build the right setting. Introducing a male and female to the setting, he noted that, by all behavioral criteria, the birds functioned very well. Unfortunately, soon after the

> birds hatched babies, they shoved the babies out of the nest, onto the ground, where they died. This cycle, beginning with mating and ending with the babies dead on the ground, repeated itself many times.
> The ornithologist tried many modifications of the setting, but none forestalled the systematic infanticide. After many hours of renewed, direct observation of tits in the wild, the ornithologist noted three patterns of behavior that had missed everyone's attention. First, throughout most of the daylight hours in the wild, the parent tits were very active at finding and bringing food for the infants. Second, the infants, with whose food demands the parents could hardly keep pace, spent the same hours with their mouths open, apparently crying for food. The third pattern was that any inanimate object, whether eggshell, leaf, or beetle shell, was quickly shoved out of the nest by the parents. With these observations in mind, the ornithologist went back to observe his captive tits and he found that, during the short time a new brood of infants lived, the parents spent only brief periods feeding them by racing between the nest and the food supply, which the ornithologists had supplied in abundance. After a short period of such feeding, the infants, apparently satiated, fell asleep. The first time they slept for any length of time during the daylight hours, the parents shoved them (two inanimate objects, after all) out of the nest. When he made the food supply *less* abundant and *less* accessible and thereby made the parents work much longer and harder to find and bring food, the ornithologist found that the infants spent more daylight time awake, demanding food, and that the tits then produced many families and cared for them to maturity (1977).

In approaching this problem, the ornithologist demonstrated the kind of ecological diagnosis Willems recommends. The ornithologist could have adopted the strategy commonly applied in psychology based on the assumption that the main determinants of behavior are inside the skin and therefore diagnosed the parent birds as crazy, sick, or otherwise in need of special help. Instead, through patient, direct observation of other representatives of the species in their natural habitat, he carefully re-examined the intact organism environment system. This enabled him to see where the delicate balance of elements within this system had been upset in the zoo; a truly ecological diagnosis of the problem.

Naturalistic Emphasis Fundamental to an ecological approach is preference for direct observation of phenomena in natural, real life situations. Willems cites Darling's suggestion that there is probably a better scientific basis for building a good environment for cows than for persons, in part because cows cannot speak our language. They are, therefore, unable to respond in interviews, fill out questionnaires, or do many experimental tasks. As a consequence, students of cow behavior have to observe what cows actually do for extended periods, usually in natural, true life circumstances. The ecologist believes that this approach has much to offer the student of human behavior as well.

Distribution of Phenomena in Nature A central task of the ecologist is to determine the distribution in nature of the phenomena of interest. He studies the range, intensity, and frequency of behavior of persons in many different kinds of life circumstances. This challenge to scientific psychology was issued in 1955 on the opening pages of Barker and Wright's first general book on ecological psychology:

> . . . we know how people behave under the conditions of experiments and clinical procedures, but we know little about the distribution of these conditions outside of laboratories and clinics. It is different in other sciences. Geologists, biologists, chemists, and physicists know in considerable detail about the distribution in nature of the materials and processes with which they deal. Chemists know something about the laws governing the interaction of oxygen and hydrogen, and they also know how these elements are distributed in nature. Entomologists

> know the biological vectors of malaria, and they also know about the occurrence of these vectors over the earth. In contrast, psychologists know little more than laymen about the frequency and degree of occurrence of their basic phenomena in the lives of men—of deprivation, hostility, freedom, friendliness, social pressure, rewards and punishments. Although we have daily records of the behavior of volcanoes, of the tides, of sun spots, and of rats and monkeys, there have been few scientific records of how a human mother cared for her young, how a particular teacher behaved in the classroom and how the children responded, what a family actually did and said during a mealtime, or how any boy lived his life from the time he awoke in the morning until he went to sleep at night. Because we lack such records we can only speculate on many important kinds of questions such as these:
>
> What changes have occurred over the generations in the way children are reared and in the way they behave?
>
> How does life differ for children in large and small families?
>
> How, in psychological terms, does life differ for rural, town, and urban families?
>
> Are American children disciplined differently from English and French children? If so, does this affect the national character of Americans, Englishmen and Frenchmen?
>
> Before we can answer these kinds of questions about behavior . . . we must know more than the laws of behavior. We must know how the relevant psychological conditions are distributed among men (1955, p. 2).

Taxonomy Along with naturalistic description of the distribution of behavioral phenomena, basic taxonomic research has been seriously neglected by psychologists (Frederiksen, 1972). What are the units of environment, of behavior, and of environment-behavior linkages? Into what types of classifications do situations, behavior, and environments fall? Ecologists believe that the development of appropriate taxonomies remains as a vast and largely unconfronted challenge to students of behavior.

Ecology and Ethology

Although a thorough, comparative analysis of ecology and ethology is beyond the scope of this paper, it is obvious that, despite some important differences, there is much in common between the ecological psychologists as discussed herein and the human ethologists such as Blurton-Jones (1972), Hutt and Hutt (1970), and Eibl-Eibesfeldt (1967).

There is a common dedication to the belief that students of behavior need to correct psychology's deficiency in neglecting the descriptive, natural history phase of scientific development. The congruence between the statements of prominent spokesmen for the two fields is striking. Barker and Wright said in 1955:

> Psychology has been predominantly an experimental science. . . . The descriptive, natural history, ecological phase of science which is so strongly represented in the biological sciences, sociology, anthropology, earth sciences, and astronomy has had virtually no counterpart in psychology. This has left a serious gap in psychological knowledge, for in leaving out ecological methods psychology has almost completely omitted a basic scientific procedure that is essential if some fundamental problems of human behaviour are to be solved (p. 1).

Only a few years later, Tinbergen (1963) expressed a similar position:

> . . . in its haste to step into the twentieth century and to become a respectable science, psychology skipped the preliminary descriptive stage that other natural sciences had gone through, and so was soon losing touch with the natural phenomena (p. 4).

Ecology and ethology share the goal of documenting in scientifically adequate ways the naturally occurring patterns of behavior as they are found in noncontrived situations of ordinary, everyday life. In 1951, Barker and Wright published *One Boy's Day,* a straightforward descriptive account of what one 7-year-old boy actually did on an ordinary day of his life from the time he awoke in the morning until he went to bed that night. Subsequent analyses of this and similar specimen records (Barker, 1963b) have generated a rich store of data on child behavior in natural situations.

For ethologists, the ethogram—a complete catalog of the behavior of a particular animal—is the starting point. Hutt and Hutt (1970) say: "It is only by repeated sampling of a child's behavior in many different situations that the consistencies in behavior emerge" (p. 29).

Substantial progress in this task is documented in several books that have appeared in recent years (e.g., Hutt and Hutt, 1970; Blurton-Jones, 1972; McGrew, 1972). Of related interest is the recent compilation and description of 73 different systems of observing young children (Boyer, Simon, and Karafin, 1973).

In both ecology and ethology, the research method of choice is direct observation by trained observers who rely chiefly upon their perceptive wit and their thorough familiarity with the organism and the main properties of its normal habitat to assure that the observational record is comprehensive and valid. If the problem requires it and circumstances permit, mechanical, photographic, and electronic aids may be employed as supplements to, but rarely as replacements for, the human observer.

The ecological and ethological approaches also agree on the need to preserve intact the phenomena of interest and the need to use research methods that do not interfere with or disturb the natural course of events. Both Barker (1963b) and Blurton-Jones (1972) among others have made the case for noninterference with the ongoing stream of behavior in its natural, true life context.

Perhaps the most fundamental and pervasive difference between the two approaches is found in ethology's derivation from evolutionary theory. Much of the work in ethology, from the formulation of the problem, through the choice of research method and definition of behavior unit, to the ultimate interpretation of the results, reflects concern for survival value or function and phylogenetic significance of the behavior. The ecological psychologists show little concern for such issues.

Ecological psychologists share with ethologists ". . . distrust of large preselected and untested categories of behavior" (Blurton-Jones, 1972, p. 1) and agree on the importance of following carefully described observational procedures that can be carried out by others at other times and in other places in order to obtain comparable data. However, the ecologists stop far short of the insistence that the observational record include only ". . . large numbers of anatomically described items of behavior" (Blurton-Jones, 1972, p. 1). This means that ethological observations often are limited to the description of molecular behavior or what Murray (1938) called "actones," e.g., behaviors of subsystems of the organism such as facial expressions, gestures, postures, locomotion, and other motor activities that occur usually outside the organism's awareness as more or less automatic implementing mediators of the larger, purposive or goal-directed actions with which the organism as a whole is cognitively occupied. In fact, Smith and Connolly assert that "Probably the most powerful tool in the ethologist's armoury is the description of specific motor patterns'' (1972, p. 74). It seems clear that for some kinds of problems, e.g., studies of correlations of behavioral and physiological measures (Hutt and Hutt, 1970, pp. 12, 13), the recording of behavior at the molecular level may be especially appropriate and fruitful. For other kinds of problems, e.g., social interaction and social relations, description of behavior in more molar terms may be more useful, as indeed some of those identified with the ethological group have suggested (e.g., Smith and Connolly, 1972, pp. 74, 75; Blurton-Jones, 1972, p. 21).

The ecologists, on the other hand, are primarily interested in molar behavior, recognizing that describing behavior at the molar level always requires some degree of inference by the observer about intrinsically unobservable psychological processes within the behaving organism such as goals, purposes, intentions, and feelings. The ecological observers are instructed to make such low level inferences but are also urged to include in their records, as much as possible, actones or molecular behaviors which often constitute the empirical basis for the inferences made about the behavior at the molar level. The ecologists believe and provide evidence (Barker and Wright, 1955; Dickman, 1963; Schoggen, 1963) that such relatively low level inferences about momentary motivation and feeling can be made in a scientifically acceptable way, but some of the ethologists (Hutt and Hutt, 1970) insist that all such inferences are intrinsically unscientific. In a recent paper, Darren Newtson (1977) provides a sophisticated discussion of some of the central issues involved here, and also summarizes a series of new and well executed experiments, the results of which do not support the pessimistic views expressed by Hutt and Hutt that people ''. . . simply are not adept at inferring . . . motivations, intentions and emotions'' (1970, p. 16).

Although workers in both groups have asserted and demonstrated their interest in environments, there is a clear difference between ecology and ethology in the amount of attention they have paid to the study of environments per se. Whereas ethologists have been primarily concerned with identifying consistencies in behavior and in behavior taxonomy, the ecologists have invested heavily in ways of describing environments and have developed a unit of environmental analysis and taxonomy—the behavior setting—which stands independent of the behavior of any particular individual. Thus human ethology continues in the organism or person-centered tradition of biology and zoology, but ecological psychology takes its inspiration from animal and plant ecology and anthropology in its effort to develop a science of the environment of molar behavior.

METHODS AND SELECTED FINDINGS IN ECOLOGICAL PSYCHOLOGY

Although the principle of noninterference by the investigator with the naturally occurring phenomena of interest has been explicitly honored by the ecological psychologists from the earliest days of their work (Barker and Wright, 1951; 1955), a more recent reformulation of the issues involved constitutes the clearest, most forceful statement to date (Barker, 1968).

In this paper, Barker notes that the *phenomena* of any science occur in nature without the benefit of any assistance from scientists but that the *data* of a science are the joint product of the phenomena and the scientist's efforts to study the phenomena via one or another of a wide range of data-generating systems. In psychology, Barker says that such data-generating systems can be divided into two broad categories depending primarily on how much control the psychologist exercises over the process.

In *transducer* data (T data) systems, there is no input from the psychologist; the phenomena are scanned by the psychologist whose functions are those of a transducer; a docile receiver, coder, and transmitter of information. "This data-generating system is, in effect, a translating machine, it translates psychological phenomena into data. The data it generates are operative images of the phenomena, prepared in retrievable form for storage and further analysis" (Barker, 1968, p. 140).

In *operator* data (O data) systems, the psychologist, in addition to functioning as a transducer, also acts as an operative part of the data-generating system by regulating input, influencing interior conditions, or constraining output. Here, the psychologist dominates the system, controlling it in order to focus upon processes that are of particular concern to him. The data refer to events that the investigator contrives. Whether the psychologist as operator achieves control via running trials in an experiment, posing questions in an interview or on a questionnaire, or setting up a problem or task to be solved on a standardized test, his operative function is equally clear; he generates the phenomena in order to study them.

Barker sees ecological psychology as:

> . . . a transducer science; in it, research psychologists function as sensors and transducers; its data record behavior and its conditions *in situ*. . . . T data refer to psychological phenomena that are explicitly excluded when the psychologist functions as operator. Indeed, the primary task of the psychologist as transducer is carefully to preserve phenomena that the psychologist as operator carefully alters, namely, psychologist-free units. . . . O data refer to phenomena that psychologists as transducers explicitly exclude, namely, psychological units arranged in accordance with the curiosities of the psychologist. The primary task of the operator is to alter, in ways that are crucial to his interests, phenomena that the psychologist as transducer leaves intact (1968, pp. 143, 144).

For example, psychologists as operators have learned a lot about intelligence and what people can and cannot do in response to the demands of standardized intelligence tests, but such methods can never tell us about the intellectual demands of everyday life. For this, transducer methods are required. Similarly, whereas operator (experimental) methods have taught us something about frustration and its consequences under the controlled conditions of the laboratory, transducer methods are needed to measure the frequency with which frustration occurs and to assess its consequences in everyday life.

Barker continues:

> The conclusion is inescapable that psychologists as operators and as transducers are not analogous, and that the data they produce have fundamentally different uses within the science. One may contend that the phenomena denoted by T data are unimportant, or that they are not psychology. One may argue that O data refer, potentially at least, to more fundamental, universal, invariant psychological processes than T data. But, however the phenomena denoted by T data are classified and evaluated, they comprise a realm of phenomena forever inaccessible via O data. The data that psychologists produce as transducers are not horse-and-buggy versions of the data they produce as operators. If one wishes to know, for example, such information as the duration of behavior units, the sources of social input, or the frequency of disturbances, only T data will provide the answers (p. 145).

The dominance of psychology by the psychologist as operator has produced a rather sophisticated armamentarium of research methods suitable for the generation of operator data: experiments, tests, interviews, and questionnaires. The lack of any similar development of transducer research methods presented the ecologists with a major methodological problem: they had to devise new tender-minded, nondestructive, nonmanipulative, phenomena-preserving research methods as they went along. The *specimen record* and the *behavior setting survey* are two such methods developed by the Kansas group and applied more extensively than any others in studies in a wide range of contexts.

The Specimen Record

This method has its roots in the earliest stage of scientific work in child psychology when Tiedemann (1787), Preyer (1888), Darwin (1877), and others made "baby biographies," anecdotal records of behavior and development of small children. The specimen record method, although inspired by these early efforts, has been developed with an effort to correct the most serious defects for which anecdotal records have been justly criticized.

A specimen record is a narrative description of the behavior of one person, usually a child, in a natural, noncontrived situation as seen by skilled observers over a substantial time period (Barker and Wright, 1955; Wright, 1967). The observer's task is to capture in plain language, without the use of psychological concepts or technical terms, a full, rich word-picture of the purposive, goal-directed behavior of the child and those aspects of the concrete situation that are relevant to the child's molar behavior. The observer tries to record as faithfully as possible everything done and said by the child and said by others with reference to the child. The description includes the manner in which the actions are carried out; the "how" of everything done and said is of great importance because it is essential for diagnosing goals, purposes and feelings. Thus specimen records are inferential and to some extent interpretive, but observers are expected to provide as much as possible in the way of concrete, observable details (e.g., volume and tone of voice, facial expression, posture, tempo, intensity), upon which their inferences often are based. Theorizing, "psychologizing," and other high level, abstract or speculative interpretations are not permitted. The inferences included are at a low level, the level of inference about feelings and motivations of others that is regularly employed by persons of normal social sensitivity in ordinary social intercourse in a culture with which they are familiar. Of course such inferences are sometimes wrong, but the ecologists believe they are right often enough to produce records that are useful for scientific work on a number of important problems (Barker and Wright, 1955; Barker, 1963b; Wright, 1967).

The early applications of the specimen record method required the observer to record handwritten notes but more recent studies have used a system of oral notes dictated during observation into a shielded microphone and portable recorder (Schoggen, 1964b).

Reproduced below is a 2-min segment from a specimen record made during a recess-time ball game lasting 15 min. The subject is Patrick Taylor, a fourth-grader, who walked on crutches with his right foot carried in a sling, due to Perthes disease. During the first 6 min of the game, Patrick's team had a turn in the field and had come to bat. As the excerpt begins, Glenn, the third batter on Patrick's team, has just made the first out.

10:22 a.m. Noticing this, Patrick jumps up, since he's the next one to bat, and swings on his crutches over toward the backstop.

As he approaches, Glenn walks toward him and says in a friendly, cheerful way, "I'll run for you."

At the same time, Harry calls over from the bank, "Hey, Patrick, can I run for you?"

Patrick turns around and, without responding directly to either of these two boys, picks up a bat from the ground.

He looks at Ken, who's standing nearby, and speaks to him in a quiet voice. I can't hear what he says.

He obviously asked Ken if he'd run for him, however, for Ken runs immediately over and takes his running stance just a few feet away from home base on the first base line.

Patrick hops with the bat directly up to the plate, leaving his crutches by the backstop.

He stands there, balancing deftly on his left foot, with the bat perched eagerly up on his shoulder, ready to bat.

Just before he reaches the plate, the pitcher calls in to him with slight impatience at the delay, "All right, let's go Patrick!"

The first pitch comes across, and Patrick swings. The bat connects, but it's a high foul ball which the catcher cannot get his hands on.

Patrick watches the ball's trajectory, then hops around, swinging the bat for practice as he waits for the pitch.

The ball goes back out, comes in again, and again Patrick connects. This hit goes down toward first base but outside the line for another foul.

The runner, not being sure, goes part way down toward first base to play safe.

10:23 a.m. The pitcher calls harshly to him, "All right, Ken, come on back."

The pitcher admonishes him to move closer in so he doesn't have such a long head start in case Patrick gets a hit.

Patrick stands up to the plate, bat cocked eagerly up on his shoulder, ready for the pitch.

The pitch comes in; it's low for ball three.

The return to the pitcher is badly overthrown, and the runners steal from second to third and from third to home. The throw to home in an attempt to put out the runner from third base is a little late, and the ump calls him safe.

As this action takes place, Patrick hops back, out of the batter's box, to avoid interfering.

Now Patrick moves back to the plate.

The pitch comes in.

Patrick swings and connects.

It's a fair ball, and Ken goes madly for first base. He easily makes it in time.

Patrick drops the bat, turns, and hops quickly over to where he left his crutches by the backstop.

He notices that Glenn has picked up his crutches and is walking around with them with his back to Patrick.

Patrick, annoyed and impatient, shouts right behind Glenn, "Give me those." He reaches out and jerks them away from Glenn.

Glenn offers no resistance but yields the crutches immediately, looking rather sheepish.

Patrick slips them under his arms and flies off toward first base using his best gait, taking a big hop with his left foot each time he comes down on it.

As Patrick reaches first base, Ken turns around and starts back toward home plate.

Patrick assumes his position on first base, ready to run. He watches the pitcher closely.

Measuring the reliability of specimen records is a difficult and complex problem. When two observers make parallel specimen records based upon watching the same child for a period of time, the problem of measuring the amount of agreement between the two records turns out to be quite a challenge because of differences between the observers in choice of words, emphasis, and amount of supporting detail provided. On this question, Wright (1967) says:

> Specimen records do not have only one reliability coefficient . . . they have as many reliability coefficients as they have attributes that mirror the subject's behavior or situation. They have different reliabilities, for example, as sources of data on the games of children, on the amounts of time children spend outdoors, on the ways children are disciplined, on the number of overlapping episodes in which children engage, and on the occurrence of daydreaming in the behavior of children. We have identified many such variables in specimen records, and each presents a separate reliability question (pp. 43, 44).

In practice, it has been necessary first to divide the specimen records into analytical units on one basis or another and then to measure agreement in terms of comparative frequencies of these units or their properties. The difficulty with this procedure, of course, is that it confounds *observer* agreement with agreement between *analysts* or *coders*. Until very recently, the ecologists have been content in their various studies using specimen records to report only agreement between analysts or coders, but a new paper by George Dreher (1975), a student of Ed Willems, describes an ingenious method for assessing observer agreement as well as analyst agreement. For those who have for so long taken the reliability of specimen records more on faith than on evidence, Dreher's new data showing very high observer agreement in records of this type are reassuring.

Because the ecologists consider specimen records to be basic, primary data useful for work on a wide range of problems in a science of molar behavior, care has been taken in all these studies to preserve copies of the specimen records in final typed form. These records are now available from a special archive recently established at the University of Kansas for scientific use by any serious investigator. The records cover hundreds of hours of behavior of children ranging in age from 2 to 10 years in a variety of life situations in several regions of the United States and in England. Their usefulness for work on many problems other than those addressed in the studies for which the records were originally made has been demonstrated many times over.

One of the first systems developed for use in analyzing specimen records is based on the identification in the records of all the behavior episodes or goal-directed, molar actions engaged in by the child subject during the period covered by the record. Independent analysts agree well in the use of the formal definition and technical criteria for identifying behavior episodes in specimen records (Wright, 1967, pp. 56–98).

Once such units of analyses have been identified in terms of their structural and dynamic properties, the next step in the analytical process is the systematic description of each episode in terms of its material and content properties, the large number of qualitative characteristics of behavior and its immediate context on which episodes differ widely, e.g., duration, source of initiation and termination, sociality, mood or affect of child and associate, outcome. Many such properties of episodes have been studied and reported in the literature (Barker and Wright, 1955; Barker, 1963b; Wright, 1967). Here are some illustrative findings mainly from analyses of 18 day-long specimen records:

1. The number of episodes occurring during a normal waking day (about 14 hr) decreases with increasing age from about 1000 for 2 and 3-year-olds to roughly half that number for 7 to 9-year-olds. There is a complementary increase over the same age range in the average duration of episodes from about ½ min to 1 min.
2. Complexity of behavior structure increases with age, i.e., the older child more often engages in more than one molar activity at a time.
3. Two-thirds of all episodes involve other persons or pets; in three-fifths of these the associate is an adult.
4. Adults dominate children in one-third of the episodes in which they are involved; children dominate the child subjects in one-sixth of the episodes in which they are involved.
5. Disturbances in the ongoing behavior stream occur at the rate of 5.4 per hr; half of these are evoked by adults.
6. Episodes of American children are of shorter duration, on the average, than those of comparable English children.
7. English adults provide children with devaluative inputs four times as frequently as American adults.

In a later study, Schoggen (1963) developed a different basic analytical unit in order to focus more directly upon environmental inputs to the stream of behavior as recorded in specimen records. The new unit, called the Environmental Force Unit (EFU), is analogous to the behavior episode except that the EFU refers to molar actions of environmental agents (other persons or pets) that are directed to the child subject of the specimen record. Thus every time anyone in the child's immediate context attempts to direct, control, modify, support, assist, respond to, or otherwise interact overtly with the child, an EFU is marked. EFU's correspond to agents' goals with respect to the child just as episodes correspond to the child's own goals.

As with the episode, the EFU is defined in terms of structural and dynamic properties and is identified in specimen records as the first stage of the analytical process. Subsequent ratings of EFU in terms of material-content properties revealed a number of interesting facts about the active social environments of the child-subjects of the 18 day-long specimen records in the Kansas archive. For example:

1. EFU's occurred at the rate of about 3 units every 5 min.
2. Most EFU's were very brief in duration (¼ min or less).
3. Mothers and school teachers were the most frequent sources of EFU's.
4. EFU's in which no conflict between the agent and the child was involved outnumbered conflict units 2 to 1.
5. Among conflict EFU's, methods used by the agent to modify the child's behavior were usually gentle and mild; offers of reward and threats of punishment were rare.
6. No differences could be found on the variables studied between the records of the four children who had physical disabilities and nondisabled children.

In his concluding paragraph to this report, Schoggen asserts:

> Perhaps the one most significant result of this study lies in the demonstration that the social environment of the child, as recorded in specimen records, displays readily recognizable properties of directedness with regard to the child, i.e., the social environment appears to have intentions with respect to the child which are easily discernible as units which can be used for descriptive and analytical studies of environmental forces acting upon children in ordinary, everyday life (p. 69).

Schoggen also used specimen records and the EFU analysis to study the social psychological environments of a larger sample of children with and without physical disabilities (Schoggen, 1964a; 1975), to pursue further the rather surprising finding of no differences in the Kansas study. Seven children with peripheral motor impairments who were regular students in ordinary public school classrooms in grades one to three were paired with similar children without physical disabilities in the same classroom. Six or eight ½-hr specimen records were made of the behavior of each child in selected settings at school and in the home for a total of 135 specimen records. In general, the EFU analysis of these records tended to support the earlier finding of no differences in the variables studied between the social psychological environments of children with and without physical disabilities.

1. The environments of the children with disabilities seemed to be neither more nor less stimulating and responsive to the child than the environments of the matched nondisabled children (as measured by frequency of EFU). The same holds true whether one counts EFU with all agents or looks separately at mother or at the classroom teacher as EFU agent.
2. The total amount of time spent by mothers and teachers does not differ between members of matched pairs.
3. There is no difference between children with and without disabilities in the amount of individual attention and help provided by EFU agents.
4. The frequency of conflict within EFU's between environmental agents and the child subjects is not different for children with disabilities.
5. There were no intrapair differences in the environmental demands placed upon the child.

These and other findings led Schoggen, after considering other possible interpretations, to conclude:

> In fact, the children with disabilities were not accorded special treatment on the dimensions considered in the analysis. We believe that disability was not a particularly potent determinant of the quality of the social action directed to these children. It appeared to be, rather, only one aspect of the relatively complex social stimulus provided by the child to his associates. The behavior of other children and adults toward these children appeared to be determined by the total complex of personal attributes of which physical disability was only one small part. The children and adults who interacted with these children appeared to be responding to the whole child as a person; physical disability seemed to be virtually disregarded or, at most, to play a very minor role in the larger context of all the child's personal qualities. People were not responding to a "crippled child" but, rather, to Nick or Patrick or Libby as persons who, almost incidentally, had a physical disability (1975, p. 144).

In another investigation (Schoggen and Schoggen, 1971; 1976), specimen records and the EFU analysis were used to study environmental forces in the home lives of 3-year-old children in three population subgroups. Eight specimen records were made on each of eight children in families representing urban and rural low income and urban middle income groups. The specimen records covered periods ranging in duration from 10 to 50 min and totaling 3 to 4 hr for each of the 24 children. The results of this analysis showed wide individual differences across the 24 children, some important similarities across the three socioeconomic groups, and some interesting intergroup differences. For example:

1. Environmental agents were most frequently female and the mother, not surprisingly, was the most active agent in the environment for most of these 3-year-old children.
2. Agents were responsive to, attentive to, and interfering with the children in one group as often as in another.
3. Children in middle income homes, compared with children in low income homes, had higher percentages of EFU's in which they were given or asked for information, engaged in more extended interaction, were given an obligation to perform some specific action, were in harmony with the goal of the agent, and received and gave messages through a verbal medium.
4. No differences could be detected on any of the variables when the sample of urban black families was compared with the urban white families.
5. Although children in low income homes received as much total input from the environment as children in middle income homes, the children in low income homes did receive less verbal input, more inhibiting behavior, and less input directed toward specific behavior of the subject.
6. Comparison of these data with those from a related study suggested that disturbances (environmental interferences with the child's pursuits) occur much more frequently at home than in nursery school and outdoor settings.

The Behavior Setting Survey

In the behavior setting survey method, the focus of research shifts from the molar behavior of particular persons as recorded in specimen records to the study of particular situations or concrete contexts of molar behavior. In this approach, the ecological psychologist studies consistencies in behavior that are associated with specific place-thing-time constellations regardless of which persons are involved. As the student of personality seeks to identify regularities or consistencies in behavior of individuals over time related to personal characteristics such as genes, prenatal conditions, early experience, and child training practices, the study of behavior settings seeks to identify regularities or consistencies in behavior across individuals over time related to the particular, concrete situations in which the behavior occurs. Although the concepts, theories, and research methods of personality psychology may be required to understand why a particular 13-year-old boy is fascinated with fire and loves to light matches, such concepts, theories, and research methods are neither needed nor appropriate to understand why lighting matches and making fires among 13-year-old boys in general occur more often on Boy Scout cookouts than in Sunday school classes. The cookout setting requires match lighting and fire making but the Sunday school class setting resists such behaviors with equal vigor and requires instead certain other kinds of behavior from 13-year-old boys, e.g., Bible reading, discussions between teacher and class members, praying, etc., regardless of the identities or individual personality characteristics of the particular persons who happen to enter these settings. The pressures and constraints of settings are so clear and so strong that occupants of the settings must conform or face vigorous sanctions, as a boy who insists on lighting matches in Sunday school or one who persists in Bible reading on cookouts will almost certainly find out. The behavior setting survey is essentially a method for studying systematically and quantitatively these environmental entities, which are the loci of such situational coërcions on the molar behavior of people. The study of settings is the study of the concrete environmental situations with respect to which people direct their molar behavior: having lunch in the Pearl Cafe; buying groceries at Reid's Grocery Store; worshipping at the Methodist Church Worship Service; working on academic activities in Fifth Grade Academic Class; rooting for the home team at the High School Basketball Game. The behavior patterns mentioned in these examples refer to the behavior of people in general in these settings; having lunch, buying groceries, worshipping, etc., are stable, extraindividual patterns of behavior which regularly and consistently occur in the settings specified. These behavior regularities or consistencies within settings are observable as characteristic of setting occupants in general and are independent of the behavior of any particular person. The behavior setting method, therefore, is a very peculiar approach to psychology, an approach that focuses not upon the behavior of an individual person nor even upon the social interaction of persons but rather upon the standing patterns of behavior of persons en masse associated with particular environmental settings. Psychology's more common preoccupation with the individual and intrapersonal behavior dynamics is abandoned in favor of concern for extraindividual patterns of behavior in concrete environmental situations. This deliberate exclusion of the individual personality is the basis for the not completely tongue-in-cheek reference to the method as "the psychology of the absent organism."

Barker explains the basic rationale for studying the ecological environment of molar behavior in the following way:

> We believe that it is very important to present a systematic account of the methods and concepts for investigating the ecological environment at this time, for the ecological environment is a more important phenomenon for the behavior sciences than it has been hitherto. When environments are relatively uniform and stable, *people* are an obvious source of behavior variance, and the dominant scientific problem and the persistent queries from the applied fields are: What are people like? What is the nature and what are the sources of individual differences? How can people be selected and sorted into the slots provided by bureaucracies, schools, businesses, armies? What are the needs and capacities of people to which highways, curricula, and laws must be adapted? But today *environments* are more varied and unstable than heretofore, and their contribution to the variance of behavior is enhanced. Both science and society ask with greater urgency than previously: What are environments like? How does man's habitat differ, for example, in developed and underdeveloped countries, in large and small schools, in glass-walled and windowless office buildings, in integrated and segregated classes? How do environments select and shape the people who inhabit them? What are the structural and dynamic properties of the environments to which people must adapt? These are questions for ecological psychology, and in particular, they pertain to the ecological environment and its consequences for men (1968, pp. 3, 4).

The concept of the behavior setting has been carefully defined and precise operations for behavior setting identification and description have been published (Barker, 1968; Barker and Schoggen, 1973). For the present purpose, it will suffice to define a behavior setting as a cluster of *standing patterns of behavior* of people en masse occurring within a *particular part of the milieu* (a specific place-thing-time constellation) and where there is a *synomorphic relation* between the behavior patterns and the milieu, i.e., the behavior and the milieu part fit together; there is a similarity of shape between the behavior and the environment.

As an example, consider the Methodist Church Worship Service which occurs every Sunday morning at 11 o'clock in the small midwestern town in which the behavior setting method was developed. The cluster of *standing patterns of behavior* in this setting includes sedate entering of the sanctuary, worshippers sitting quietly in their pews, the playing of appropriate organ music, the rising and singing of hymns on signal from the minister, the collection of the offering, giving and listening to the sermon, etc. The *particular milieu part* is the main sanctuary of the Methodist church in the town of Midwest, Kansas, U.S.A., together with its component parts and objects, e.g., pews, chancel, choir loft, organ, pulpit holding the big Bible, hymn books, attendance register, etc. The *synomorphic relation* between the milieu parts and the behavior patterns is seen, for example, in the fact that the pews face the chancel and are the proper size and height to support sitting and listening; the pulpit has a surface which slants away from the pews to support the Bible and notes or references for the minister as he speaks when facing the congregation.

The ecologists did not invent or create behavior settings, they merely discovered them, gave them a name, and studied them systematically. Settings are objective, hard, empirical realities, with a prior and continuing existence quite independent of the possible interest of scientists in studying them. The settings of Midwest—the Rotary Club Meeting, the High School Basketball Game, Mrs. Trackett's First Grade Academic Class, and several hundred more—are well known to the residents of the town for whom the settings are as visible and objective as rivers, trees, and tornadoes. Settings are natural units in the sense that they have self-generated as opposed to investigator-imposed boundaries, i.e., the ecologist has nothing to say about when a setting begins and ends or where it takes place; other forces both within and outside the setting regulate these events. A related and important characteristic of behavior settings as ecological units is that each setting has a particular, denotable locale in space and time. Thus, unlike the processes designated by some abstract concepts in social science, behavior settings are easily locatable, observable, enterable, and studiable occurrences.

A behavior setting survey is a comprehensive inventory and description of all the behavior settings occurring within a particular community or institution during a stated period of time, usually a calendar year. Settings are identified in terms of their intrinsic structural and dynamic properties. Equivalence across units is obtained by procedures that recognize as settings only those that display a given degree of internal interdependence of interior parts and independence from external events (see Barker, 1968, chapters 3 and 4 for details).

The data obtained in a behavior setting survey are secured using a variety of methods including extensive direct observation by trained field workers who spend many hours in settings as participant observers; reference to public records such as newspapers, directories, school schedules, organization programs and bulletins, and membership rosters; and consultation with informants selected for their knowledge of particular areas of community life. These sources provide data sufficient to enable independent analysts to identify and describe behavior settings and many of their characteristics with an acceptable degree of agreement.

In most of the applications of the behavior-settings method to date, the studies have arbitrarily limited themselves to consideration of the behavior settings that occur in the public areas of a town or an institution, i.e., homes and other areas for private or personal use have been omitted. Except for this limitation, a behavior setting survey of a town or an institution includes all the behavior that occurs within the town or institution during the survey year because behavior settings are ubiquitous. All behavior occurs in one or another behavior setting; there are no gaps or interstices between settings and anyone within the town or institution studied is always in one or another of its behavior settings.

Once all the public settings in a town or institution have been identified, the final step in making a behavior setting survey is to describe the settings in terms of whichever of their many attributes and characteristics may be of interest. In studies reported so far, these have included dimensions such as the characteristics of the setting inhabitants in terms of age, sex, and social class; how much time inhabitants spend in the setting; which inhabitants exercise control over the operation of the setting; which population subgroups the setting is intended to serve primarily; and a variety of other habitat qualities.

Studies of communities and institutions in terms of behavior settings have been completed in small midwestern towns (Barker and Wright, 1955; Barker, 1968), in an English village (Barker and Schoggen, 1973), in high schools of varying size (Barker and Gump, 1964), in an institution for handicapped children (Newton, 1953), in churches varying in size (Wicker, 1969), and in preschool programs (Schoggen, 1973).

The most recent and extensive of these reports (Barker and Schoggen, 1973) describes a study of two small towns, Midwest, Kansas, and Yoredale, Yorkshire, England, on two different occasions separated by a decade, 1954–55 and 1963–64. Midwest was selected originally for its manageable size, its cultural vitality and its geographic location (proximity to the University of Kansas and independence from larger metropolitan centers). Yoredale was chosen later for its similarity to Midwest on dimensions of obvious importance. Both towns are seats of local government and centers for trade and educational, recreational, and cultural activities for the surrounding rural areas.

From the great wealth of findings about Midwest and Yoredale as environments for molar behavior, only the one with the greatest significance for the present purpose is summarized here in truncated and simplified form.

Although the towns were quite similar in terms of overall habitat extent and many other respects, there was one major difference which seems to be important. This difference is in the number of *habitat-claims,* a term which requires some explanation. The behavior settings that comprise the towns' habitats specify human components for certain loci (slots, positions) within them. These are called habitat-claims for human components. The instructor's position in Yoredale's Evening Institute German Class is such a habitat-claim; this position requires a human component, one with the necessary knowledge and skills, in order to become operational. Habitat-claims are stable, structural, and dynamic features of a town's habitat. The number of habitat-claims for operatives of a behavior setting is the number of positions of responsibility that must be filled for the normal occurrence of the setting. For example, Presbyterian Church Worship Service in Midwest requires 20 operatives (one minister, one organist, twelve choir members, two ushers, two candle lighters, two greeters); thus there are 20 habitat-claims in this setting. The town's habitats are highly dependent upon human components for their operation and maintenance.

In 1963–64, the 884 behavior settings of Midwest had a total of 10,220 habitat-claims for operatives, many more than the 7,764 found in Yoredale's 758 behavior settings (Barker and Schoggen, 1973, chapter 3). Thus there were in Midwest many more positions of responsibility (chairmen, hostesses, entertainers, cooks, speakers, etc.) to be filled than there were in Yoredale, 132% as many altogether. Midwest's habitat called for more proprietorships, captaincies, chairmanships, and presidencies, and had more positions that are important and difficult than Yoredale's habitat.

The impact of this very substantial difference is compounded by the fact that Midwest had a smaller total number of town residents available to serve as human components in filling the greater number of habitat-claims. Midwest had a total of 830 human components available to staff its 10,220 habitat claims: Yoredale had 1,310 human components to fill its 7,764 habitat claims. Thus Midwest had 2,456 more habitat-claims to be filled by 480 fewer town inhabitants. This works out to an average of 12.3 habitat-claims per Midwesterner compared to 5.9 per Dalesman. Thus, in 1963–64 the average Midwesterner was about twice as likely as the average Dalesman to be called upon to accept responsibility for operation of the town's public settings. It should also be noted that habitat-claim is the property of a behavior setting that may occur on one or a number of days in the survey year. In fact, the mean numbers of occurrences of behavior settings in 1963–64 were 60.4 in Midwest and 86.0 in Yoredale; hence there were 743 *occurrences* of claims for operatives per Midwesterner and 507 per Dalesman.

Thus Midwest, relative to Yoredale, appeared to be shorthanded; there was a manpower shortage in Midwest in that fewer people were available to do the existing jobs. Relative to Yoredale, the behavior settings of Midwest were undermanned. Additional data documenting this difference are also reported (Barker and Schoggen, 1973, chapter 8).

These and similar data obtained in several ecological studies over the years (Barker and Wright, 1955; Barker, 1960; Barker and Barker, 1961; Barker and Gump, 1964; Barker and Schoggen, 1973) led Barker to develop a behavior setting theory with special reference to the consequences on the behavior of the inhabitants of undermanning, this property of the ecological environment which has emerged so regularly as characteristic of small towns and institutions. This theory is presented in detail elsewhere (Barker, 1968) and can only be summarized here in terms of a few of its main features. A recent statement captures the key notion:

> The basic idea of behavior setting theory is that the inhabitants of behavior settings are one class of components, among other classes (nonhuman behavior objects), that make up the internal media of behaviour settings. The number of available inhabitants of a behaviour setting, relative to the optimal number, affects its operation—including, via sensors and feedback circuits, the strengths and directions of forces acting upon its human components. One critical relationship is between number of inhabitants and the strength and range of directions of the forces acting upon them; *forces upon a town's inhabitants toward participation in the program and maintenance circuits of its behavior settings vary in mean strength per inhabitant, and in mean range of direction per inhabitant, inversely with the number of available inhabitants*. This relation holds when the number of inhabitants varies between the

> minimum number required to operate and maintain it at its lowest operating level and the optimal number required to operate and maintain it at its most effective level. To the degree, therefore, that Midwest and Yoredale differ within these limits in number of human components, there are predictable differences for their inhabitants (Barker and Schoggen, 1973, p. 251).

In less technical language, the main point of this statement is that undermanned settings, i.e., settings with unfilled habitat-claims, exert more pressure on potential participants to enter and take part in the operation and maintenance of the setting than adequately manned or overmanned settings. If the Junior class play has parts for 12 actors and there are only 15 members of the Junior class, no member of the class is likely to be exempt from pressure to take a part or at least to help backstage but if there are 50 Juniors, only the more talented or highly motivated are likely to become involved.

Concretely, the theory predicts that Midwest's habitat with its relatively undermanned settings will generate the following differences in the behavior output of Midwesterners as compared with Dalesmen: a) Midwesterners will, on the average, spend more time per person in the public setting of the town; b) Midwesterners will, on the average, more frequently assume positions of responsibility in the operation of the town's behavior settings; and c) Midwesterners will, on the average, carry out many more actions of highest leadership responsibility in the town's behavior settings.

The findings of the study (Barker and Schoggen, 1973, chapter 8) strongly support all three of these predictions: a) the average Midwesterner spent 125% as many hours per year in the public behavior settings of the town (Midwest = 1,356; Yoredale = 1,089 person hours per year per person); b) the average Midwesterner occupied positions of responsibility in the operation of the town's behavior settings 250% as frequently as Dalesmen (Midwest = 8.0; Yoredale = 3.2 positions per year per person); c) the average Midwesterner carried out 257% as many actions of highest leadership responsibility in the town's behavior settings (Midwest = 1.8; Yoredale = 0.7 leader acts per year per person).

The theory of undermanning has also been tested in a series of studies of high schools differing in size (Barker and Gump, 1964). One of these studies (Gump and Friesen, 1964) compared one large (2,287 students) high school with four small schools (83 to 151 students) in eastern Kansas in terms of student participation in the voluntary nonclass behavior settings of the schools. They found that, as expected, the settings of the small schools were in fact undermanned relative to the settings of the large school (mean number of persons per behavior setting was 12 in small schools and 36 in the large school).

The results showed that students in the small schools participated in just as many extracurricular settings as large school students despite the larger total number of such settings available to the large school students. Also consistent with the theoretical expectations was the finding that, on the average, small school Juniors occupied positions of responsibility in twice as many behavior settings as did large school Juniors (small school, 8.6; large school, 3.5 positions per student). Here are the data:

	Large	*Small*
Total number of Juniors	794	23
Total number of settings	189	48
Mean positions per Junior	3.5	8.6

where "Small" is the average data from four small schools. Thus, whereas the large school provided a richer habitat in terms of total number of settings available, the small schools co-opted students into positions of responsibility in operating their settings much more often.

In a follow-up study, Willems (1964a) attempted to assess the psychological significance of these differences in behavioral participation. Samples of the Junior students were interviewed using both open-ended and card-sorting techniques intended to identify psychologically experienced forces toward participation in the nonschool settings. The data are reported in terms of own forces (attractions) and induced or external forces (pressures) reported by the students as reasons for participating in the voluntary activities. Results are given for both *regular* (ordinary, average) students and for students designated *marginal,* i.e., students at high risk for dropping out of school because of low academic aptitude and other background factors.

Small school regular students reported significantly more forces toward participation in settings than did large school students in terms of both own forces and foreign forces. This was indicated by both card-sort and open-ended data. Regular students and marginal students within the small schools did not differ appreciably in either the number of pressures or the number of attractions reported. However, in the large school, marginal students reported both fewer attractions and fewer pressures, but only the latter difference was statistically significant. Willems comments on these findings as follows:

> The data on forces and responsibilities are relevant to the question of the comparative efficacy of personal variables and ecological variables in influencing behavior. The absence of differences between regular and marginal students in the small schools and the presence of such differences in the large school indicates that school size, as well as the kind of person, is a determinant of forces toward participation. The fact that marginal students of the small schools reported more forces than did the regular students of the large school is relevant too. In the large school, the academically marginal student appeared to be truly an outsider, while in the small schools being marginal made no apparent difference on the experience of pressures, attractions, and responsibilities (Willems, 1964a).

In an altogether independent investigation, Baird (1969) subjected the central hypothesis of the *Big School, Small School* report to critical examination and obtained relevant new data from a very large national sample of 21,371 students drawn randomly from the 712,000 who took the ACT (American College Test) and Student Profile for college admission. High school size was studied in relation to number of high school achievements and activities. Baird reports that, consistent with behavior setting theory, students in small schools participated to a greater extent in a variety of areas than did students in large schools.

Wicker and his students have addressed the theory of undermanned behavior settings in a series of studies of churches varying in size (Wicker, 1969; Wicker and Mehler, 1971; Wicker, McGrath, and Armstrong, 1972) and report findings that are generally consistent with the theory.

Further data relevant to the issue of institutional and organizational size in relation to resident and member behavior in highly varied arenas ranging from high school music festivals and Rotary Clubs to coal pits and Air Force bases are reviewed in other reports (Barker, 1960; Barker and Gump, 1964; Willems, 1964b; Barker, 1968). Most of these studies provide findings which are generally supportive of behavior setting theory and none report conflicting results.

Beyond the derivations from behavior setting theory reported and documented above, a number of probable psychological consequences of undermanned behavior settings have been suggested (Barker and Gump, 1964; Barker, 1968; Barker and Schoggen, 1973). Although not derived from the theory of undermanning in any strict sense, these are psychological consequences on inhabitants of undermanned ecological environments which seem reasonable to expect on the basis of common observation and some empirical evidence.

1. Persons in undermanned habitats have *less sensitivity to and are less evaluative of individual differences*; they are more tolerant of their associates. When the supply is short and the demand is high, it is necessary to accept those persons who are available to do the job even if their skills and experience are limited. In Midwest, with its severe manpower shortage relative to Yoredale, less experienced and less able persons (children, adolescents, and old people) are accepted into settings and given leadership responsibilities more commonly than their English counterparts. Discrimination on the basis of appearances and superficial traits is less likely in undermanned settings. When there is a manpower surplus, on the other hand, competition among many possible contenders for the limited number of available opportunities to participate sometimes becomes so keen that many persons with appropriate experience and excellent functional skills are excluded, sometimes on the basis of superficial personality traits or other largely irrelevant considerations.
2. Persons in undermanned habitats *see themselves as having greater functional importance*. The greater relative scarcity of setting inhabitants actually makes them more important people and they experience this directly without needing to be told. It is obvious that a setting, to operate, must have a minimum number of participants, and each person's contribution therefore is seen as more valuable. In a small church choir with only two tenors, both feel a strong obligation to attend rehearsals and performances because they understand the serious consequences of their absence for the tenor section and the threat to the choir as a whole. Small school students expressed similar feelings about being needed to help make the setting go.
3. Persons in undermanned habitats have *more responsibility*. Responsibility is experienced by a person when a behavior setting and what others gain from it depend upon his actions. A setting that is optimally populated does not burden itself with indispensable personnel; people are too unreliable, so substitutes, vice presidents, a second team, are regular features of optimally manned or overmanned settings.
4. Persons in undermanned habitats have *greater functional identity,* i.e., they are seen in terms of what they can do in the setting. A person with an essential function is seen as more than a person, as a person-in-context. The concern is with getting the job done, rather than what kind of person is doing the job.
5. Persons in undermanned habitats *experience greater insecurity*. Faced with the need to perform more difficult and more varied actions often without "proper" training or appropriate experience, a person in an underpopulated setting is in greater jeopardy of failing to carry through his tasks. The problem is exacerbated by the lack of reserves to turn to for help. This amounts to increased dependence upon every other person to

carry through on his responsibilities. But this risk of failure also implies the possibility of success if the person is able to carry through his tasks in the setting. This gives meaning and personal significance to the activity.

IMPLICATIONS FOR MENTAL RETARDATION

Almost none of the theory and research reviewed in this paper was directed toward improving our understanding of problems in mental retardation or toward designing better programs for preventing or ameliorating the negative consequences of limited intellectual abilities. Yet the ecological approach described above has many facets that seem to have significance for the field of mental retardation.

Implications of the Ecological Perspective

The most basic or fundamental suggestion arising from the ecological perspective is its insistence on abandoning the often unrecognized assumption, which has tended to dominate thinking in psychology, that behavior is to be understood and explained primarily in terms of person-centered, "under the skin" personality factors. Instead, it would adopt as a guiding principle the concept of behavior in context, i.e., behavior and environment as interdependent elements in a unitary, dynamic system. This shift in emphasis away from psychodynamic, psychometric, and other preoccupations with intrapersonal processes to emphasis on behavior and situation as an interactive process calls for much more research on mentally retarded persons in a wide variety of natural, real life situations. From the ecological point of view, much of the work attempting to improve measures of individual intelligence in psychologists' offices over the past 50 years would better have been directed toward ways of assessing environmental demands and behavior-situation transactions in the arena of everyday life.

In mental retardation, such person-centered assumptions were reflected in the view of the retarded as suffering from individual deficits. A recent statement by Begab makes the point:

> For the major part of our history, we have been guided by the credo that the individual is in essence master of his destiny. Ambition, hard work, the rational and efficient use of time, morality and independence were the gateways to success and the door of opportunity was open to all who possessed these virtues. Values of rugged individualism and self-reliance served as cornerstones for public school teaching and social policy. Failures in this presumed open-ended system were attributed to personal weaknesses and deficiencies [Levine and Levine, 1970]. With this perspective, solutions had to be person centered and oriented toward the remediation of individual deficits . . . (Begab, 1975, p. 4).

However, emphasis on sociocultural factors in mental retardation is not new, as Nihira (1973) has recently pointed out. Even though there have been calls for many years to include cultural factors and ability to cope with environmental demands in the assessment of adaptive behavior (e.g., Howe, 1858; Berry and Gordon, 1931; Doll, 1966; Heber, 1961; Nihira, 1973), efforts to develop concrete, objective, and precise measures of such factors are rare. Even the work of Nihira and his colleagues was limited primarily to verbal reports and paper and pencil techniques. The ecologist commends these efforts but prefers direct observation in natural situations.

But in mental retardation, as elsewhere in behavioral science, methods of studying behavior in real life situations are, despite encouraging progress in recent years, still in a rather primitive stage of development relative to the sophisticated tools of experimental, personality, and social psychology. Methods for describing, classifying and conceptualizing the ecological environments of behavior are even less well developed. Brunswik's (1957) admonition that psychology must be concerned with the texture of the environment as it extends in depth away from its boundary with behavior applies with equal force in mental retardation. But we know little more about how to do this today than we did when Brunswik suggested it almost 20 years ago. Researchers in mental retardation as well as in psychology and other behavioral sciences who take the ecological perspective seriously should give high priority to the development of methods for studying environments of behavior.

The ecological orientation suggests that those responsible for programs of service to retarded persons should strive to practice the kind of ecological diagnosis demonstrated by the ornithologist mentioned earlier who solved the problem of infanticide in captive bearded tits by careful observation and analysis of the total ecosystem in which the problem occurred. Just as the ornithologist found that the bizarre behavior of the parent birds reflected his own inadvertent disturbance of the balance of elements in the ecological environment and not some mysterious, bird-type psychopathology, problem behavior in mentally retarded persons may reflect an analogous ecological problem.

The Re-Ed Program developed by Nicholas Hobbs (1966) and his associates in Nashville, Tennessee, as a new approach to treatment for emotionally disturbed children is one of the most sophisticated efforts ever made to apply systematically ecological concepts in a service program.

Implications from the Specimen Record Method

The work to date in making and analyzing specimen records of behavior has been little more than illustrative of the usefulness of such methods for reducing our vast ignorance of the structure, dynamics, and manifold qualitative attributes of molar human behavior in noncontrived circumstances of everyday life. Although methodological work has necessarily required a heavy investment in the past, the value of the method has been established and extensive applications are needed.

The specimen record method seems especially well suited to studies of the behavior of mentally retarded children whose disability renders the use of research instruments requiring verbal and symbolic responses somewhat problematical at best. Experience with the method suggests that, properly used, it can record with minimal distortion the naturally occurring molar behavior of children in the 2 to 10-year-old range. The method preserves for later analysis the natural continuity and sequence of the behavior stream for relatively extended time periods.

Applications of this method to behavior studies of retarded children promise to give us a much better understanding of some important questions that bear upon the planning of programs for the retarded. For example, the studies mentioned earlier have provided some baseline or normative type data on the behavior of fairly normal children in typical situations of home and school. An important question then becomes obvious: how does the behavior of children called retarded differ? For example: How many episodes per min do they undertake? How is the structure of their behavior different, e.g., is it more similar to structural patterns characteristic of younger children? Are success, frustration, indulgence, and conflict more or less frequent in their everyday lives? How do answers to these and other questions differ for retarded children in different life situations, e.g., institutions, group homes, large and small families? How do answers to such questions change for a given retarded child over long time periods, e.g., from age 3 to age 10; and more generally, how are developmental trends in the behavior of retarded children different from those of children called normal? Just as observational studies relevant to such questions seem to be essential to a better understanding of child development in general, our ignorance of such phenomena in retarded children is a serious impediment to good program planning and the formulation of sound social policy for the retarded. The specimen record method would seem to be helpful in addressing this need.

Implications of the Behavior Setting Method

If the study of the naturally occurring molar behavior of retarded persons is in an underdeveloped state, the study of the ecological environment of such behavior has been even more seriously neglected. The person-centered orientation in psychology has left the environment of behavior almost entirely in the domain of other social sciences, which have properly dealt with it at the levels of their primary interest and competence: demographic, cultural, and institutional. Studies of the concrete intact environments, the immediate contexts of the molar behavior of retarded persons, seem to be all but nonexistent. Yet the need for information such studies could provide and the great value of such information in mental retardation scarcely seems open to question.

For example, one of the clearest findings of the behavior setting analysis in small towns is that accessibility to the ecological environment at the level of behavior setting operative increases with age from infancy through childhood and adolescence to a peak at adulthood (Barker and Wright, 1955; Barker and Schoggen 1973). As a child grows up in these small towns, ever more of the settings of the towns open up to him; they become a part of his territory over which he has some say. If freedom of movement and influence across ever larger proportions of the community are valued, then it is fair to say that it pays to grow up in these towns. However, the only reported study of this process in a residential institution for handicapped children (Newton, 1953) found that the ecological environment for these children was largely constant in size across the age range from early elementary school age to early adolescence and that children in the younger age groups occupied operative level positions almost as frequently as older children. Increasing maturity in the small towns was accompanied by benefits in the way of opportunities and status which did not accompany maturity in the institution (Barker and Wright, 1955, p. 118). Apparently it did not pay to grow up in the institution.

Although this is only one small study of one institution, it suggests the kind of insight into the development of retarded children which studies of ecological environments could provide.

Finally, the implications of the theory of undermanning for mental retardation seem to be substantial and call urgently for empirical investigation. The evidence sketched above from studies of high schools and small towns suggests that ecological environments with surplus manpower exert stultifying and debilitating pressures on their human inhabitants whereas undermanned ecologies tend to enhance growth and development by providing opportunities and challenges for meaningful participation in important activities. High schools, churches, towns, and other ecological environments that have manpower surpluses seem to be ruthless in excluding or limiting primarily to spectator positions all but the most able of the available inhabitants. But undermanned settings reach out to almost any potential participant with encouragement to enter and take an active part in the operation of the setting even though his skills may be limited.

The question, of course, is what are the properties of the ecological environments of the mentally retarded? The case made by Bernard Farber (1968) that the retarded in the United States comprise a major part of a surplus population is convincing, but his evidence is chiefly at the demographic and institutional levels. The theory of undermanning requires data more closely tied to the level of molar actions of persons; studies of the ecological environments of molar behavior, of behavior settings, are needed.

There is reason to anticipate, however, that such studies will in fact show that most people identified as mentally retarded, both children and adults, live in overmanned ecological environments which deprive them of responsible participation in activities that they regard as important; opportunities to do things for themselves, to set goals and try to reach them, to risk failure (Perske, 1972) and relish success, and to join with friends and avoid enemies. The current movement toward normalization (Nirje, 1969) is probably based in part on an intuitive understanding that the ecological environments provided for residents of large institutions are likely to be the overmanned ecology carried to an extreme.

Behavior setting theory seems to be consistent with the goal of normalization to treat the retarded as nearly normal as possible, but the above data relevant to the theory of undermanning show that the critical phrase "as normal as possible" may have very different meanings in undermanned as opposed to overmanned settings. The same behavior that gains acceptance and approval in an undermanned setting may be the basis for rejection and disapproval in an overmanned setting. Studies of traditional residential institutions with the behavior setting method could provide the needed empirical evidence. Similar studies of alternative residential programs, e.g., group homes, are needed with equal urgency.

To the ecological psychologist interested in programs for the retarded, perhaps the ultimate challenge is to use the behavior setting technology to help design practical, workable environments for the retarded that capitalize on the growth enhancing properties of undermanned behavior settings.

REFERENCES

Baird, L. L. 1969. Big school, small school: a critical examination of the hypothesis. J. Educ. Psychol. 60:253–260.

Barker, R. G. 1960. Ecology and motivation. In: M. R. Jones (ed.), Nebraska Symposium on Motivation. University of Nebraska Press, Lincoln.

Barker, R. G. 1963a. On the nature of the environment. J. Soc. Issues 19:17–38.

Barker, R. G. 1963b. The Stream of Behavior. Appleton-Century-Crofts Inc., New York.

Barker, R. G. 1968. Ecological Psychology: Concepts and Methods for Studying the Environment of Human Behavior. Stanford University Press, Stanford, California.

Barker, R. G., and Barker, L. S. 1961. Behavior units for the comparative study of cultures. In: B. Kaplan (ed.), Studying Personality Cross Culturally. Harper and Row, New York.

Barker, R. G., and Gump, P. V. 1964. Big School, Small School. Stanford University Press, Stanford, California.

Barker, R. G., and Schoggen, P. 1973. Qualities of Community Life: Methods of Measuring Environment and Behavior Applied to an American and an English Town. Jossey-Bass, Inc., San Francisco.

Barker, R. G., and Wright, H. F. 1951. One Boy's Day. Harper & Brothers, New York.

Barker, R. G., and Wright, H. F. 1955. Midwest and Its Children. Harper and Row, New York. (Reissued by Archon Books, Hamden, Connecticut, 1971).

Begab, M. 1975. The mentally retarded and society: trends and issues. In: M. Begab and S. A. Richardson (eds.), The Mentally Retarded and Society: A Social Perspective. University Park Press, Baltimore.

Berry, R. J. A., and Gordon, R. G. 1931. The Mental Defective: A Problem in Social Inefficiency. McGraw-Hill Book Company, New York.

Blurton-Jones, N. G. 1972. Ethological Studies of Child Behaviour. Cambridge University Press, Cambridge, England.

Boyer, E. Gil, Simon, A., and Karafin, G. R. 1973. Measures of Maturation: An Anthology of Early Childhood Observational Instruments. Research for Better Schools, Inc., Philadelphia.

Bruner, J. A. 1965. The growth of the mind. Am. Psychol. 20:1007–1017.

Brunswik, E. 1952. The conceptual framework of psychology. International Encyclopedia of Unified Science, Vol. 1, Pt. 2. University of Chicago Press, Chicago.

Brunswik, E. 1956. Historical and thematic relations of psychology to other sciences. Sci. Monthly 83:151–161.

Brunswik, E. 1957. Scope and aspects of the cognitive problem. In: H. Gruber, R. Jesser, and K. Hammond (eds.), Cognition: The Colorado Symposium, pp. 5–31. Harvard University Press, Cambridge.

Darwin, C. R. 1877. A biographical sketch of an infant. Mind 2:285–294.

Dickman, H. 1963. The perception of behavioral units. In: R. G. Barker (ed.), The Stream of Behavior. Appleton-Century-Crofts Inc., New York.

Doll, E. A. 1966. Recognition of mental retardation in the school-age child. In: L. Philips (ed.), Prevention and Treatment of Mental Retardation. Basic Books Inc., New York.

Dreher, G. F. 1975. Reliability assessment in narrative observation of human behavior. Masters thesis, University of Houston.

Eibl-Eibesfeldt, I. 1967. Concepts of ethology and their significance in the study of human behavior. In: H. W. Stevenson, E. H. Hess, and H. L. Rheingold (eds.), Early Behavior: Comparative and Developmental Approaches. John Wiley & Sons Inc., New York.

Farber, B. 1968. Mental Retardation: Its Social Context and Social Consequences. Houghton Mifflin Company, Boston.

Frederiksen, N. 1972. Toward a taxonomy of situations. Am. Psychol. 27:114–123.

Gump, P. V., and Friesen, W. 1964. Participation in nonclass settings. In: R. G. Barker and P. V. Gump (eds.), Big School, Small School. Stanford University Press, Stanford, California.

Hawley, A. H. 1944. Ecology and human ecology. Soc. Forces 22:398–405.

Heber, R. A. 1961. A manual on terminology and classification in mental retardation. Am. J. Ment. Defic., Monogr. Suppl. 2nd Ed.

Heider, F. 1959. On perception, event structure, and the psychological environment: selected papers. Psychol. Issues 1:1–123.

Hobbs, N. 1966. Helping disturbed children: psychological and ecological strategies. Am. Psychol. 21:1105–1115.

Howe, S. G. 1858. On the Causes of Idiocy. McLachlin and Stewart, Edinburgh. (Arno Press, New York, reprinted in 1972).

Hutt, S. J., and Hutt, C. 1970. Direct Observation and Measurement of Behavior. Charles C Thomas Publisher, Springfield, Illinois.

Jolly, A. 1972. The Evolution of Primate Behavior. The Macmillan Company, New York.

Kluckhohn, F. R. 1940. The participant observer technique in small communities. Am. J. Sociol. 46:331–343.

Leeper, R. W. 1966. A critical consideration of Egon Brunswik's probabilistic functionism. In: K. R. Hammond (ed.), The Psychology of Egon Brunswik. Holt, Rinehart & Winston, New York.

Levine, M., and Levine, A. 1970. A Social History of the Helping Services: Clinic, Court, School, and Community. Appleton-Century-Crofts Inc., New York.

Lewin, K. 1935. Dynamic Theory of Personality. McGraw-Hill Book Company, New York.

Lewin, K. 1936. Principles of Topological Psychology. McGraw-Hill Book Company, New York.

Lewin, K. 1938. The conceptual representation and the measurement of psychological forces. Contributions to Psychological Theory, Vol. 1, no. 4. Duke University Press, Durham, North Carolina.

Lewin, K. 1951a. Behavior and development as a function of the total situation. In: D. Cartwright (ed.), Field Theory in Social Science. Harper & Brothers, New York.

Lewin, K. 1951b. Defining the "field at a given time." In: D. Cartwright (ed.), Field Theory and Social Science. Harper & Brothers, New York.

Lewin, K. 1951c. Frontiers in group dynamics. In: D. Cartwright (ed.), Field Theory in Social Science. Harper & Brothers, New York.

Lewin, K. 1951d. Psychological ecology. In: D. Cartwright (ed.), Field Theory and Social Science. Harper & Brothers, New York.

McDougall, W. 1923. Outline of Psychology. Charles Scribner's Sons, New York.

McGrew, W. C. 1972. An Ethological Study of Children's Behavior. Academic Press, New York.

Mead, M. 1928. Coming of Age in Samoa. William Morrow & Co. Inc., New York.

Muenzinger, K. 1942. Psychology: The Science of Behavior. Harper & Brothers, New York.

Murray, H. A. 1938. Explorations in Personality. Oxford University Press, New York.

Newton, M. R. 1953. A study in psychological ecology: The behavior settings in an institution for handicapped children. Masters thesis, University of Kansas.

Newtson, D. 1977. Foundations of attribution: The perception of ongoing behavior. In: J. Harvey, W. Ickes, and R. Kidd (eds.), New Directions in Attribution Research.

Nihira, K. 1973. The importance of environmental demands in the measurement of adaptive behavior. In: G. Tarjan, R. K. Eyman, and C. E. Meyers (eds.), Sociobehavioral Studies in Mental Retardation. American Association on Mental Deficiency, Los Angeles.

Nirje, B. 1969. The normalization principle and its human management implications. In: R. Kugel and W. Wolfensberger (eds.), Changing Patterns in Residential Services for the Mentally Retarded. pp. 179–195. President's Committee on Mental Retardation, Washington D.C.

Perske, R. 1972. The dignity of risk and the mentally retarded. Ment. Retard. 10(1):24–27.

Preyer, W. 1888. The Mind of the Child. D. Appleton Co. (Arno Press, New York, reprinted in 1973).

Schoggen, M. 1973. Characteristics of the environment of three classrooms: An exploratory study. J. F. Kennedy Center, George Peabody College, Nashville, Tennessee (preprint).

Schoggen, M., and Schoggen, P. 1971. Environmental forces in the home lives of three-year-old children in three population subgroups. George Peabody College, DARCEE Papers and Reports, Nashville, Tennessee 5:2.

Schoggen, M., and Schoggen, P. 1976. Environmental forces in the home lives of three-year-old children in three population subgroups. JSAS Catalog of Selected Documents in Psychology 6:8 (Manuscript No. 1178).

Schoggen, P. 1963. Environmental forces in the everyday lives of children. In: R. G. Barker (ed.),

The Stream of Behavior. Appleton-Century-Crofts Inc., New York.

Schoggen, P. 1964a. Environmental forces in the everyday lives of children with physical disabilities. (Mimeo report on Vocational Rehabilitation Administration Project No. 714).

Schoggen, P. 1964b. Mechanical aids for making specimen records of behavior. Child Dev. 35:985–988.

Schoggen, P. 1975. An ecological study of children with physical disabilities in school and at home. In: R. Weinberg and F. Wood (eds.), Observation of Pupils and Teachers in Mainstream and Special Education Settings: Alternative Strategies. Leadership Training Institute in Special Education, University of Minnesota, Minneapolis.

Smith, P. K., and Connolly, K. 1972. Patterns of play and social interaction in pre-school children. In: N. Blurton-Jones (ed.), Ethological Studies of Child Behaviour. The University Press, Cambridge, England.

Tiedemann, D. 1897. Beobachtungen über die Entwickelung der Seelenfähigkeiten bei Kindern. Oscar Bande, Altenberg (first published in 1787).

Tinbergen, N. 1963. On aims and methods of ethology. Z. Tierpsychol. 20:410–433. (Quoted in Hutt and Hutt, 1970, p. 4).

Tolman, E. C. 1932. Purposive Behavior in Animals and Men. Century, New York.

Whiting, J. W. M., and Child, I. 1953. Child Training and Personality. Yale University Press, New Haven.

Wicker, A. W. 1969. Size of church membership and members' support of church behavior settings. J. Pers. Soc. Psychol. 13:278–288.

Wicker, A. W. 1972. Processes which mediate behavior-environment congruence. Behav. Sci. 17:265–277.

Wicker, A. W. 1973. Undermanning theory and research: Implications for the study of psychological and behavioral effects of excess human populations. Representative Res. Soc. Psychol. 4:185–206.

Wicker, A. W., McGrath, J. E., and Armstrong, G. E. 1972. Organization size and behavior setting capacity as determinants of member participation. Behav. Sci. 17:499–513.

Wicker, A. W., and Mehler, A. 1971. Assimilation of new members in a large and small church. J. Appl. Psychol. 55:151–156.

Willems, E. P. 1964a. Forces toward participation in behavior settings. In: R. G. Barker and P. V. Gump (eds.), Big School, Small School. Stanford University Press, Stanford, California.

Willems, E. P. 1964b. Review of research. In: R. G. Barker and P. V. Gump (eds.), Big School, Small School. Stanford University Press, Stanford, California.

Willems, E. P. 1965. An ecological orientation in psychology. Merrill-Palmer Q. 11:317–343.

Willems, E. P. 1969. Planning a rationale for naturalistic research. In: E. P. Willems and H. L. Raush (eds.), Naturalistic Viewpoints in Psychological Research. Holt, Rinehart & Winston, New York.

Willems, E. P. 1977. Behavioral ecology as a perspective in psychology. In: C. W. Deckner (ed), Perspectives for Methodology in Behavioral Research. Charles C. Thomas Publisher, Springfield, Illinois.

Wright, H. F. 1967. Recording and Analyzing Child Behavior. Harper and Row, New York.

Conceptualizations and Applications of Observational Methods to the Study of Retarded and Nonretarded Individuals

PARENT-INFANT INTERACTION STUDIES

Introduction

Kathryn Barnard

The methodology and context of the chapters in this section relate especially to early identification of at risk infants in the area of mental retardation. These papers highlight the value of parent-infant research for illuminating the as yet "mystical role" of the child's early environment in shaping development. Each study presents data suggesting that reciprocal interaction between caregivers and young children is a critical variable in maximizing the "normalcy" of development. For example, the work of Vietze et al. in chapter 5 showed that mothers of developmentally delayed children had higher vocalization rates than mothers of nondelayed children; however, the vocalization levels of delayed infants at 24 months of age were at the level of 12-month-olds in the nondelayed group. This suggests that one reason for the developmental delay may reside in inappropriate patterning of the mother's vocalizations, rather than deficits in the infant's vocal capacities. A study by Morio (1976) found that mothers of normal infants markedly change their temporal patterning of verbalization when the infant reaches 8 months of age. Before 8 months, these mothers had only occasional pauses within bouts of vocalization. At 8 months the amount of pause time increased considerably. These pauses provided the infant with time to respond vocally in temporal correlation with the mother's utterances. If mothers of delayed infants failed to emit such pauses, they might well shape their infants in an abnormal fashion.

The question of understanding temporal or sequential relationships was also stressed by Parke in chapter 3. His work suggests that simple counts of behavioral occurrences or measures of total duration are inadequate for understanding the nature of parent-child interactions. A methodology is needed for measuring interactions in terms of the timing and intensity of behaviors occurring between interactors, both simultaneously and across finite time periods. Although quantitative measurement of sequences, rhythms, and cycles is necessary, Parke also suggests that other types of quantitative and qualitative information are necessary for a full understanding of parent-child relationships. Thus parent reports, attitude measures, and measures of social perception are important data that must be correlated with direct behavioral observations in order to understand cause and effect in parent-child interactions. In this context, Parke cites the work of Borussard and Hartner (1971) showing that maternal perceptions of 30-day-old infants are highly correlated with later behavior and development.

Parke's chapter also presents quantitative data illustrating the fact that fathers as well as mothers can be important in determining the developmental course of at risk infants. This work seems especially pertinent to issues concerning prevention of mental and social retardation in infants identified as high risk. Males have traditionally played only a minor role in the care and training of young retarded children and infants. With the current trend toward deinstitutionalization and normalization programs for retarded children, studying the role of "fathers" may take on great importance.

In chapter 4, Thoman and Becker stress the concept of uniqueness of each individual parent-child unit. Their emphasis is on developing observational methods that measure interaction as a system of interdependent responses among the participants. The basic assumption underlying Thoman and Becker's model is that continuities and predictability of developmental processes can be understood only by measuring how infant, parent, and environmental factors operate together as a system supporting development of adaptive individual, social, and intellectual behaviors of the child.

Central to this systems approach is the recording of behaviors in a sequential fashion so that emerging behavior patterns can be identified. As in many biological systems, Thoman and Becker's data suggest that individual dyads exhibit much less behavioral variability than that seen when measures are averaged between dyads. Thus, regardless of the specific behaviors comprising a mother-infant interaction, Thoman and Becker's work suggests that *social interaction* occurs for any particular dyad only when 1) the infant is in an awake state, 2) the infant is held or carried by the mother, and 3) the mother is not involved in simple caregiving activities. Although mother, infant, and environmental factors might be measured separately in an observational scoring system, Thoman and Becker suggest that the behaviors can only be understood conceptually when all three of these sources of variation are considered as a total system. The denied end product of this approach is a description of the rules which explain the timing, sequences, and intensity of behaviors occurring in an interaction. This view, along with those expressed by Parke and Vietze et al., underscores the idea that identification of infants at risk for developmental behavioral disabilities must focus not only on the characteristics of the individual child, but also on the immediate social and nonsocial environment in which each child is developing.

REFERENCES

Borussard, E. R., and Hartner, M. S. S. 1971. Further consideration regarding maternal perception of the first born. In: J. Hellmuth (ed.), Exceptional Infant: Studies in Abnormalities. Vol. 2. Bruner/Mazel, New York.

Morio, M. 1976. An investigation of verbal behavior of maternal-infant pairs during feeding at 1, 4, 8 and 12 months of age. Unpublished master's thesis, University of Washington.

chapter 3

Parent-Infant Interaction: Progress, Paradigms, and Problems

Ross D. Parke

In recent years, increasing effort has been devoted to understanding the nature of early parent-infant interaction. The assumption is that an understanding of the processes governing the patterns of interaction between infants and parents will yield early clues to the general problem of social and cognitive development. In this chapter, a critical evaluation of the assumptions underlying our current research strategies in the area of parent-infant interaction is provided. A second goal is to isolate directions for future research. Specifically, a cognitive mediational paradigm in which parental cognitions, attitudes, and values are given a more explicit role in the parent-infant interaction process is advocated. In contrast to a dyadic analysis of parent-infant interaction, larger units of analysis, such as the family triad, should be examined. A final aim of this chapter is to specify the implications of parent-infant interaction for the study of mental retardation.

A HISTORICAL OVERVIEW

A number of factors have shaped the direction of both theory and methodology in this area. First, the emergence of parent-infant interaction as an active area of inquiry stems partly from the general revival of interest in infancy and early experience. It is noteworthy that the discovery of the infant as a perceptual, cognitive, and information-processing organism preceded the intensive investigation of parent-infant interaction. Studies by Fantz (1961), Kessen (1963), Lipsitt (1963), and others clearly indicated that from an early age the infant was capable of a variety of perceptual and cognitive feats making it a viable partner in an interaction context. Similarly, a host of laboratory experimental studies indicated that the social repertoire of the infant could be modified by environmental feedback. For example, Brackbill (1958), Weisberg (1963), and Rheingold, Gewirtz, and Ross (1959) demonstrated that smiling, crying, and vocalizing could be altered by social cues in the environment. Another influence was, of course, the concern for isolating the early experimental antecedents of later development, with the aim of intervention to improve subsequent cognitive functioning. In light of the limited success of intervention programs aimed at modifying the preschool child (Bronfenbrenner, 1975), there has been a re-awakening of interest in infancy as a period for intervention and an increased interest in the identification of infants at risk for later cognitive and social retardation. This combination of earlier research and current concerns is, in part, responsible for the re-awakened interest in the topic of parent-infant interaction. By now, this is a familiar history.

The enthusiastic endorsement of a naturalistic observational methodology for a large share of the early research in this area, however, stems from a slightly different source. In the past decade there has been a general concern about the limited ecological validity of our traditional methodologies, particularly our reliance on the laboratory experiment as the sine qua non of the student of social development and socialization. In fact, a "mythology of childhood," to borrow Baldwin's (1967) phrase, has evolved in which a set of effects noted in the laboratory is assumed to actually occur in naturalistic socialization contexts and be an accurate account of how the child is socialized. As a result there has been a confusion between necessary and sufficient causality; the laboratory experiments tell us only that certain variables are possible contributors to the child's social-cognitive development. However, the extent to which these hypothesized processes are, in fact, necessary techniques for adequate socialization is left unanswered. To the extent that the aim is a technological one, in which the most effective techniques for modifying behavior in clinical and educational contexts are sought, the ecological validity issue can be ignored. However, if the actual developmental processes are to be elucidated, the problem cannot be dismissed. This concern has led to the increased use of observational methodologies in order to assess ongoing interaction patterns in naturalistic settings (cf. Moss, 1967; Yarrow, Rubinstein, and Pedersen, 1975).

There is another noteworthy shift in research and theorizing in the area of parent-infant interaction. Traditionally, most approaches to social development assumed a unidirectional model whereby the parent influences the child's development; the child's contribution to his own socialization was rarely recognized. In a second phase, under the influence of Bell's (1968) classic paper, the historical imbalance was corrected and the infant's contribution to his own socialization is now widely accepted. In part, this shift occurred because of the experimental analyses of infant competencies of the 1960's, which demonstrated the wide range of capacities as well as the readiness of the infant for social interaction. A third phase is now being increasingly recognized. In our enthusiasm to correct a historical imbalance we focused on the infant's impact on the parent instead of the more appropriate focus on the reciprocal nature of the interactive process. The current zeitgeist, however, has clearly shifted to a study of the reciprocity of interaction: the ways in which parents and infants mutually regulate each other are of central interest.

Finally, the focus of parent-infant interaction studies has increasingly concentrated on the earliest stages of interaction with observations often beginning in the hospital and continuing in the home, in order to track the developmental changes in parent-infant interaction patterns. This noteworthy shift in emphasis is in contrast to earlier research guided by attachment theory (Bowlby, 1969). Under the influence of attachment theory, the focus was largely on the period after 6 months of age, because it was assumed that the infant could only form an attachment with the parent after achieving object permanence. The current emphasis recognizes that the process of mutual regulation begins much earlier and that processes whereby the parent becomes familiar with and responsive to the infant are a necessary aspect of the paradigm. Of course, it is hardly necessary for the parent to wait 6 months for the cognitive achievement of object permanence! These considerations have increasingly supported the study of early parent-infant interaction as well as an emphasis on the processes of social interaction.

MODELS OF PARENT-INFANT INTERACTION

There are a variety of approaches to the study of parent-infant interaction and each makes certain assumptions about a) the nature of the infant and parent and b) the nature of the interactive process. (For a detailed discussion of these issues, see Lewis and Lee-Painter, 1974.)

Some of the common approaches that have been used in this area are illustrated. One of the simplest levels of analysis involves the examination of the behaviors displayed by two individuals (e.g., mother and infant) when they are together. Typically, the frequencies of a variety of behaviors are scored. For example, Moss (1967) scored the occurrence or nonoccurrence of parental behavior in each 60-sec interval over an 8-hr period in the home. Similarly, infant behavior was recorded in the same fashion. Time sampling approaches have been used by a wide range of investigators of parent-infant interaction (cf. Hofer, 1975; Lewis and Rosenblum, 1974). However, the data collected in this fashion are *not* truly interactive because they permit no statements concerning the manner in which the infant and parent activities are coordinated. One simply knows that parents and infants behave in certain ways when they are in each other's presence. The implicit assumption underlying this approach is that the infant or parent is a stimulus for certain partner behaviors, but not in a specific regulatory fashion. Rather, it is assumed that there is a repertoire of behavior elicited by the presence of an infant, but the moment-to-moment modifications in either the elements of the behavioral repertoire or the timing or intensity of the behaviors in the repertoire are not specified.

A closer examination of interaction is derivable from this type of data, by examining either a) correlations between parent and infant behaviors or b) the co-occurrence of a parent and infant behavior in the same time interval. Both are hazardous and only partial solutions to describing interaction. First, correlations between the frequency of occurrence of parental and infant behaviors indicates only that the overall level of a parent behavior is related to the overall level of infant behavior. No information is yielded concerning how closely the parent and infant behaviors were in fact related in time. Although one may interpret the correlation between infant fussing and maternal rocking as an indication that parental rocking is in response to the infant fussing, this is only a suggestive hypothesis because this type of data yields no information concerning the sequence of the parent and infant behaviors.

Of course, the co-occurrence of parent and infant behaviors may yield interactive data; again, this is not necessarily true, because the degree of temporal separation of behaviors within a time interval is not known. For example, a parent may vocalize at 1 sec after the beginning of a 30-sec time frame, whereas the baby may not vocalize until the 23rd sec of the 30-sec interval. It is questionable whether we can legitimately argue that the parent and infant vocalizations are, in fact, interactive, i.e., in response to the partner's behavior. A related problem noted by Altmann (1974) concerns the violation of behaviors that persist; by using this time-sampling approach, discrete behaviors such as touch or move and nondiscrete behaviors such as hold or look, which typically continue over some time period, are treated in a similar fashion.

Alternative approaches to interaction are available and come closer to providing a more truly interactive picture of the parent-infant dyad. One common approach is the use of sequential analyses; because Bakeman (1977) has reviewed these approaches, only brief mention of these strategies is made here. The following example illustrates this approach.

In a recent study, Parke and Sawin (1975) examined the interaction patterns between parents (both mother and father) and their 2 to 4-day-old infants during feeding. A wide range of parental and infant behaviors was recorded during the feeding observations. These include hold patterns (hold close), visual (e.g., look), auditory (vocalize), and tactual (touch, rock) stimulation, as well as specific feeding behaviors (stimulate, feed, and caregiving, e.g., wipe face). Similarly for the infant, a range of visual (look), auditory (vocalize), and feeding (sucking) behaviors were recorded.

All behaviors were assigned a 3-digit numerical code and were recorded in sequence along a continuous time line using a Datamyte keyboard recording device. The Datamyte is a 10-key device that permits behaviors with assigned numerical values to be punched into the system. The keys are tone-related and record the auditory pattern on a cassette tape; in turn, this produces a printout of numerical values (i.e., behaviors in their order and time of occurrence). Two sets of sequences are derived from the interaction data: a) infant elicited parent behavior, whereby the probability of occurrence of various parental behaviors is determined in response to an infant-signal (e.g., crying, moving, sucking); b) parent-elicited infant behavior whereby the probability of occurrence of various infant behaviors are determined in response to a parental stimulus input (touch, rock, vocalize, etc.).

To illustrate, let us examine the changes in probability of a particular parental behavior in the 10-sec interval following an infant behavior. In other words, if an infant emits behavior, what happens in the next 10-sec interval in terms of the parent's behavior? A powerful infant signal in the feeding context is an auditory distress signal, such as a cough, spit up, or sneeze. The main reaction of parents to this signal is, quite sensibly, to stop feeding and the parent does this with a conditional probability of 0.33. However, the unconditional probability of this parent behavior—stop feeding—is quite low (0.05). Similarly, parents vocalize with an unconditional probability of 0.27, but vocalize with a probability of 0.45 when the infant sneezes, spits up, or coughs. In addition, the parent unconditional probability of looking closely is 0.12, which doubles to 0.25 whenever the infant spits or coughs. Touching, on the other hand, is inhibited slightly by this type of infant signal (see Figure 1). Next, consider the impact of an infant vocalization. As Figure 2 illustrates, the most likely occurrence is that the caregiver will, in turn, emit a positive vocalization and touch the infant; the parent is less likely to look more closely at the infant. As a final illustration, consider the modifying impact of mouth movements. Parents of both sexes increase their vocalizing, touching, and stimulation of feeding activity in response to mouth movements (Figure 3).

However, there are certain assumptions underlying our approach to interaction that merit exploration. This approach assumes that the behavior of the two individuals in a

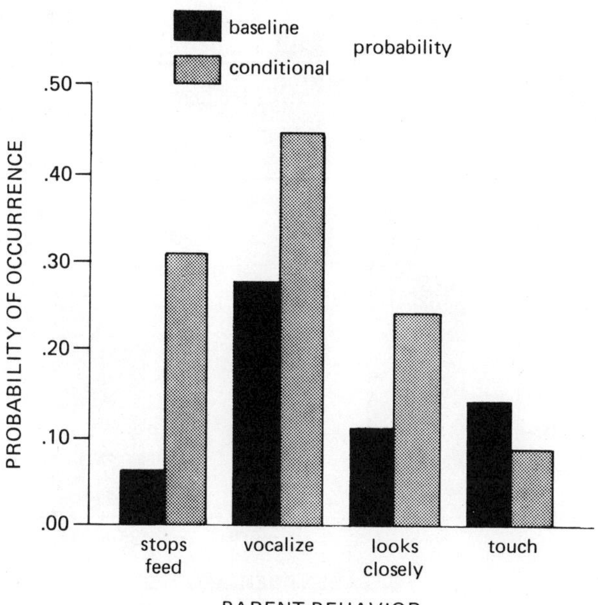

Figure 1. Infant modifier of parental behavior: sneeze, spit up, cough.

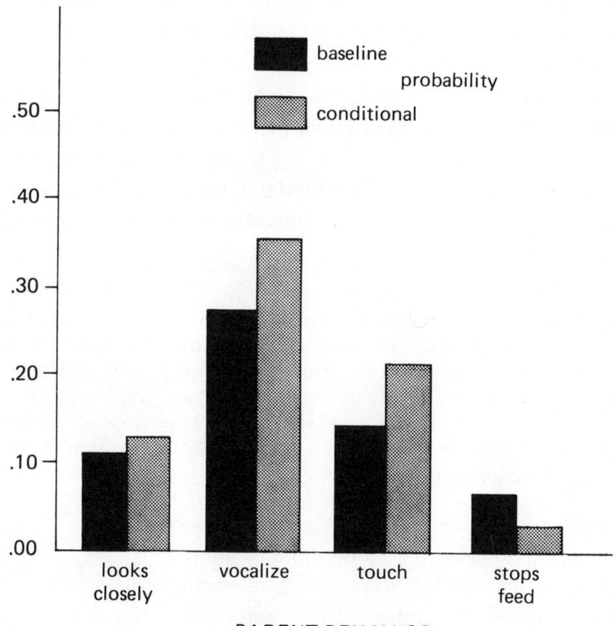

Figure 2. Infant modifier of parental behavior: positive vocalization.

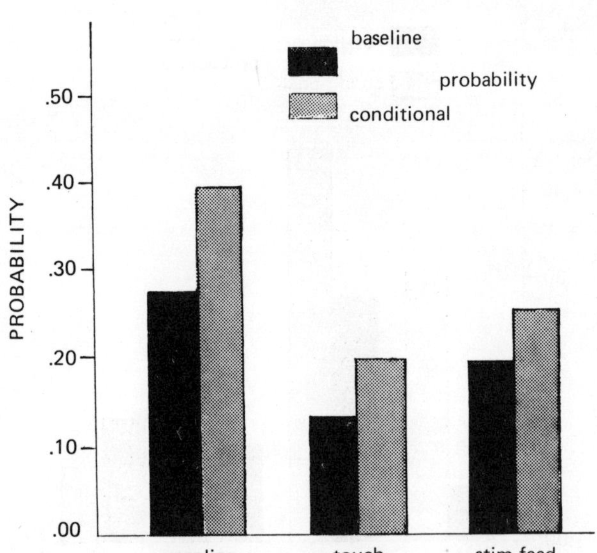

Figure 3. Infant modifier of parent behavior: mouth movements.

dyad can be best characterized by the immediately preceding behavior. To a large degree we are still victims of the stimulus-response (S-R) heritage whereby it is assumed that discrete chains of parent-infant behaviors function in much the same fashion as older and less fashionable S-R relationships. There are, of course, some modifications of these traditional assumptions because no rigid classification of an event as either a stimulus or response is adhered to; rather, it is recognized that any behavior can serve as either stimulus or response. It seems to be more the inadequacies of conceptual and analytic schemes than the nature of the interactive process that had dictated this S-R approach to interaction.

Two research programs have attempted to describe the interactive process in cyclic or rhythmic terms. Brazelton, Koslowski, and Main (1974), for example, note that:

> When the infant was interacting with his mother, there seemed to be a constant cycle of attention (A), followed by withdrawal of attention (W)—the cycle being used by each partner as he approached and then withdrew and waited for a response from the other participant. . . . The behavior of any one member becomes a part of a cluster of behaviors which interact with a cluster of behaviors from the other member of the dyad. No single behavior can be separated from the cluster for analysis without losing its meaning in the sequence. The effect of clustering and sequencing takes over in assessing the value of particular behaviors and in the same way the dyadic nature of interaction superseded the importance of an individual member's clusters and sequences (pp. 55, 56).

These authors have made tentative suggestions concerning the phases that a cycle of attention-nonattention between a mother and infant may follow: a) imitation b) orientation c) state of attention d) acceleration e) peak of excitement and f) deceleration—repeat.

One of the important features of this approach is that it may permit a content free analysis of the nature of the interaction process itself. That is, the formal rules that govern the rhythmic nature of interaction may be revealed through this approach. Developmental shifts could then be described in terms of the changing values associated with a variety of parameters associated with the interaction process. By implication, this approach suggests that the specific behaviors such as looking, vocalizing, moving, etc., which are the main data for more traditional approaches including sequential analyses, are of less importance for understanding the nature of interaction than the timing and intensity of the behavior in relation to the behavior of the partner.

Although this approach is intuitively appealing, to date most of the work has been descriptive case studies; the problem of quantifying this type of cyclic behavior pattern between two partners has remained outside the realm of the traditional statistical models. A technique that seems to hold considerable promise for providing a quantitative representation of cyclic interaction patterns is time-series analysis (Glass, Willson, and Gottman, 1975; Campbell and Stanley, 1966). For an excellent illustration of the application of time-series to parent-infant data, see Thomas and Martin (1976). Time-series analyses should prove useful not simply for *describing* developmental changes in parent-infant interaction, but interrupted time-series designs (e.g., simple intervention, reversal design variations of multiple baseline designs) could be helpful in evaluation of the impact of interventions on patterns of parent-infant interaction (Gottman, 1973; Gottman, McFall, and Barnett, 1969).

Another statistical approach that could be used in the analyses of the rhythmic or cyclic properties of interaction patterns is Sackett's (1974) sequential lag technique. The advantage of this strategy over time series is that fewer assumptions concerning the properties of the data distributions are made and meaningful analyses can be executed with fewer observations than in the case of a time-series approach. In short, statistical techniques are available that make this type of analysis of parent-infant interaction increasingly viable.

In the final analysis, however, the basis for selecting data collection strategy and for choosing level of analysis should be dictated by the nature of the problem, the status of theory in the area, and the stage of development of the research program. In the early stages of an investigation or in a theoretically underdeveloped area, a time-sampling strategy may be most appropriate. After preliminary work has been completed, selection of a more detailed and sophisticated but more expensive sequential analytic strategy may be appropriate. Similarly, techniques that focus on a content free analysis of interaction patterns (cf. Bakeman, 1977) may be inappropriate for certain types of problems. In our own research, where the concern is to describe the similarities and differences in father versus mother-infant interaction, the particular kinds of stimulation (e.g., auditory versus tactual) as well as the patterns of interaction are viewed as theoretically important discriminators between parents. It is clear that simply moving to a more molecular or more abstract level of analysis should not be our goal; rather comparative analysis of the usefulness of different strategies for particular problems needs to be carefully done before any particular level or type of analysis is preferentially advocated.

A COGNITIVE MEDIATIONAL APPROACH TO PARENT-INFANT INTERACTION

A general issue that has been largely ignored in recent studies of parent-infant interaction is the impact of parental cognitions, perceptions, attitudes, and knowledge on the interaction process. Implicit in many models of interaction is the assumption that the parent reacts to the behavior of the infant in a mechanical or unthinking fashion. Again, this is, in large measure, a legacy of the S-R heritage which has caused the role of subjective events to be ignored in an effort to develop an objective analysis of interaction patterns. Nor has the recent trend of replacing S-R language with the assumptions of a biologically derived ethological approach resulted in any correction of this denial of cognitive factors in social interaction. Another explanation may be that in our enthusiasm to give the infant proper recognition as a contributor to the interactive process, the assumptions have been oversimplified concerning the partner's relative capacities in the dyadic exchange by treating them as co-acting equals. Unfortunately, it may have inadvertently been assumed that the cognitive capacities of the infant and parent could functionally be treated as similar. Although no one would seriously support such a view, we have in fact been treating the parent as a black box reactor in the parent-infant interaction context. This failure to treat parents as information-processing organisms is particularly surprising in light of the general cognitive revival with psychology in the past 15 years.

One reason for the limited recognition of cognitive variables in current theoretical conceptualization of parent-infant interaction is the failure to adequately distinguish between *parental reports as objective measures of parental behavior* and *parental reports as indices of parental knowledge, attitudes, stereotypes, and perceptions*. These latter classes of variables are legitimate and important sources of data and are not easily derived from observation alone. These types of parental reports provide information about ways in which parents perceive, organize, and understand both their infants and their roles as parents. The assumption is that these cognitive sets serve as filters through which the objective behaviors of the infant are processed. It is not assumed that parent perceptions of infant behavior are short-hand routes to circumvent the task of directly observing the infant. Rather, it is assumed that these perceptions, attitudes, and values *are* different and to some degree independent sources of data. In fact, it is probably a mistake to assume that actual and perceived behaviors are necessarily similar and can be treated as parallel sources of information.

In this section, some of the ways in which these classes of verbal behavior, including parental knowledge, perceptions, stereotypes, and attitudes, may alter parent and infant behavior in the interaction context are discussed.

Parental Knowledge of Infant Behavior

An important determinant of parent-infant interaction is the agent's own assumptions about the infant's capacities. There are wide individual differences in adults' knowledge of the sensory and perceptual capacities of the newborn. These parental differences will have an important impact on the nature of the infant behaviors that are responded to *and* the types of behavior that the parent will engage in. Parents who assume that human newborns are similar to kittens with only a little less fur and no tail and can't see for 10 days are hardly likely to be very responsive to the infant's eye-to-eye contact and are not very likely to provide visual stimulation. Some support for this speculation derives from Kilbride, Johnson, and Streissguth (1971) who found that lower class mothers, who provided less visual stimulation for their 2-week-old infants than middle class mothers, were less likely to assume that infants could see at birth. Much more information concerning the ways in which parental knowledge about perceptual, motor, and cognitive capacities affect the nature of their interaction is necessary. Direct testing of the proposition that this type of knowledge alters parent-infant interaction is possible by providing new and accurate information and then evaluating changes in the interaction patterns.

Parental Perceptions of Infant Behavior

It is not simply parental knowledge of infant abilities, but also perception of infant behavior that may alter parental behavior in the parent-infant interaction context. In contrast to earlier approaches, which treated actual and perceived behaviors as equivalent sources of information (e.g., Thomas et al., 1963), the recent development of questionnaires aimed at tapping parental perception of infant temperament (e.g., Carey, 1970; Scarr and Salapatek, 1970; Pedersen, Andersen and Cain, 1976) recognizes the independent contribution of parental perceptions to the interaction process. The important issue that merits underscoring in the present context is this: do objective or subjective accounts of infant characteristics provide the most leverage in understanding parent-infant interaction? A more thorough investigation of the degree of discrepancy between objective scoring schemes and parental perceptions is needed.

Another dimension should be distinguished. It is not simply parental perceptions of infant characteristics that are important, but the parent's evaluation of these particular traits. The important lesson of the work of Thomas et al. (1963) was that neither the individual characteristics of the child nor the individual characteristics of the parent could be considered alone. Of the original 136 children in their study, 39 later showed behavior problems of varying degrees (Chess, 1971). In each case, the problem could be traced back to an unfavorable interaction of the child with a particular temperament and various features of the environment, but children with similar temperaments were found in both normal and problem groups. The important issue is the parent's perception and evaluation of the particular behavior patterns.

Parental Stereotypes as Determinants of Parent-Infant Interaction

Parental stereotypes of behaviors that they expect from infants of different sex is another illustration of the way in which cognitive factors may influence interaction patterns. In a recent study, Rubin, Provenzano, and Luria (1974) asked mothers and fathers to rate their newborn sons or daughters in the first 24 hr after birth. Although male and female infants did not differ in birth length, weight, or Apgar scores, daughters were significantly more likely than sons to be described as little, beautiful, pretty, and cute, and as resembling their mothers. Fathers, who had seen but not handled their infants, were more extreme in their ratings of both sons and daughters than were mothers. Sons were rated as firmer, larger featured, better coordinated, more alert, stronger, and hardier and daughters as softer, finer featured, more awkward, more inattentive, weaker, and more delicate by their fathers than by their mothers. As the authors note, "the central implication of the study, then, is that sex-typing and sex role socialization appear to have already begun their course at the time of the infant's birth, when information about the infant is minimal. The

Gestalt parents develop and the labels they ascribe to their newborn infant may well affect subsequent expectations about the manner in which their infant ought to behave as well as parental behavior itself.'' (Rubin et al., 1974, pp. 518, 519).

Nor is this sex stereotyping restricted to parents and newborn infants. Condry and Condry (1976) asked male and female college subjects to rate an infant's videotaped emotional reactions to four different arousing stimuli. Of interest was the sex label attributed to the 9-month infant, so half of the subjects were told that they were observing a ''boy'' and the other half a ''girl.'' In one sequence, in which the infant was presented with a jack-in-the-box and over a series of presentations cried and screamed, the results were dramatically influenced by the labels. Observers rated the ''boy'' as expressing ''anger,'' and the ''girl'' as expressing ''fear.'' Although their study was not designed to reveal treatment differences, Condry and Condry (1976) note, ''It seems reasonable to assume that a child who is thought to be afraid is held and cuddled more than a child who is thought to be angry'' (p. 16). Finally, the ''boy'' was viewed as more ''active'' and ''potent'' than the female infant on semantic differential ratings.

Together these two studies emphasize the importance of a social mediation approach to early parent-infant interaction, in which stereotypes are recognized as playing a role in shaping parental behavior.

The issue, of course, is whether these early perceptions of sex differences are based on detectable differences in the newborn. In addition, if there are behavioral differences, which sets of factors—behavioral or perceptual—yield the most predictive power in understanding parent-infant interaction? First, as a number of recent reviews have indicated, there are detectable sex differences as early as the newborn period (Korner, 1974; Maccoby and Jacklin, 1974). However, they are neither large in number nor very impressive in terms of magnitude and, in general, offer scant support for the parental stereotypes noted by Rubin et al. First, there are no sex differences in alertness, as indexed by visual tracking of moving objects (Korner, 1970; Brazelton, 1974) or in the frequency and duration of the state of alert inactivity (Korner, 1970). Similarly, there have been no sex differences demonstrated in auditory receptivity (Korner, 1974). Neither activity level nor neonatal crying show sex differences (Korner, 1974). However, females exhibit more reflex smiles than males (Korner, 1969; Freedman, 1971) whereas males exhibit more startles (Korner, 1969).

There are, of course, sex differences in parental treatment. For example, Thoman, Liederman, and Olson (1972) reported that mothers vocalized more to girls than to boys. Parke and O'Leary (1976), on the other hand, found that fathers were more discriminating in terms of their treatment of infants of different sexes than mothers; they touched and vocalized to boys (particularly first born) more than to girls of either ordinal position, an exaggeration that parallels the more extreme father ratings of Rubin et al. (1974). At present, the source of these parental differences in treatment of boys and girls is largely unspecified. Attempts to monitor the behavior of boys and girls in the interaction situation generally have revealed few clear sex differences (Parke and Sawin, 1975). Nor have attempts been successful to use independent assessments of infant behavior (e.g., Brazelton Scale) as explanatory links between infant sex differences and parental reactions to boys and girls in an interaction context. The next obvious step has not yet been systematically taken, namely, to assess directly both parental stereotypes concerning sex differences in infants *and* to measure parent-infant interaction patterns. By measuring both of these across time, as well as measuring actual detectable behavioral differences in the infant, some clues concerning the ways in which parental sex role stereotypes are maintained and modified may be forthcoming.

Just as parents and other caregivers have sex role stereotypes, they also have stereotypes concerning the features that constitute the attractiveness of an infant. As Bell (1974) has speculated, the morphological characteristics such as an infant's protruding cheeks may contribute to launching parental behavior. Recent research has indicated not only that physical attractiveness can be reliably rated in infants, but that these ratings may affect caregiver-infant interaction.

First, let us turn to the issue of judgment of infant attractiveness. To determine whether nurses could make reliable judgments of the attractiveness of premature infants was the aim of a recent study by Corter, Trehub, Boukydis, Ford, Celhoffer, and Minde (1976); nurses rated the attractiveness of pictures of premature infants and also rated the prognosis for each infant's future intellectual development. First, there was good agreement among the nurses in judging individual differences in the attractiveness of premature infants. The potential importance of physical attractiveness for the infant's social experience is suggested by the significant correlation between the experienced nurses' judgments of attractiveness and their guesses about future intellectual prognosis. If the nurses believe that the more attractive infants have a greater chance for normal or better intellectual development, they might invest more effort in interacting with and stimulating these infants. The authors note that:

> Whether or not nurses really believe that appearance might predict later IQ, it is reasonable to assume that the amount of nonmedical attention they pay to infants might vary partly as a function of how "pleasant looking" a particular infant is. Although physical attractiveness may be an important variable only in the "first stages of interaction," infant-nurse interaction may not go much beyond the first stages in many hospitals. For example, it was found that premature infants were attended to by an average of 71 different nurses during an average stay of 49 days. Under such conditions it may be that "first impressions" based on physical attractiveness have substantial weight in determining the social environment experienced by premature infants (Corter et al., 1976, pp. 9, 10).

In light of recent evidence (Cornell and Gottfried, 1976) that extra stimulation does have beneficial effects on the development of premature infants, it would be worthwhile to determine whether infant attractiveness does, in fact, alter the frequency and quality of infant-caregiver interactions.

Some preliminary although suggestive data comes from our own studies of interaction patterns between normal, full term infants and their parents (Parke and Sawin, 1975). An observer rated the physical attractiveness of the infant on a 10-point scale. These independent ratings were correlated with the parent behaviors and revealed that the interaction patterns of both mothers and fathers were related to the attractiveness measures. Mothers maintain more eye and ventral contact, and kiss more frequently more attractive infants. Fathers stimulate attractive infants more than less attractive infants; they touch, kiss, and move highly attractive infants more frequently (Figure 4). As Harlow's previous work has demonstrated, "to a baby all maternal faces are beautiful and a mother's face that will stop a clock will not stop an infant" (Harlow and Suomi, 1970). Unfortunately,

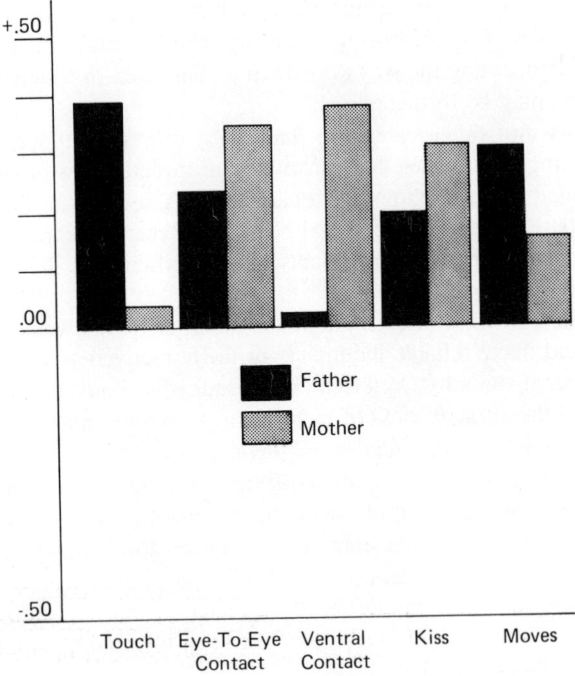

Figure 4. The impact of infant attractiveness on parent-infant interaction.

parents do not seem to follow this rule and "to a parent some babies are more beautiful than others and a baby's face that may stop a clock may also stop a mother."

It is clear that more research on the ways in which parents develop concepts of infant attractiveness may be profitable.

Parents as Personality Theorists

Although personality traits are under attack in favor of situationally based explanations of behavior (cf. Mischel, 1968, 1973), there is another aspect of the trait attribution process that may be of importance for understanding the process of parent-infant interaction. Although parental behavior cannot be explained through the application of a series of personality traits, the parental process of applying trait labels to their infants may be an important factor in understanding their behavior and treatment of infants. With Mischel (1973), "the traditional personality paradigm views traits as the intrapsychic causes of behavioral consistency, the present position sees them as summary terms (labels, codes, organizing constructs) applied to observed behavior" (1973, p. 264).

Over time, parents develop stable expectations in the form of labels. In turn, these labels may be important for determining the types of interaction patterns. The labels, of course, may take a variety of forms including clinical-medical terms such as hyperactive, colicky, or premature *or* may include more common adjectives such as happy, contented, difficult, or playful.

Change in a mother's view of her infant as a factor in later vulnerability is nicely demonstrated by Borussard and Hartner (1971). Using a questionnaire, they assessed how a mother saw her child in relation to her view of the average infant. The infants were divided into high and low risk samples on the basis of whether their mothers saw them as worse or better than the average child. At 4 years of age, they were given a clinical assessment and divided into categories according to the apparent need for therapeutic intervention. The infants identified as high risk on the bases of the mothers' labeling at 1 month were significantly more likely to require clinical intervention at 4 years of age. Borussard and Hartner concluded that the process of a successful or unsuccessful mother-infant relationship was already well established at 1 month of age and that mothers were instrumental in, as well as predictive of, their children's later mental health. The important issue, of course, is the extent to which mothers are simply accurate in their reading of their infant's behavioral difficulties or whether their perception and labeling of their infants results in a self-fulfilling prophecy. Studies in which parental expectations and parental attitudes are modified and their impact on parent-infant interaction are clearly necessary.

Many questions remain. How do parents develop stable impressions or traits about their infants? What types of cues are used by parents in designating one label versus another? How consistent and how discriminable do the cues have to be for this trait assignment process to emerge? Are there differences in mothers in their tendency to assign trait labels and how stable are the mothers in their use of these labels? How do these labels become communicated to other caregivers? For example, a father's interaction with his infant may be affected by his wife's labeling of the infant. Similarly, nurses may communicate labels to a parent that may alter their interactions with the infant. The implications of early labeling of children who are at risk for mental retardation have recently been noted by Hobbs (1975), Mercer (1973), and others. The processes by which this labeling happens, however, warrant more attention from researchers of parent-infant interaction.

Nor are the effects of labeling restricted to the infant; the parent may be labeled early by hospital personnel as "insensitive" or "indifferent." Even though these labels may not be directly communicated to the mother, they nevertheless may affect the nurses' treatment of the mother, the type of support they offer and even the opportunities they provide for mother-infant interaction. Although labeling of parents as high risk for child abuse, for example, may be in the interests of protecting children, the positive prediction rate from early screening is so low as to raise serious doubts about the wisdom of early labeling (cf. Light, 1973; Parke and Collmer, 1975).

Finally, it is likely that recent social psychological research on the influence of attribution theory on behavior will prove useful in understanding both the origins and implications of parental labeling of infants (cf. Kelley, 1972; Weiner and Kun, 1976).

Implications of a Cognitive Mediational Approach to Parent-Infant Interaction

The main argument of this section is clear: Direct observations of parent-infant interaction need to be supplemented with systematic measures of parental perceptions and attitudes concerning their infants. These additional measures should be of value in three ways. First, this information could be the source of new hypotheses and insights. Second, these verbal report data my serve as a guide in the selection of coding categories. For example, knowledge of the specific dimensions that underlie sex-role sterotypes may aid in building a sensitive observational scheme for detecting infant sex differences. Third, parental reports may serve an explanatory function. The explanation of a variety of observed differences such as social class or cultural differences in the type or amount of stimulation may often be found in parental belief systems, attitudes, and expectations. Finally, this approach has very clear-cut implications for modification of parent-infant interaction patterns. As illustrated in this section, parental behavior is, to some degree, controlled by knowledge of infant behavior, expections about behavior differneces, and early diagnostic labels. One component of a modification program should involve the alteration of parental attitudes, expectations, and knowledge about their infants. Evaluating the success of a cognitive modification strategy through direct observation will yield information about the practical value of this approach, and will permit an evaluation of the theoretical value of a cognitive mediational approach to parent-infant interaction as well.

ON THE IMPORTANCE OF CONTEXT: A COGNITIVE INTERPRETATION

One of the least studied but probably most important classes of factors that influence parent-infant interaction patterns is the immediate *context* or *setting* in which the interaction takes place. Not only do contexts vary in terms of their degree of structure, but also the same responses adopt a very different meaning in various contexts. Recently, Brazelton, Tronick, Adamson, Als, and Wise (1975) presented a typology outlining the amount of constraint and structure in different types of situations (Figure 5). Although the feeding situation may be a reasonable choice for studying parent-infant interaction because it is an ecologically important interaction context, other contexts that are less structured may yield a rich picture of the extent to which the infant is able to control and direct the flow of

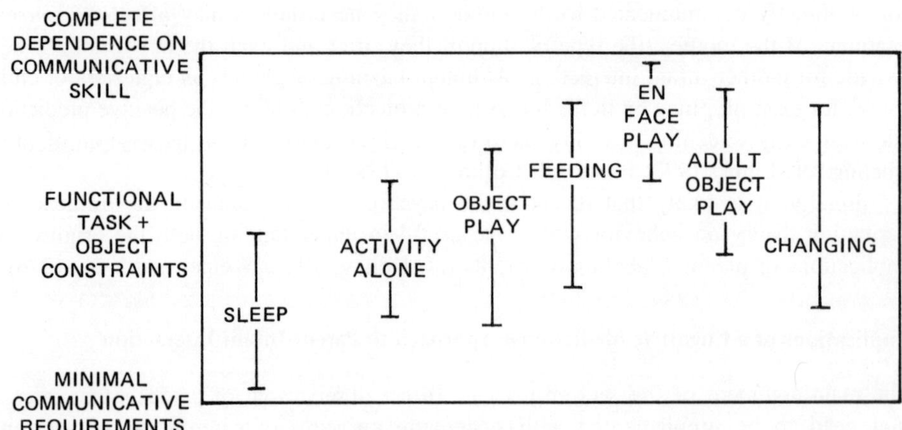

Figure 5. Relative communicative requirements of different infant activities (from Brazelton et al., 1975, p. 138).

the interaction. Although Brazelton et al. organized situations in terms of their relative communicative requirements for the participants, the meaning associated with various contexts for different adult caregivers needs to be systematically explored. Just as the same type of adult stimulus (e.g., a masked face) may elicit fear in one context and laughter in another (Sroufe, Waters, and Matas 1974), so adults attach different meanings to the same infant cues in different contexts. For example, parents are likely to react to arm waving and laughing in very different ways in feeding and play contexts. What do adults perceive as the principal goals of interaction in different situations and how do these cognitive organizing sets modify the subsequent behaviors of the adult? Comparisons across types of contexts would be necessary in order to specify the *degree* to which parental reactions to infant behaviors are influenced by different contexts. Second, it is necessary to specify the *types* of infant cues that adults respond to in different contexts. Third, what is the nature of the adult behaviors that are emitted in response to the same types of infant cues in different settings?

Physical Environment and Culture as Contexts

A distinction needs to be made among various uses of the term "context." In studies of parent-infant interaction, the term usually refers to the immediate interaction setting, such as feeding, playing, diapering, etc. This use should be distinguished from the larger physical environment in which the immediate interaction context is embedded; in turn, the larger physical setting should be distinguished from the cultural context in which both of these more delimited settings exist. Let us briefly examine each of these two alternative uses of context.

Physical Environment as Context The emergence of an environmental psychology (Ittelson et al., 1974) has focused our attention on the structural organization of the physical environment as a determinant of social behavior, including parent-infant interaction patterns. For example, the physical organization, layout, and size of the house will dictate the types and amount of parent-infant interaction. Arrangements that permit the infant to have its own room will reduce the amount of parent-infant contact in contrast to arrangements in which the infant sleeps in the same room as the parents or in the main adult activity area. Similarly, the types of transportation devices (e.g., slings, backpacks, carriages) will make a difference in the amount and type of parent-infant contact. (cf. Rheingold and Keene, 1965; Goldberg, 1972). Another determinant of parent-infant interaction is the type and availability of toys in the infant's physical environment. As Quilitch and Risley (1973) have demonstrated, the properties of different kinds of toys elicit varying degrees of social interaction. In short, the characteristics of the physical environment in which parent-infant interaction takes place need to be systematically described as a first step in determining its impact on the interaction patterns.

Culture as Context An examination of cross cultural variations in parent-infant interaction is another way of illustrating the important role that cognitive factors play in social behavior; parent-infant interaction patterns are clearly determined and shaped by the values, beliefs, and goals of the culture, and only by recognizing these cognitive elements can cross cultural variability in interaction styles be understood. Moreover, it serves as a reminder of the relativity of our own particular styles of parent-infant interaction and at the same time forces us to articulate a set of broadly shared cultural attitudes concerning infants and the nature of the parent-infant interaction. In turn, these assumptions and attitudes within our own culture are undergoing continuing revision, as new knowledge about infants and the impact of different types of environmental interventions emerge. Consider this 1928 advice of John B. Watson:

> There is a sensible way of treating children. Treat them as though they were young adults. Dress them, bathe them with care and circumspection. Let your behavior always be objective and kindly, [but] never hug and kiss them, never let them sit in your lap. If you must, kiss them once on the forehead when they say good night.

In contrast, consider Benjamin Spock's advice in 1968:

> Don't be afraid to love and enjoy him. Every baby needs to be smiled at, talked to, played with, fondled—gently and lovingly—just as much as he needs vitamins and calories . . . Be companionable with your baby. Be quietly friendly with your baby whenever you are with him. When you hug him or make noises at him, when you show him that you think he's the most wonderful baby in the world, it makes his spirit grow . . .

In fact, far too little attention has been paid to the task of monitoring the secular shifts in child-care practices and to the equally important task of specifying the mechanisms by which new trends are initiated. The current zeitgeist in our culture assumes that the child and even perhaps the adult is shaped by infant experiences. Moreover, it is increasingly assumed that the earliest experiences in the postpartum period are important. Second, it is assumed that a responsive, contingent environment is important. The caregiver should be responsive and sensitive to a baby's signals and cues. Third, it is assumed that a stimulating, varying, and novel physical environment is important for infant development. In short, there is a set of presumably shared cultural expectations concerning the appropriate tactics for parent-infant interaction which are the first level of influence in shaping parent-infant interaction.

A few examples illustrate the culture-bound nature of our assumptions. Kagan and Klein's (1973) recent report of infancy in Guatemala indicates that not all cultures share our assumptions about the importance of early stimulation and responsive, sensitive caregivers. Guatemalan infants were spoken to or played with only 6% of the time, in contrast to 25% in American middle class homes. No toys were available and the infants were permitted little opportunity to crawl and explore their environment.

"The mothers in these settings seem to regard their infants the way an American parent views an expensive cashmere sweater: Keep it nearby and protect it but do not engage it reciprocally" (Kagan and Klein, 1973). Kagan and Klein's interpretation is noteworthy because it emphasizes the mediating role of parental cognitions in shaping their interaction patterns: "The mother's lack of active manipulation, stimulation, or interactive play with her infant is not indicative of indifference or rejection, but is a reasonable posture given her knowledge of child development" (Kagan and Klein, 1973). Nor are these violations of our American expectations limited to primitive cultures.

Although it is often assumed that European and American cultures are very similar, recent comparisons of Dutch and American infant caregiving patterns dispel this myth. Rebelsky (1967) notes a variety of differences:

> American mothers looked at, held, fed, talked to, smiled at, patted and showed more affection to their babies and more often than did Dutch mothers. U.S. and Dutch mothers did

> not differ in the amount of time spent adjusting, rocking, nodding or playing with the baby. The rank order of the behaviors was similar across cultures, though the frequencies differed. . . . In general, U.S. mothers spent more time with their babies than did Dutch mothers. In addition, Dutch mothers spent less time in interaction with their babies at 3 months than at 2 weeks, unlike American mothers who spent more time with their baby, especially increasing in talking to the baby, at 3 months than at 2 weeks.

Similarly, their reactions to crying differed:

> U.S. mothers tended to hear their babies crying and responded to the cry, whereas in Holland mothers often couldn't hear the crying (since the bedroom door was shut and the mother was in another room with the door shut) or didn't respond if the crying was heard. The cultural views differ: crying meant a call for help for U.S. mothers; they often reported lactating when they heard the cry. In Holland crying was considered a part of a baby's behavior, good for the lungs and not always something to stop. In addition, though a mother might hear the cry in Holland and interpret it as a hunger cry she still would not respond if it was not time for a scheduled feeding (Rebelsky, 1967, p. 390).

These examples provide further demonstration of the necessity for considering cognitive variables such as beliefs, values, and expectations in our efforts to understand parent-infant interaction patterns. Just as assessments of individual cognitive variables may be useful in accounting for variability in individual parent-infant dyads, assessments of cultural belief systems will prove useful in understanding cross cultural variations in interaction patterns.

BEYOND THE MOTHER-INFANT DYAD: THE FATHER AND THE FAMILY

Father-Infant Dyad

To date we have largely restricted ourselves to the study of the parent-infant dyad, typically, the mother-infant dyad. The historical and theoretical reasons for this emphasis on the mother-infant relationship are well known (Schaffer, 1971), and generally attributed to both our cultural attitudes concerning the mother as primary caregiver (Josselyn, 1956) and as the first and most important attachment figure (Bowlby, 1951). The other influence of course is our psychoanalytic and our Hullian heritage, both of which emphasize the importance of the feeding situation as the critical context for the development of social responsiveness (Walters and Parke, 1965). This exclusive emphasis on the mother-infant relationship has recently been challenged by revised theory and cultural shifts (Lynn, 1974) as well as by empirical findings at both the animal (Mitchell, Redican, and Gomber, 1974) and human levels (Parke and O'Leary, 1976; Parke and Sawin, 1976).

A brief review of this recent work will serve as a corrective to our exclusive emphasis on the mother-infant dyad. In a series of studies of father-newborn interaction (Parke, O'Leary, and West, 1972; Parke and O'Leary, 1976), it was found that fathers are highly involved and interested in newborn infants. A time-sampling approach yielded results indicating that mothers and fathers did not differ in the degree of touching, looking, vocalizing, or kissing when alone with the infant. There were only two behaviors, smiling and feeding, in which the mother surpassed the father. However, even though the mother and father differ in terms of their involvement in the feeding context they are both equally sensitive in slightly different ways to the infant's cues. Recall our earlier description of the parental reactions to infant distress cues. Mothers and fathers differ only slightly: mothers have a probability of stopping their feeding activity of 0.27 whereas fathers cease feeding with a probability 0.35 in response to the infant cluster of spit up, sneeze, and cough. Similarly, both mothers (0.28) and fathers (0.21) look more closely in response to this infant cue in the feeding context. Although the father may spend less time overall, he is as *sensitive as the mother to infant cues in the feeding contexts.*

These studies indicate that fathers are interested and competent actors in the early parent-infant interaction drama. Their potential roles in the care and stimulation of high risk infants, however, remains to be examined. To date nearly all of the work on father-infant interaction has involved normal, healthy, full term infants. The ways in which fathers interact with high risk infants clearly need to be systematically examined. The father could play an important role in reducing some of the detrimental effects of the social isolation that often accompanies the premature infant. The father may be available as a social stimulator before the mother, particularly in the case of high risk infants who are often being cared for at a central high risk nursery that is, typically, separated physically from the delivery hospital. The father's role in the care and stimulation of the high risk infant needs not only further study but institutional support as well. Hospital visiting arrangements need to be modified to encourage paternal participation, paternity leaves need to be more easily available, and hospital-based training in caregiving and stimulation needs to be provided for fathers as well as mothers. To date, little is known about the long term effects of early father involvement with newborn infants. However, recent work by Lind (1974) in Sweden, who was heavily influenced by the work of Klaus and Kennell (1970; Kennell, Trause, and Klaus, 1975) in the U.S. on the effects of early extended contact between infants and their mothers, is suggestive. Lind found that fathers who were provided the opportunity to learn and practice basic caregiving skills during the postpartum hospital period were more involved with their infants in the home at 3 months. It would appear that opportunities for fathers to take an active role with their newborn infants is an important antecedent to fuller father participation in the caregiving of the baby in later infancy.

Mother-Father-Infant Triad

It is necessary to expand our observations to include not only the father alone with his infant, but to analyze the family triad of mother, father, and infant.

In two of our earlier studies, we examined the triad and compared the behavior of mother and father both alone with the infant and in the family triad (Parke, O'Leary, and West, 1972; Parke and O'Leary, 1976). In both studies the father was a highly involved participant in the family context and either equaled or excelled the mother in stimulating and nurturing the infant. Of greatest interest were comparisons of the parents in the dyadic and triadic settings. The presence of the spouse significantly altered the behavior of the other parent; specifically, both father and mother expressed more positive affect (smiling) toward their infant and showed a higher level of exploration when the other parent was also present. The family context, in short, appeared to elicit greater affective and exploratory behavior on the part of both parents. Our hypothesis is that the parents verbally stimulate each other by focusing the partner's attention on aspects of the baby's behavior, and by commenting on the infant's appearance, which in turn elicits either positive affect directed to the baby or exploration to check out an aspect of behavior noted by their spouse. These results indicate that parent-infant interaction patterns are modified by the presence of another adult; in turn, the implication is that we have assumed prematurely that parent-infant interaction can be understood by our sole focus on the parent-infant dyad alone.

Moreover, other recent investigations emphasize the importance of studying the family triad by illustrating the impact of the husband-wife relationship on the parent-infant interaction process and the influence of the birth of a high risk infant on the cohesiveness of the family.

Pedersen (1975) assessed the influence of the husband-wife relationship on the mother-infant interaction in a feeding context. Ratings were made of the quality of the mother-infant relationship in connection with two time-sampling home observations when the infants were 4 weeks old. Of particular interest was "feeding competence," which refers to the appropriateness of the mother in managing feeding. "Mothers rated high are able to pace the feeding well, intersperse feeding and burping without disrupting the baby and seem sensitive to the baby's needs for either stimulation of feeding or brief rest periods during the course of feedings" (Pedersen, 1975, p. 4). In addition, the husband-wife relationship was assessed through an interview; and finally, neonatal assessments (Brazelton, 1974) were available.

Pedersen summarized his results as follows:

> The husband-wife relationship was linked to the mother-infant unit. When the father was more supportive of the mother, that is, evaluated her maternal skills more positively, she was more effective in feeding the baby. Then again, maybe competent mothers elicit more positive evaluations from their husbands. The reverse holds for marital discord. High tension and conflict in the marriage was associated with more inept feeding on the part of the mother (Pedersen, 1975, p. 6).

The picture is even more complex, however, as indicated by the observation that the status and well being of the infant, as assessed by alertness and motor maturity, is also related to the marital relationship. With an alert baby, the father evaluated the mother more positively; with a motorically mature baby, there appeared to be less tension and conflict in the marriage. In Pedersen's (1975) view "a good baby and a good marriage go together."

Both Parke and Pedersen used "normal" healthy, full term infants. However, one would expect that the impact of a high risk infant would have an even more profound impact on the family interaction patterns. Of relevance to this issue is the earlier work of Leiderman (Leiderman and Seashore, 1975; Leifer, Leiderman, Barnett, and Williams, 1972).

These investigators examined the impact of the separation that often occurs between parents and premature infants on subsequent mother-infant interaction and family functioning. Two groups of premature infants and their families as well as a sample of normal infants participated. The parents of premature infants in one group had contact with their infants during the separation period, while a second group had little contact over a period of approximately 3 weeks postpartum. Although the study demonstrated the importance of contact for the development of the mother-infant relationship (cf. Kennell, Trause, and Klaus, 1975), the finding of particular interest for this chapter concerned the impact of the premature infant on family cohesiveness. When the infants were 21 months old, eight divorces had occurred in the original sample of 66 families: five divorces occurred in families of the separated group, two in the contact group, and one in the full term group. Leiderman and Seashore suggest, "that separation in the newborn period does have an effect, albeit non-specific, by acting through the family as a stress that creates disequilibrium in the nuclear family structure" (1975, pp. 229, 230).

The importance of these findings is clear: in order to understand either the mother-infant or father-infant relationship, the total set of relationships among the members of the family needs to be assessed. Although interviews are likely to be helpful, they are not sufficient; rather, direct observations of both mother *and* father alone with their infants as well as the mother, father, and infant together are necessary.

Beyond the Parent: The Usefulness of the Nonparent Caregiver

It is unlikely that the bidirectional effects in parent-infant interaction are best understood by restricting oneself to the parent-infant dyad. Strategies are necessary that permit greater control over both sides of the interaction; ideally, one should be able to manipulate both the adult and child sides of the interaction independently.

Although the use of parents—both mother and father—is highly desirable in the interests of ecological validity, this strategy may not be the most effective one for understanding the contribution of the infant to the interaction sequence. Part of the problem is that *both* parent and infant may vary in their characteristics. Therefore, in any parent-infant dyad the unique characteristics of the infant may be masked by the parental characteristics; the result, of course, is the modification by a unique infant of a particular parent. To illustrate, take the case of obstetrical medication that is administered to the mother during labor and delivery, but which passes the placental barrier and, therefore, also affects the infant; any infant behaviors which effect a change in maternal behavior may, in part, be due to the medication received by the mother. An alternative is the use of a standard caregiver, which would permit a more sensitive assessment of the impact of behavioral variations across infants on the behavior of a caregiver; but in the situation where the behavior or style of responding on the part of the caregiver is less variable.

There is a further reason for using nonparent caregivers, namely as a comparison point against which to assess the uniqueness of the adult as "parent." Are there behaviors associated with the position of parent that are unique and different from a nonparent male or female?

IS NATURALISTIC OBSERVATION SUFFICIENT?

Although many investigators prefer naturalistic observation in the interests of maintaining a high degree of ecological validity, it is clear that sole reliance on a single strategy would be a serious error. A variety of strategies are necessary at this stage of our understanding of parent-infant interaction processes. One popular strategy involves a series of steps. First, observation in the naturalistic environment is undertaken to generate hypotheses and isolate meaningful variables followed by systematic manipulation of these variables in a more controlled context. This strategy is nicely illustrated in a pair of recent studies of the impact of infant cues on parental behavior. A number of earlier studies have revealed some of the cues that apparently affect parental responsiveness in naturalistic settings (Gewirtz and Gewirtz, 1969; Moss, 1967); on the basis of this work, one could make sensible choices concerning the particular infant cues to manipulate systematically.

Moss (1974) experimentally explored the impact of infant crying and fussing on parental responsiveness. At 3½ months of age, infants were studied in a laboratory while their mothers were interviewed in a separate room. The mothers were able to monitor the behavior of their infants through a panel of lights which, the parents were told, would be turned on if their babies fussed or cried. Each mother was given the option to check her infant any time during the procedure. The light signal was turned on according to a prearranged schedule, thus providing an opportunity to determine the mother's responsiveness to her infant's protesting in the absence of any noxious auditory input. Moreover, the use of this experimental arrangement permitted the investigators to determine whether their naturalistically observed maternal reactions to protest were due to "a sympathetic desire to soothe and comfort the infant or more from a desire to terminate an auditory stimulus that she finds aversive and intolerable" (Moss, 1974, p. 187). In addition to noting that protest behavior does induce maternal action, Moss related maternal responsivity to the light signals and the mother's latency in responding to crying in the home situation. His results indicated positive and significant correlation between the lab and home measures, at least for male infants. The importance of this study stems from two sources: one, the authors used experimental analysis to establish the causal link between infant cue and maternal behavior. Second and most importantly, the authors related the lab measure back to the naturalistic context in which it was originally observed.

In another recent study, Gewirtz and Boyd (1975) arranged an experimental situation in which mother and infant interacted, but which permitted control over the infant's behavior. The infant and mother were on opposite sides of an observation window so the mother could not see that she was not actually responding to her own infant but rather a simulation of an infant turning his head and vocalizing. These investigators showed that these infant behaviors were capable of modifying smiling and vocalizing in the mother.

Another approach which has not been investigated is to train parents to read baby cues and signals. It is becoming increasingly recognized that parents differ in their ability to recognize and respond to infant cues. Isolating techniques for modifying parental responsiveness to infant signals may not only be an important intervention strategy, but may yield insight into the ways that parental responsivity to infant signals develops.

In any case it is clear that no single strategy, method, or level of analysis will suffice. Eventually it may be possible to go beyond the descriptive statement that infants do affect their caregivers, to specify when, how, and with what consequence for both the infant and the caregiver.

SIGNIFICANCE OF PARENT-INFANT INTERACTION RESEARCH FOR THE STUDY OF MENTAL RETARDATION

The implications of the research in this area for the field of mental retardation can be best appreciated by a brief review of the long term outcomes of premature and other types of high risk infants. Recently, Sameroff and Chandler (1975) reviewed studies of the long term impact of various perinatal risk factors such as prematurity, anoxia, and other newborn status indicators on later cognitive and social functioning. In general, their review found little support for a traditional model of development which assumes that the contributions of constitutional and environmental factors are independent of each other. The assumption was not supported that "a defect in the constitution of an individual will produce a defective adult irrespective of environmental circumstance and a pathogenic environment will produce a defective adult independent of his constitution" (Sameroff and Chandler, 1975, p. 232). Knowledge of either set of factors alone yielded poor prediction. Knowing only that an infant was premature or anoxic was a poor predictor of later status. Similarly, knowing only that the environment was insufficient was an equally poor predictor. Rather, the review suggested that the long term prognosis of infants at risk for later cognitive and social retardation could only be understood in the context of an understanding of the environment. High risk infants raised in stimulating and supportive environments, in fact, were not different from low risk infants. Unfortunately the task of specifying the nature of the environment has only begun. However, it is likely that one of the keys to understanding the long term prognosis of children at risk is through an intensive study of the manner in which parent-infant dyads adapt to one another over the course of development. Through a better understanding of the dynamics of the interactional process, a better understanding of the ways in which the environment supports or dilutes the child's cognitive and social capacities may be revealed.

However, it should be stressed that there is no substitute for the direct assessment and investigation of the target population. It is attractive to generalize from studies of normal parent-infant interaction to various types of retarded infants. In spite of our current paucity of knowledge, the few recent studies of the interaction patterns between retarded infants and their parents (e.g., Greenberg, 1971; Kogan and Wimberger, 1966) clearly indicate that each target group merits detailed investigations, and no easy generalizations from normal parent-infant investigations are possible.

As Fraiberg's (1971) work has clearly demonstrated, this step of direct and tetailed observational assessment is a critically important prelude to the development of adequate intervention programs aimed at promoting more satisfactory motor, social, and cognitive development in developmentally delayed infants.

Finally, the study of developmentally delayed infants is a useful but underutilized approach to the evaluation of the theoretical importance of certain capacities and abilities for social and cognitive development. Fraiberg's (1971) work on the development of blind infants is representative; by investigating infants without sight, Fraiberg has furthered our understanding of the role that distance receptor stimulation plays in regulating parent-infant interaction. Similarly, Freedman's (1964) studies of the smiling of deaf-blind infants yielded data on these capacities for eliciting and maintaining this type of affect. Or consider Decarie's (1969) work on thalidomide infants; her investigations contributed to our understanding of the role of sensory-motor capacities in the development of cognition in infancy.

Through parallel studies aimed at understanding both the general processes that govern parent-infant interaction and the specific regulatory cues that modulate the interaction patterns of particular kinds of retarded, disabled, and handicapped infants, we will move closer to our goal of understanding and, it is hoped, modifying these interaction patterns to facilitate the cognitive and social development of these infants.

REFERENCES

Altmann, J. 1974. Observational study of behavior sampling methods. Behaviour. 49:227-265.

Bakeman, R. 1977. Untangling streams of behavior: sequential analyses of observation data. In: G. P. Sackett (ed.), Observing Behavior. Vol. 2. Data Collection and Analysis Methods. University Park Press, Baltimore.

Baldwin, A. 1967. Theories of Child Development. John Wiley & Sons Inc., New York.

Bell, R. Q. 1968. A reinterpretation of the direction of effects in studies of socialization. Psychol. Rev. 75:81–95.

Bell, R. Q. 1974. Contributions of human infants to caregiving and social interaction. In: M. Lewis and L. A. Rosenblum (eds.), The Effect of the Infant on Its Caregiver. John Wiley & Sons Inc., New York.

Borussard, E. R., and Hartner, M. S. S. 1971. Further consideration regarding maternal perception of the first born. In: J. Hellmuth (ed.), Exceptional Infant: Studies in Abnormalities. Vol. 2. Bruner/Mazel, New York.

Bowlby, J. 1951. Maternal Care and Mental Health. World Health Organization.

Bowlby, J. 1969. Attachment and Loss. Vol. 1. Hogarth Press Ltd., London.

Brackbill, Y. 1958. Extinction of the smiling response in infants as a function of reinforcement schedule. Child Dev. 29:115–124.

Brazelton, T. B. 1974. Neonatal Behavioral Assessment Scale. Spastics International Medical Publications, Heinemann Ltd., London.

Brazelton, T. B., Koslowski, B., and Main, B. 1974. The origins of reciprocity: the early mother-infant interaction. In: M. Lewis and L. A. Rosenblum (eds.), The Effects of the Infant on Its Caregiver. John Wiley & Sons Inc., New York.

Brazelton, T. B., Tronick, E., Adamson, L., Als, H., and Wise, S. 1975. Early mother-infant reciprocity. In: M. A. Hofer (ed.), Parent-Infant Interaction. Elsevier, Amsterdam.

Bronfenbrenner, U. 1975. Is early intervention effective? In: B. Freidlander, G. M. Sterrit, and G. E. Kirk (eds.), Exceptional Infant: Assessment and Intervention. Bruner/Mazel, New York.

Campbell, D. T., and Stanley, J. C. 1966. Experimental and Quasi-experimental Designs for Research. Rand McNally & Company, Chicago.

Carey, W. B. 1970. A simplified method for measuring infant temperament. J. Pediatr. 77:188–194.

Chess, S. 1971. Genesis of behavior disorder. In: J. G. Howells (ed.), Modern Perspectives in International Child Psychiatry. Bruner/Mazel, New York.

Condry, J., and Condry, S. 1976. The development of sex differences: a study of the eye of the beholder. Child Dev.

Cornell, E. H., and Gottfried, A. W. 1976. Intervention with premature infants. Child Dev. 47:32–39.

Corter, C., Trehub, S., Boukydis, C., Ford, L., Celhoffer, L., and Minde, K. 1976. Nurses' judgments of the attractiveness of premature infants. Unpublished manuscript, University of Toronto and Hospital for Sick Children.

Decarie, T. G. 1969. A study of the mental and emotional development of the thalidomide child. In: B. Foss (ed.), Determinants of Infant Behavior, pp. 167–187. Vol. 4. Methuen & Co. Ltd., London.

Fantz, R. 1961. The origin of form perception. Sci. Am. 204:66–72.

Fraiberg, S. 1971. Intervention in infancy: A program for blind infants. J. Am. Acad. Child Psychiatry 10:381–405.

Freedman, D. G. 1964. Smiling in blind infants and the issue of innate vs. acquired. J. Child Psychol. Psychiatry 5:171–184.

Freedman, D. G. 1974. Human Infancy: An Evolutionary Perspective. Lawrence Erlbaum Associates, Publisher, Hillsdale, New Jersey.

Gewirtz, J. L., and Gewirtz, H. B. 1969. Stimulus conditions, infant behaviors and social learning in four Israeli child-rearing environments. In: B. M. Foss (ed.), Determinants of Infant Behavior. Methuen & Co. Ltd., London.

Gewirtz, J. L., and Boyd, E. F. 1975. The infant conditions his mother: experiments on directions of influence in mother-infant interaction. Paper presented at meetings of the Society for Research in Child Development, Denver.

Glass, G. V., Willson, V. L., and Gottman, J. M. 1975. Design and Analysis of Time-series Experiments. Colorado Assoc. University Press, Boulder.

Goldberg, S. 1972. Infant care and growth in urban Zambia. Human Dev. 15:77–89.

Gottman, J. M. 1973. N-of-one and N-of-two research in psychotherapy. Psychol. Bull. 80:93–105.

Gottman, J. M., McFall, R. M., and Barnett, J. T. 1969. Design and analysis of research using time-series. Psychol. Bull. 72:299-306.

Greenberg, H. 1971. A comparison of infant-mother interactional behavior in infants with atypical behavior and normal infants. In: J. Hellmuth (ed.), The Exceptional Infant, Vol. 2. Bruner/Mazel, New York.

Harlow, H. F., and Suomi, S. J. 1970. The nature of love—simplified. Am. Psychol. 25:161–168.

Hobbs, N. 1975. The Futures of Children. Jossey-Bass, Inc., San Francisco.

Hofer, M. A. (ed.). 1975. Parent-infant Interaction. Elsevier, Amsterdam.

Ittelson, W. H., Proshansky, H. M., Rivlin, L. G., and Winkel, G. H. 1974. An Introduction to Environmental Psychology. Holt, Rinehart & Winston, New York.

Josselyn, I. M. 1956. Cultural forces, motherliness and fatherliness. Am. J. Orthopsychiatry 26:264–271.

Kagan, J., and Klein, R. E. 1973. Cross-cultural perspectives on early development. Am. Psychol. 28.

Kelley, H. H. 1972. Causal Schemata and the Attribution Process. General Learning Press, Morristown, New Jersey.

Kennell, J. H., Trause, M. A., and Klaus, M. H. 1975. Evidence for a sensitive period in the human mother. In: M. A. Hofer (ed.), Parent-infant Interaction. Elsevier, Amsterdam.

Kessen, W. 1963. Research in the psychological development of the infant. Merrill-Palmer Q. 9:83–94.

Kilbride, H., Johnson, D., and Streissguth, A. P. 1971. Early Home Experiences of Newborns as a Function of Social Class, Infant Sex and Birth Order. Unpublished manuscript, University of Washington, Seattle.

Klaus, M. H., and Kennell, J. H. 1970. Mothers separated from their newborn infants. Pediatr. Clin. North Am. 17:1015–1037.

Kogan, K. L., and Wimberger, H. C. 1966. An approach to defining mother-child interaction styles. Percept. Mot. Skills 23:1171–1177.

Korner, A. F. 1969. Neonatal startles, smiles, erections, and reflex sucks as related to state, sex and individuality. Child Dev. 40:1039–1053.

Korner, A. F. 1970. Visual alertness in neonates: individual differences and their correlates. Percept. Mot. Skills 31:67–78.

Korner, A. F. 1974. The effect of the infant's state, level of arousal, sex and ontogenetic stage on the caregiver. In: M. Lewis and L. A. Rosenblum (eds.), The Effect of the Infant on Its Caregiver. John Wiley & Sons Inc., New York.

Leiderman, P. H., and Seashore, M. J. 1975. Mother-infant separation: some delayed consequences. In: M. A. Hofer (ed.), Parent-infant Interaction. Elsevier, Amsterdam.

Lewis, M., and Lee-Painter, S. 1974. An interactional approach to the mother-infant dyad. In: M. Lewis and L. A. Rosenblum (eds.), The Effect of the INfant on Its Caregiver. John Wiley & Sons Inc., New York.

Lewis, M., and Rosenblum, L. A. 1974. The Effect of the Infant on Its Caregiver. John Wiley & Sons Inc., New York.

Leifer, A. D., Leiderman, P. H., Barnett, C. R., and Williams, J. A. 1972. Effects of mother-infant separation on maternal attachment behavior. Child Dev. 43:1203–1218.

Light, R. 1973. Abused and neglected children in America: a study of alternative policies. Harvard Educ. Rev. 43:556–598.

Lind, R. 1974. Observations after delivery of communication between mother-infant-father. Paper presented at the International Congress of Pediatrics, Buenos Aires.

Lipsitt, L. 1963. Learning in the first year of life. In: L. P. Lipsitt and C. Spiker (eds.), Advances in Child Development and Behavior, pp. 147–196. Vol. 1. Academic Press, New York.

Lynn, D. B. 1974. The Father: His Role in Child Development. Brooks Cole, Monterey.

Maccoby, E. E., and Jacklin, C. N. 1974. The Psychology of Sex Differences. Stanford University Press, Stanford.

Mercer, J. 1973. Labeling the Mentally Retarded: Clinical and Social System Perspectives on Mental Retardation. University of California Press, Berkeley.

Mischel, W. 1968. Personality and Assessment. John Wiley & Sons Inc., New York.

Mischel, W. 1973. Toward a cognitive social learning reconceptualization of personality. Psychol. Rev. 80:252–283.

Mitchell, G. D., Redican, W. K., and Gomber, J. 1974. Males can raise babies. Psychol. Today 7:63–67.

Moss, H. A. 1967. Sex, age and state as determinants of mother-infant interaction. Merrill-Palmer Q. 13:19–36.

Moss, H. A. 1974. Communication in mother-infant interaction. In: L. Kramer, P. Pliner, and T. Alloway (eds.), Advances in the Study of Communication and Affect, Vol. 1. Nonverbal Communication. Plenum Press Inc., New York.

Parke, R. D., and Collmer, D. A. 1975. Child abuse: an interdisciplinary analysis. In: E. M. Hetherington (eds.), Review of Child Development Research, Vol. 5. University of Chicago Press, Chicago.

Parke, R. D., and O'Leary, S. E. 1976. Father-mother infant interaction in the newborn period: some findings, some observations and some unresolved issues. In: K. Riegel and J. Meacham (eds.), The Developing Individual in a Changing World. Mouton & Co., The Hague.

Parke, R. D., O'Leary, S. E., and West, S. 1972. Mother-father-newborn interaction: effects of maternal medication, labor and sex of infant. Proc. Am. Psychol. Assoc. 85–86.

Parke, R. D., and Sawin, D. B. 1975. Infant characteristics and behavior as elicitors of maternal and paternal responsivity. Paper presented at the Biennial Meeting of the Society for Research in Child Development, Denver.

Parke, R. D., and Sawin, D. B. 1976. The father's role in infancy: a re-evaluation. The Family Co-ordinator.

Pedersen, F. A. 1975. Mother, father and infant as an interaction system. Paper presented at the Annual Convention of the American Psychological Association, Chicago.

Pedersen, F. A., Anderson, B. J., and Cain, R. L. 1976. A methodology for assessing parental perceptions of infant temperament. Paper presented at the 4th Biennial Southeastern Conference on Human Development.

Quilitch, H. R., and Risley, T. R. 1973. The effects of play materials on social play. J. Appl. Behav. Anal. 6:573–578.

Rebelsky, F. 1967. Infancy in two cultures. Ned. Tijdschr. Psychol. 22:379–385.

Rheingold, H. L., Gewirtz, J. L., and Ross, H. W. 1959. Social conditioning of vocalizations in infants. J. Comp. Physiol. Psychol. 52:68–73.

Rheingold, H. L., and Keene, G. C. 1965. Transport of the human young. In: B. Foss (ed.), Determinants of Infant Behavior, pp. 87–106. Vol. 2. Methuen & Co., London.

Rubin, J. Z., Provenzano, F. J., and Luria, Z. 1974. The eye of the beholder: parents' view on sex of newborns. Am. J. Orthopsychiatry 43:518–519, 720–731.

Sackett, G. P. 1974. A Nonparametric Lag Sequential Analysis for Studying Dependency Among Responses in Observational Scoring Systems. Unpublished manuscript, University of Washington, Seattle.

Sameroff, A. J., and Chandler, M. J. 1975. Reproductive risk and the continuum of caretaking casualty. In: F. D. Horowitz (ed.), Review of Child Development Research, pp. 187–244. Vol. 4. University of Chicago Press, Chicago.

Scarr, S., and Salapatek, P. 1970. Patterns of fear development during infancy. Merrill-Palmer Q. 16:53–90.

Schaffer, H. R. 1971. The Origins of Sociability. Penguin Books Ltd., London.

Spock, B. 1968. Baby and Child Care. Simon & Schuster Inc., New York.

Sroufe, A., Waters, E., and Matas, L. 1974. Contextual determinants of infant affective response. In: M. Lewis and L. A. Rosenblum (eds.), The Origins of Fear. John Wiley & Sons, New York.

Thoman, E. B., Liederman, P. H., and Olson, J. P. 1972. Neonate-mother interaction during breast-feeding. Dev. Psychol. 6:110–118.

Thomas, A., Chess, S., Birch, H. G., Hertzig, M. E., and Korn, S. 1963. Behavioral Individuality in Early Childhood. New York University Press, New York.

Thomas, E. C. A., and Martin, J. A. 1976. Analyses of parent-infant interaction. Psychol. Rev. 83:141–156.

Walters, R. H., and Parke, R. D. 1965. The role of the distance receptors in the development of social responsiveness. In: L. P. Lipsitt and C. C. Spiker (eds.), Advances in Child Development and Behavior, pp. 59–96. Vol. 2. Academic Press, New York.

Watson, J. B. 1928. Psychological Care of the Infant and Child. W. W. Norton & Company Inc., New York.

Weiner, B., and Kun, A. 1976. The development of causal attributions and the growth of achievement and social motivation. In: S. Feldman and D. Bush (eds.), Cognitive Development and Social Development. Lawrence Erlbaum Associates, Publishers, Hillsdale, New Jersey.

Weisberg, P. 1963. Social and nonsocial conditioning of infant vocalization. Child Dev. 34:377–388.

Yarrow, L. J., Rubinstein, J. L., and Pedersen, F. A. 1975. Infant and Environment: Early Cognitive and Motivational Development. Hemisphere, Washington.

chapter 4

Individual Patterns of Mother-Infant Interaction

Evelyn B. Thoman, Patricia T. Becker, and Margaret P. Freese

In recent years there has been a growing number of studies described by investigators as "naturalistic." This trend has aroused concern among some developmental psychologists who assert that ultimate answers are to be found only through rigorously controlled experimental studies in the laboratory. There is a tendency to view studies as either experimental *or* naturalistic, and to emphasize differences in the procedures, assumptions, and interpretations for these two types of research. However, the distinctions between experimental and naturalistic models are not generally made clear either with respect to their procedures or to their guiding theoretical assumptions. Experimental studies involve conditions and behaviors that are more or less naturalistic, and many naturalistic studies include experimental manipulations. The issue of the relative merits of experimental and naturalistic studies may be dissipated if the application of these terms to procedures is distinguished clearly from their application to the models or assumptions that guide procedures.

In this paper are presented examples from the literature on infancy and mother-infant interaction to demonstrate that research procedures may vary along a continuum from more to less naturalistic with respect to the behaviors observed and the conditions under which they are observed. At one extreme of the continuum are the rigorously controlled laboratory conditions and highly artificial types of interventions used for controlling the occurrence of response; at the other extreme are procedures involving observations in the home—the natural habitat—without any interventions whatsoever. This chapter indicates how the experimental model with its causal assumptions can provide the context for studies at any point along the continuum of naturalness in procedures. Also presented is a perspective of procedures at the extreme naturalistic end of the continuum, indicating that these can be guided by very diverse models of behavioral development. A systems approach is presented as the framework for our own research. Finally, observations of three developmentally delayed infants are used to illustrate data analyses and interpretations within a systems approach.

THE CONTINUUM OF NATURALNESS IN STUDIES OF EARLY DEVELOPMENT

First, let us amplify a point just made: experimental studies involve behaviors that are more or less natural, and naturalistic studies may include environmental manipulations.

The research described in this chapter was supported by The Grant Foundation, Inc., NICHD Grant HD 08195-01A2, and NIMH Predoctoral Fellowship 5268-81-13645.

We are dealing with a continuum of methodologies rather than with two distinctly different methodologies, one experimental-manipulative, and the other naturalistic-observational. For any given study, the methodology of choice will depend upon what kinds of questions the investigator wants to ask.

In examining the procedures typically employed in research on infant development, considerable variation along the least to most naturalistic continuum is found. The sensory, perceptual, motor, and learning capabilities of infants have typically been explored using a rigorous experimental method to determine what the infant can do under a specified set of circumstances in the laboratory. The infant's natural repertoire of behaviors has been exploited effectively in these studies. Observations of behaviors such as sucking, visual attention, head turning, movement, generalized activity, and changes in state have been used as indicators of what the infant has perceived or learned. Obviously, the infant's capabilities so determined have implications for his/her functioning in the environment. However, the nature of those implications is not certain.

The infant's interactions with the environment, especially with the mother, have also been explored using rigorous experimental designs. For example, Korner and Thoman (1970, 1972) studied changes in state of the newborn as a function of vestibular and contact stimulation given in the context of maternal-type interventions. Eckerman and Rheingold (1974) studied the responses of 10-month-old infants to an unfamiliar adult as a function of whether or not the adult smiled at the baby. The naturally occurring vocalizations of the infants, attention to the unfamiliar adult, and the infant's spontaneous exploration of available toys were the dependent variables observed. In a slightly more naturalistic approach, a number of investigators have manipulated conditions in order to affect the nature of the mother-infant interaction, for example, by instructing the mother to behave in an unusual or unexpected manner (Brazelton, Tronick, Adamson, Als, and Wise, 1975; Papousek and Papousek, 1975). The subsequent behaviors of the infant and mother were recorded in as much detail as possible. For this type of study, one can examine sequences of elicited behaviors as a function of the experimental manipulations performed.

Progressing along the continuum from least to most naturalistic procedures, some studies have involved experimental manipulations that are as minimal as placing the infant at a predetermined distance from the mother in a home-like laboratory situation (Lewis and Goldberg, 1969). In still others (Brody, 1956), mothers and infants have been observed in the laboratory in a home-like setting with no interventions whatsoever.

Finally, the most natural of naturalistic observations are considered to be those made in the home without any interventions. These studies vary widely with respect to their objectives, the mode of observation and recording, data analyses, and inferences. They have in common the fact that observations are actually made in the natural habitat, and they typically include familiar aspects of the infant's environment: the mother, the father, other caregivers, or inanimate features such as toys (Moss and Robson, 1968; Gewirtz and Gewirtz, 1969; Escalona and Corman, 1971; Richards and Bernal, 1971; Ainsworth, Bell, and Stayton, 1972; Tulkin and Kagan, 1972; Clarke-Stewart, 1973; Lewis and Lee-Painter, 1974; Cohen and Beckwith, 1975; Yarrow, Rubenstein, and Pedersen, 1975).

Does the absence of intervention in studies described as naturalistic imply a major difference in approach? We believe the answer depends upon whether the procedures or the assumptions that underlie the research designs are focused upon. Procedures clearly vary along a continuum of naturalness. Another factor, the assumptions underlying the procedures, contributes to the answer to this question. In particular, the assumption of causality figures heavily in any conclusions that might be drawn with regard to this issue. We will therefore examine the causal approach and its implications in more detail.

THE CAUSAL APPROACH TO MOTHER-INFANT INTERACTION

A basic assumption within the experimental model is the possibility of identifying specific events or factors that have a direct and identifiable impact on the course of development. This assumption does not preclude the use of naturalistic conditions and naturally occurring behaviors. The question is under what circumstances is it reasonable to assume causality in the same sense that it is assumed within the experimental model.

Even in naturalistic studies carried out without any intervention whatsoever, investigators may assume that it should be possible to identify factors in either the mother or the infant that produce changes in the other member of the dyad. Rosenthal (1973) clearly reflects this assumption when she concludes, from a review of the literature on infant-environment interaction, that studies made in the natural habitat are generally used in lieu of an experimental design when the investigators wish to obtain information on variables which they feel are not open to experiment because of practical or ethical considerations. She describes various research designs and statistical analyses that have been employed to permit inferences with respect to the direction of mutual effects. In some instances, investigators have made the analysis of direction of effects an explicit objective (e.g., Lewis and Lee-Painter, 1974; Clarke-Stewart, 1973). In other cases, however, adherence to the causal assumption and its use as a focus for research questions is only implied in conjunction with statements of the limitations of correlational data.

There are two major issues with regard to experimental designs that adhere to the causal assumption. One is the question of generalizability. Causality can most clearly be demonstrated in a carefully controlled laboratory situation. It is inferred that events observed in the laboratory have relevance for those that occur in the infant's everyday environment. However, the validity of this assumption has not been tested.

The second major issue involving causality pertains to the question of whether any set of causal relations could ever account for the dynamic qualities of the developing mother-infant relationship. Schroedinger expressed doubts about the validity of the principle of causality in 1935: "The relation of cause and effect, as Hume pointed out long ago, is not something that we find in nature, but is rather characteristic of the way in which we regard nature. We are quite free to maintain this principle of causality or to alter it according to our convenience, in the sense of taking it in whatever way makes for a simpler description of natural phenomena" (p. 116).

This statement suggests that we can adopt either causal or noncausal assumptions, whichever seem most appropriate for our research objectives. Schroedinger additionally stated, ". . . it must be pointed out here that not only are we free to drop a long accepted principle when we think we've found something more convenient from the viewpoint of physical research, but that we are free to readopt the rejected principle when we find we've made a mistake in laying it aside. . . . A developing empirical science need not and must not be afraid of being taunted with the lack of consistency between its announcements at subsequent epochs'' (Schroedinger, 1935, p. 116).

In summary, the causal assumption can be applied anywhere along the continuum of naturalness in procedures. At the naturalistic end of the continuum, either causal or noncausal assumptions may be the guide for research. These assumptions are truly dichotomous, because they result in two distinctly different conceptualizations of the developing infant and the mother-infant relationship.

NONCAUSAL APPROACHES TO MOTHER-INFANT INTERACTION

A number of investigators have proposed models of mother-infant interaction in which this relationship is viewed as a system. Recognition that mothers and infants influence each other's behavior and that the ongoing process of mutual change is probably the essence of the relationship makes it essential that the dynamic characteristics of the interaction be considered. When mother and infant are viewed as a system, there are too many interacting factors to take seriously the causal impact of any single form of behavior.

General systems theory (Bertalanffy, 1968; Weiss, 1971) provides a perspective that incorporates the interdependence of the mother and infant as systems subunits. The relationship can be viewed within the framework of the following summary definition of a system: a system is a whole or a unit composed of hierarchically organized and functionally highly interdependent subunits that may themselves be systems. As with any organization, the overall organization has characteristics that are not apparent in the behavior of either of the components.

Several investigators have promoted systems conceptualizations of the mother-infant relationship. Sander's commitment to this point of view is long-standing. He has stated, ''The interplay of active tendencies in infant and mother in reaching a reciprocal quality of relationship forms the unifying thread around which interactional accounts will be organized. The reciprocal quality in interaction is an achievement which is marked by harmony. It represents a fit or fitting together of active tendencies in each partner'' (Sander, 1964, p. 233). Sander and his associates have experimentally manipulated the pairing of infants with different caregivers (Sander, Stechler, Burns, and Julia, 1970; Burns, Sander, Stechler, and Julia, 1972). This design is an example of experimental manipulations within a noncausal framework. Sander has clearly not interpreted his findings in terms of the effects of the caregiver on the infant or of the infant on the caregiver. He has focused on the total relationship and the nature of the mutual adaptation in the process of interaction.

Stern (1971, 1974) has depicted the mutuality of the mother-infant system in a somewhat different way, by providing a very fine grained analysis of instant-by-instant events in play interactions. Play provides a particularly clear illustration of the necessity for an interactive model because, as Stern (1974) has noted, ''During the play activity both members are almost constantly making readjustments in their behavior so as to achieve the goal of the activity'' (p. 210). In the analysis of his data, Stern has used transitional matrices to show patterns of probabilities ''. . . of any dyadic state proceeding to any other dyadic state, including itself'' (p. 191). Lewis and Lee-Painter (1974) have also explored a systems approach; they emphasize the limitations of our current models, which cannot yet adequately depict the nonstatic flow of interaction apart from its elements.

Our own model for viewing the mother-infant system emphasizes the ongoing reciprocity in the relationship. If one adheres to an interactional framework, it becomes difficult to conceive of either partner as ''causing'' the behavior of the other. The baby may cry and cause the mother to pick it up; or by picking the baby up, the mother may cause it to stop crying and become alert. However, the identification of these apparent causal relations becomes trivial within the context of an ongoing series of sequences, and it is doubtful that any isolated form of maternal behavior will by itself have a specifiable effect on the infant's overall development. The effect of the mother's behavior will instead be a function of the individual characteristics of the infant and the interaction patterns of the mother-infant pair. It is necessary, of course, to identify the components of a series of sequences, such as the mother picking up the infant when it cries, but it is simplistic to look at isolated two-step mother and infant behaviors as interaction. The consequences of the characteristics of the relationship must be analyzed in some way if the process by which the infant and the mother-infant relationship develops is to be understood.

The noncausal research approaches described have several important similarities. They all involve conceptualizations of mother and infant as a dyadic system. Each depends upon the collection of naturalistic observational data. Additionally, none of them has emphasized the identification of early predictors which are causally related to behavioral measures at some later point in time.

The research approaches described also share some major obstacles. Systems conceptualizations require examination of the developmental process. However, there is not currently available either a language for labeling interactive processes or statistics that are appropriate for translating elemental data into systems data that change over time. Although some investigators have made use of Markov sequence analyses in looking at interactive process, as Lewis and Lee-Painter (1974) have pointed out, the determination of a point of entry into an ongoing system is always a problem.

In order to depict important processes in ongoing mother-infant systems, it is necessary to observe and record behaviors sequentially, but it is also necessary to study the changes in behaviors over time. Only with successive or longitudinal observations can the development of patterns in an ongoing relationship be identified. As Wohlwill (1973) has argued, inherent in developmental research are questions of rates and patterns which do not lend themselves to analyses based on essentially linear models of change as an index of the effects of independent variables. This is especially true when development is seen as occurring within a system. These arguments lead directly to an emphasis on the naturalistic and longitudinal study of individual mother-infant pairs.

INTRODUCTION TO A NATURALISTIC STUDY OF MOTHERS AND INFANTS

One major premise for our research is that individual patterns of infant and mother behaviors can be identified. A second premise is that these patterns either persist over time or serve as the basis for later patterns of behavior in the infant or the mother-infant relationship. We have studied mother-infant pairs intensively during the first weeks of life, with follow-up observations and assessments at later ages. Our objectives are to describe individual mother-infant pairs and to identify consistencies or continuities in their behaviors over time. The data for the total group of subjects provide the starting point from which information on individual pairs is derived. Where patterns of change in more than one dyad are similar, we can combine that portion of their data and thus begin to have the basis for making generalizations about the interactive process.

A critical step enabling one to draw conclusions regarding consistencies and continuities is to identify variables that reliably discriminate individual mother-infant pairs. Many researchers, although placing a great deal of emphasis on interobserver reliability in carrying out naturalistic studies, often assume, rather than assess, the reliability of the measures they use. In this study, data from the weekly observations during the first month of life for the total group of subjects permit analyses for repeated measures to identify those variables that do reliably discriminate among dyads.

Given measurement reliability, the data from the total group of babies provide a mean or baseline with which individual subjects or groups of subjects can be compared. In addition, the relative level of any mother-infant pair on a group of measures provides a reliable picture or profile pattern for that dyad. Thus, the group means, as normative data, are not the primary focus in this study. The data for the individual are depicted within the context of that for the group. This is a very different approach to arriving at generalizations than the use of group means, which cannot take into account individual patterns. Individual patterns, or descriptions of individual processes, are the essence of the systems approach. The results reported here are intended to demonstrate the use of individuals and commonalities among them to go beyond the case study approach and to explore the possibilities of generalities within a systems conceptualization.

Although the specific patterns of behaviors of each mother-infant pair may be unique, the process of interaction and of the infant's development is, in essence, expressed only in the individual infant or mother-infant pair. The developmental process is not a group phenomenon. The study of the unique ways in which different mother-infant pairs express the interactive process will ultimately provide the basis for an understanding of this process. Thus, the study of individual mother-infant pairs must precede generalizations, rather than generalizations being derived from studies of the normative behavior of groups, which may or may not indicate what is typical for any individual.

This is a report from a naturalistic study of 20 mother-infant pairs who were observed intensively during the infants' first 5 weeks of life. From follow-up assessment of these infants, three individuals were identified who showed marked developmental delays. The purposes of the present report are first, to define procedures by which the earliest mother-infant interactions can be reliably described; second, to identify some relationships between early mother-infant interactions and the later development of the three selected infants; and finally, to illustrate one approach to exploring patterns of interaction within an individual mother-infant pair.

METHODS

Subjects

The subjects for this study were 20 healthy, full term infants and their mothers. The mothers, all primipara, were enrolled in the project during their last trimester of pregnancy. Thirteen of the mothers delivered males and seven delivered females.

General Procedures

Prenatal assessments of the mothers and observations of the mothers and infants in the hospital during the early postpartum period were made (Freese, 1975). These procedures are not described in detail in the present report, which focuses on observations made in the homes when the infants were 2, 3, 4, and 5 weeks old. However, it should be mentioned that each mother fed and interacted with her infant in the presence of an observer on at least two occasions during her postpartum hospital stay and thus was familiar with the intensive observation procedures and the presence of a noninteracting observer prior to the first home observation.

The first home observation was made when each infant was 8 to 14 days old, with subsequent home observations made at approximately weekly intervals. Each observation consisted of a continuous 7-hr period. Two observers participated in the observation, each recording for 3½ hr. The changing of observers in the middle of the observations was accomplished without interruption of either the observational procedures or ongoing household activities.

During the observational period, the observer avoided interaction with anyone in the household. She selected locations that gave her a clear view of the infant's face but were as unobtrusive as possible in the household setting. Whenever the infant was moved, the observer followed. During long sleep periods when the infant was in the crib, the observer remained with the infant and recorded sleep patterns in great detail.

Recording Procedures

The occurrence of any of 75 mother or infant behaviors was code-recorded every 10 sec throughout the 7-hr observation. The behaviors recorded are listed in Table 1. A small electronic timing device provided observers with a signal through an ear microphone every 10 sec. At each signal the necessary codes were recorded, with no formal pause in the observational process. In this way, nearly continuous recording of the occurrence of each variable was possible.

Several factors made it possible to reliably record this large number of mother-infant behaviors. First, many of the coded behaviors occurred only in limited contexts. For example, suck stimulation, not sucking, and not attached only occurred when the infant was feeding or had been given a pacifier. Second, the detail with which certain variables were recorded varied within the observation. For instance, distinctions among the sleep states were made only when the infant was alone in the crib; when the mother was holding the infant these distinctions were not always possible, so only the fact that the infant's

Table 1. Mother and infant variables

Mother location[a]
- Out
- Far
- Near
- In contact
- Hold
- Carry

Infant location[a]
- Crib
- Cradle board
- Other

Infant position[a]
- Prone
- Supine
- Up
- Up at shoulder

Mother-infant activity[a]
- Feed
- Change
- Bathe
- Noncaregiving

Feeding subcategories[a]
- Breast or bottle
- Water
- Solids

Bathing subcategories[a]
- Head
- Immersion

Maternal behaviors
- Provide pacifier
- Suck stimulation
- Vis-à-vis
- en Face position
- Look
- Talk
- Talk to other
- Noise
- Smile or laugh
- Pat
- Caress
- Move
- Rock

Infant behaviors
- Not attached
- Not sucking
- Rhythmic mouthing
- Hand-mouth
- Spit up
- Suck
- Mouth
- Smile
- Frown
- Grimace
- Yawn
- Breath-hold
- Vocalize
- Noise
- Grunt
- Sigh
- Sigh-sob
- Cough
- Bowel movement
- Eyes open
- Rapid eye movement
- Stretch
- Large movement
- Small movement
- Startle
- Poor startle
- Jitter
- Jerk

Infant behavioral states[a]
- Quiet sleep (2 categories)
- Active sleep (3 categories)
- Uncertain
- Drowse
- Daze
- Alert inactivity
- Waking activity
- Fuss
- Cry

[a] These are mutually exclusive categories for code-recording purposes.

eyes were closed was recorded. Also, the variables include a number of sets of totally inclusive and mutually exclusive categories of behavior that were recorded only when a change of category occurred within the set. For example, an infant's position was coded as prone, up, up at shoulder, or supine. Once a position was recorded, it was not recoded until the position changed. Finally, economy in recording was aided by the use of standard inferences that eliminated the actual marking of some variables. For instance, if the mother carried the infant, this implied that the infant was being moved, and consequently the move category was not coded.

Reliabilities among the three observers were calculated for each variable using the following formula: 2 (number of agreements)/number of occurrences recorded by both observers. Agreement within the same epoch was required for mutually exclusive behavior categories, which are so indicated in Table 1. Agreement within adjacent 10-sec epochs was required for the remainder of the mother and infant behaviors. Reliability was assessed on an ongoing basis: both feedings given by all but one mother while in the hospital were observed by two observers. The interrater reliabilities among the three observers for the variables to be reported in the present study ranged from 0.75 to 0.99.

Follow-up Assessments

Follow-up procedures have been completed for all available infants from the observational study. These include home observations of sleep state behaviors, later mother-infant interactions, neurological assessments, and administrations of developmental scales. Only the developmental scales are relevant to the present report.

The Bayley Scales of Infant Development (Bayley, 1969) and the Uzgiris-Hunt Ordinal Scales of Psychological Development (Uzgiris and Hunt, 1975) were administered twice, at 7 months and again at 12 months. At about 2½ years, the McCarthy Scales of Children's Abilities (McCarthy, 1972) were administered. The 7-month and 12-month assessments were done in the infants' homes; the 2½-year assessment was done either in the home or at the laboratory, whichever the family preferred.

RESULTS

For the 20 infants, there was a total of 209,751 10-sec epochs recorded over the four weekly home observations, with presence-absence information on 75 behaviors during each epoch. From this quantity of data, innumerable questions could be asked and innumerable relationships, both reliable and unreliable, could be discovered. However, we have chosen to use analyses only to answer specific questions about individual or groups of mother-infant pairs. During the course of the observations for this project, a large number of hypotheses were generated concerning the nature of continuities in mother-infant relationships. In view of the theme of the present conference, questions about the interaction patterns of three developmentally delayed infants were explored for this report.

Variables Analyzed

From the list of recorded behaviors presented in Table 1, behaviors that could be grouped together under a general heading were combined. Definitions of the combined variables are as follows.

Total observation is the number of epochs in any home observation.

Looking occurs when the mother is engaged in any of the following maternal variables: look, en face, vis-à-vis.

Stimulation occurs when the mother is engaged in any of the following maternal stimulation variables: pat, caress, move, rock.

Awake occurs when the infant is in one of the following infant behavioral states: drowse, daze, alert inactivity, waking activity, fuss, cry.

Caregiving occurs when the mother-infant pair is engaged in one of the following mother-infant activities: feed, change, bathe.

Change or bathe occurs when the mother-infant pair is engaged in either of the following mother-infant activities: change, bathe.

Hold or carry occurs when the mother is in either of the following mother locations: hold, carry.

Fuss or cry occurs when the infant is in either of the following infant behavioral states: fuss, cry.

Social interaction occurs when all of the following conditions are met: 1) infant state is awake; 2) mother location is hold or carry; 3) mother-infant activity is noncaregiving.

Noncaregiving interaction occurs when both of the following conditions are met: 1) mother location is hold or carry; 2) mother-infant activity is noncaregiving.

State changes are changes in infant state category of at least three consecutive epochs. (Categories for this determination were: 1) quiet sleep; 2) active sleep; 3) awake, uncertain.)

This set of combined variables actually encompasses 22 of the individual mother and infant behaviors recorded. All of these behaviors are regarded as characteristics of the mother-infant system, even though for convenience some are recorded as mother behaviors and some as infant behaviors. The activities of each member of the dyad are a function of the behaviors of the other member. For this reason and because there is obviously overlap in the recorded behaviors included in the combinations of variables, the combined variables cannot be considered independent.

Individual Differences in Behaviors: Reliability of Variables

It was first necessary to establish the reliability of the selected variables in discriminating among the individuals before using them to describe individual infants. The four successive weekly observations permitted the assessment of reliability, or individual differences, among mother-infant pairs for each measure over the 4 weeks. Absolute frequencies of occurrence were not appropriate for analyses, as the total number of epochs for each home observation was never exactly equivalent to the 2520 that make up a 7-hr period ($\bar{X}$ = 2495; s.d. = 110). In most instances, the total number of occurrences of a variable was expressed as a percentage of the total number of epochs in the observation. In some cases,

Table 2. Mean percent of epochs for each variable over the four weeks, F values for individual differences, total test reliability (r_{tt}), and standard error of measurement

Variable	Mean %	F (df = 18, 54)	r_{tt}	SE
Social interaction/total	10.38	3.703[a]	0.730	2.39
Look and social interaction/total	7.95	3.914[a]	0.745	1.85
Stimulation and social interaction/total	8.41	3.136[a]	0.681	2.07
Caregiving/hold or carry	43.17	5.404[a]	0.815	5.74
Awake/total	34.51	2.009[b]	0.502	4.82
Fuss or cry/total	3.84	3.670[a]	0.728	0.95
Hold or carry/total	26.93	6.077[a]	0.835	3.95
Feed/total	10.93	6.269[a]	0.840	1.96
Social interaction/awake	29.46	4.977[a]	0.799	4.86
State change/hour of sleep[c]	5.88	2.585[a]	0.613	1.55
Open-eyed REM/REM	16.21	6.263[a]	0.840	3.52

[a] $p < 0.01$
[b] $p < 0.05$
[c] Based on the longest period of sleep within each observation.

however, we were interested in the number of epochs of a behavior that occurred as a percentage of another variable. For example, if the amount of time an infant spent crying was of interest, it was useful to know not only how much of the total observation time he spent crying, but also how much crying occurred as a percentage of the time he was held or was alone in the crib. The combination variables used for analyses and the portion of the observation used as the base for percentage values are presented in Table 2.

The mean percentage value for each of the 11 combination variables across the four home observations for the 20 mother-infant pairs is also presented in Table 2. The mean percentage values were used in an analysis of variance to assess change in mean percentages over weeks for the entire group, differences between pairs having male and female infants, and individual differences. Table 2 also presents the F values and significance levels of assessment of individual differences and the r_{tt} values indicating the reliability of assessment of each variable over the four weekly observations. There were no sex differences found on any of these comparisons, nor were there any significant changes over the time of the four home observations. Each of the measures gives a reliable estimate of the behavior of individual mother-infant pairs, and for all of the variables there were highly significant individual differences. Thus, the mean score across observations depicts for each mother-infant pair its relative position on each variable, and is a potential predictor of later behavior.

Comparisons of Three Individual Pairs Within the Total Group

Infants 3, 12, and 16 were selected for comparison with the total group because for each there were indications of developmental delay at a later age. At 7 months, their scores on the mental development index (MDI) of the Bayley Mental Scale were 86, 83, and 86, respectively. Only Infant 16 was available for a regularly scheduled assessment at 12

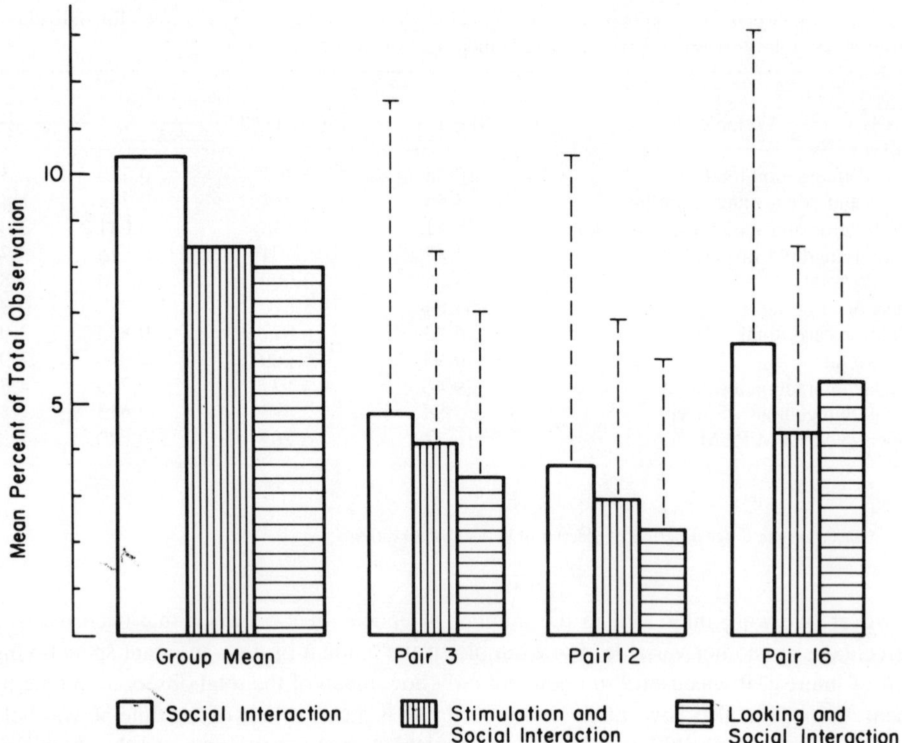

Figure 1. Mean percentage of time over weeks 2, 3, 4, and 5 spent in social interaction, stimulation with social interaction, and looking with social interaction: Group mean (20 infants) and mother-infant pairs 3, 12, and 16. Dashed lines show 95% confidence limit.

months: her MDI at that time was 74. Infant 12 was assessed using the Bayley Mental Scale at 21 months, and obtained an MDI of 64. Infant 3 was seen briefly and assessed informally at 24 months. At that time, his language development appeared delayed. In the report of a neurological examination at 2½ years, the language deficit was again noted, and the neurologist further stated that the child's behavior made him impossible to test. This is consistent with the child's performance on the McCarthy Scales of Children's Abilities, which were administered in the home at 34 months. The examiner reported that the child performed at the average level on four of the 17 scales. It was not possible to assess him on the remaining 13 scales because he refused to participate in the testing procedures. His current level of functioning is therefore uncertain.

The behavioral measures from the home observations were used to compare the three individual mother-infant pairs with the total group. Since the reliability of the measures was based on the four home observations and since there were no changes over weeks for the total group, mean percentage values across weeks were used to compare subject pairs. In all comparisons, the data for pairs 3, 12, and 16 were included in those of the total group since their selection and separation from the group was made post hoc.

The first question of interest was whether the three infants and mothers had interac-

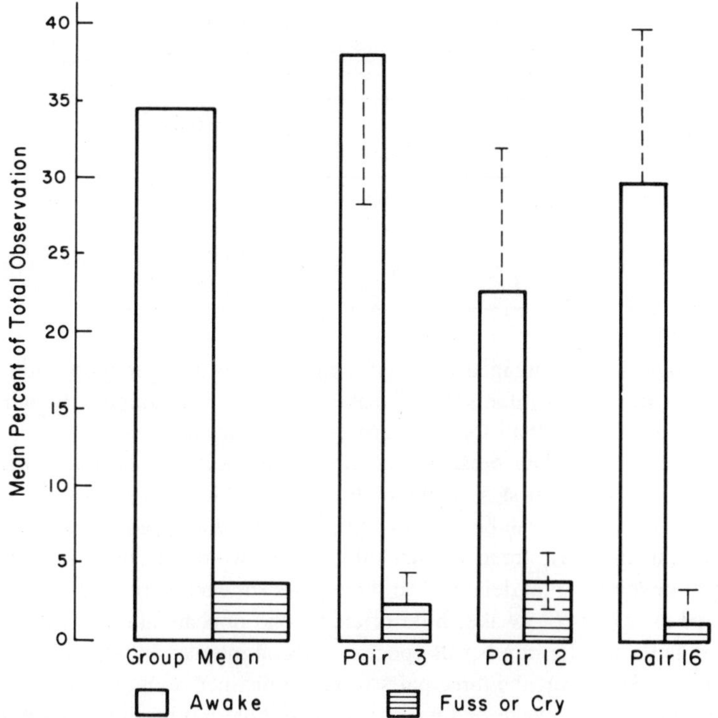

Figure 2. Mean percentage of time over weeks 2, 3, 4, and 5 spent in awake and fuss or cry: Group mean (20 infants) and mother-infant pairs 3, 12, and 16. Dashed lines show 95% confidence limit.

tion characteristics that differentiated them from the overall group. Three variables, social interaction, stimulation, and looking, were selected for examination with respect to this question. In Figure 1, the mean percent of social interaction in the total observation over the 4 weeks is presented for the group of 20 infants and for each of the three individual infants. In addition, the percentages of looking and stimulation in conjunction with social interaction are indicated. Finally, the upper limit of the 95% confidence interval for the measures for each of the individual infants is indicated. It can be seen that all three mother-infant pairs have markedly less social interaction than the mean of the total group. Concurrently, the percentage of epochs the mothers spent looking at and stimulating their infants during social interactions was also lower for these three mother-infant pairs.

A number of variables could be relevant for elaboration of the low levels of social interaction that were observed in these three dyads. A first consideration was the amount of wakefulness and crying exhibited by the three infants. Figure 2 presents the comparisons for the variables awake and fuss or cry. As it shows, the percentages of time that the three infants were awake and fussing or crying did not differ markedly from those of the group.

Another question was asked regarding the distribution of the time mothers held or carried their infants between caregiving and noncaregiving interactions. Table 3 presents the relevant data, indicating the percentage of caregiving in hold or carry. The three

Table 3. Mean percent of hold or carry devoted to caregiving by total group and mother-infant pairs 3, 12, and 16 in four home observations

Subject	Mean	Confidence interval
Group	43.2	
Pair 3	54.9	43.41–66.37
Pair 12	57.7	46.24–69.20
Pair 16	57.4	45.88–68.84

individual mothers were engaged in caregiving activities a larger proportion of the time they held and carried their infants than the average mother, although only pairs 12 and 16 were significantly higher than the total group in this measure.

To summarize the data presented so far, it has been demonstrated that the mean scores averaged over the first 5 weeks of life are reliable measures of the behaviors of mother-infant pairs which can be used to compare individual dyads with the larger group. For the present analyses, three mother-infant pairs were selected because the infants showed later developmental delays. The three pairs showed markedly less social interaction, defined as epochs of awake, hold or carry, and noncaretaking. These mothers and infants also had a smaller number of epochs of social interaction which included looking and stimulation. However, the three pairs were not distinctive in the total amount of time the infants' states were awake or fuss or cry. The three mother-infant pairs had a much higher proportion of caregiving during hold or carry than did the entire group, two of them beyond the 95% confidence range.

The Interactive Process in One Mother-Infant Pair

The data just described clearly indicate that the three mother-infant pairs differed from the total group in certain aspects of their interaction. However, no data have been presented on the patterning of these interactive behaviors. Examination of sequential data is necessary to depict the nature of the interactive process.

One mother-infant pair, pair 3, was selected for analyses of the interaction process. The data were examined to answer questions with respect to some unique characteristics of the infant's state cues and the intensity of the mother's efforts to respond to the infant's cues. Briefly, the infant gave mixed signals about his behavioral states, even about whether he was awake or asleep. His mother appeared eager to respond, and yet uncertain about when a response was appropriate. Description of an incident during the home observation at 4 weeks can illustrate this interpretation of their behaviors:

> The episode began with the infant asleep in the crib. During the 3 min prior to the mother's intervention, there were six epochs during which open-eyed rapid eye movements (REM) occurred. The mother picked the baby up, undressed him, and gave him an immersion bath which lasted for 5 min. Throughout the bath the infant's eyes did not open. As she talked to him, one of the mother's comments was that she did not understand why the infant kept his eyes closed. As she dressed her infant after the bath, he began to waken. She put him to the

breast and after several efforts to get him to feed, she put him back into the crib and left the room. While in the crib alone, the infant remained awake and primarily alert for 15 min.

In order to determine whether the incident described was an isolated one or was typical of this mother-infant relationship, the data were examined for all 20 infants to answer the following questions about the state of the infant prior to an intervention, and the nature of the activities that constitute an intervention:

1. What infant behavioral states preceded interventions in which the mother initiated physical contact with her infant?
2. Beginning when the mother established physical contact with her infant following a period of at least 2 min of noncontact, what was the nature of her interventions over the next 5 min?

These questions were first approached by identifying every instance in which a mother touched her infant in some way following a period of at least 2 min (12 epochs) in which the infant had not been touched. Thus, we have a sequence which can be described as follows: no intervention → physical contact. For this analysis, the states of the infant during the 12 epochs preceding the intervention were tabulated using the following categories:

1. *Sleep* (quiet sleep, active sleep) *or transition* (uncertain, drowse, daze)
2. *Quiet wakefulness* (alert inactivity or waking activity without vocalization)
3. *Fussy vocalizations* (fuss, cry, alert inactivity, or waking activity with vocalization).

The activities of the mother were tabulated for 5 min (30 epochs) succeeding the intervention, using the following categories: stimulation, hold or carry, change or bathe, and feed.

The nature of the sequences for mother-infant pair 3 was consistent with the incident described above. The total frequency of the mother's interventions was higher than that for the total group. She initiated contact with her infant, following at least 2 min without contact, on 36 occasions over the 4 weeks; the mean for the entire group was 26.4 (s.d. = 9.9). More notable was the fact that mother 3 initiated feeding within 5 min following an initial intervention more often than any other mother; 18 times over the 4 weeks in comparison to a mean of 7.4 (s.d. = 4.5) for the total group.

On the infant's side, the picture is consistent with the earlier description of mixed signals. He gave about as many fussy vocalizations during the 2 min preceding the interventions as the total group of infants (27.2% of the epochs compared with a mean of 25.8% for the group). However, he also had the highest percentage of epochs spent in sleep or transition during the same time period (19.3% of the epochs compared with 6.6%, s.d. = 5.9 for the entire group). Thus, he was giving both waking and sleeping signals during the 2-min preintervention periods.

Additional Data Analyses of Mother-Infant Pair 3

Additional data analyses were carried out to describe mother-infant pair 3 in order to further elucidate the nature of the interactive process.

As indicated in the previous section, mother 3 picked her infant up somewhat more frequently than the average mother. This raised the question of how much of the total

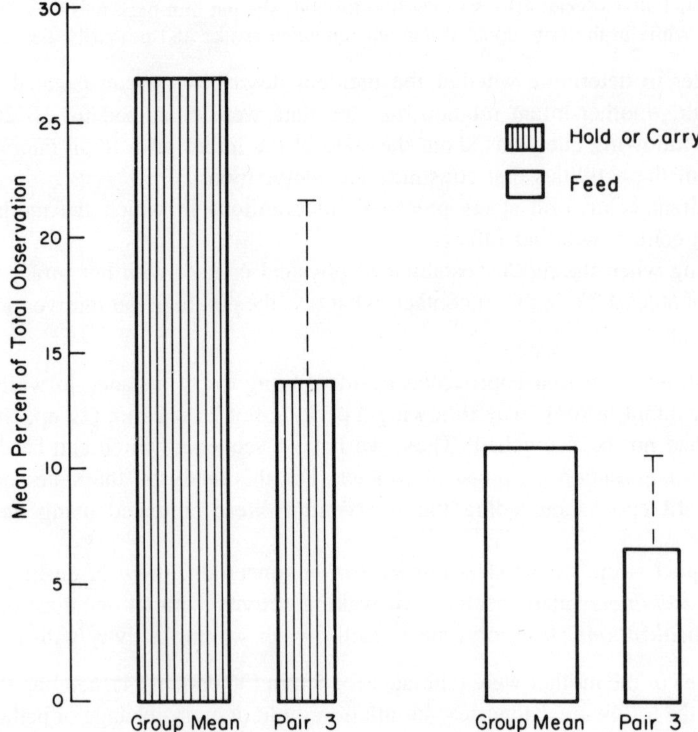

Figure 3. Mean percentage of time over weeks 2, 3, 4, and 5 spent in hold or carry and feed: Group mean (20 infants) and mother-infant pair 3. Dashed lines show 95% confidence limit.

observation she held or carried her infant, including caregiving and noncaregiving activities when the infant was either awake or asleep. As shown in Figure 3, hold or carry was a significantly smaller portion of the total observation for pair 3 than for the entire group.

Since the number of times mother 3 began feeding her infant within 5 min of an initial contact with him was greater than that of any other mother, we were also interested in knowing whether she was distinctive in the total amount of time she spent feeding her infant. A summary of these data are also presented in Figure 3, which shows the mean amount of time spent feeding by the total group and by pair 3, along with the upper limit of the 95% confidence interval for pair 3. Pair 3 spent less time feeding than the mean for the group, with the difference approaching significance at the 94% limit.

In the analyses of the three selected infants, it was shown in Figure 1 that mother 3 spent less time in social interaction than the mothers in the entire group. Furthermore, it was shown in Figure 2 that her infant was awake during as much of the observation day as the other infants. It follows that this mother was using less of her infant's awake time for social interaction than was the case for the total group. The data to support this conclusion are presented in Table 4.

Our major interest with respect to infant 3 was his rapid shifts in behavioral states. Evidence of rapid state changes was reported in the previous section, where it was shown

Table 4. Mean percent of awake time that total group and mother-infant pair 3 engaged in social interaction in four home observations

Subject	Mean	Confidence interval
Group	29.46	
Pair 3	11.88	2.16–21.60

that this infant exhibited an average amount of fussing and crying and a high proportion of sleeping or drowsing during the 12 epochs preceding interventions by his mother. To provide additional confirmation of the infant's state variability, several analyses were carried out.

First, the number of periods of sleep lasting 5 min or longer were recorded for each infant. It was found that infant 3 had 16 sleep periods during the four weekly observations compared with the group mean of 10.8 (s.d. = 2.4). Thus, the infant was changing from sleep to wakefulness with greater frequency than the other infants.

The next question was whether the infant's state lability was apparent within sleep periods. For all infants, using the longest sleep period during each of the four observa-

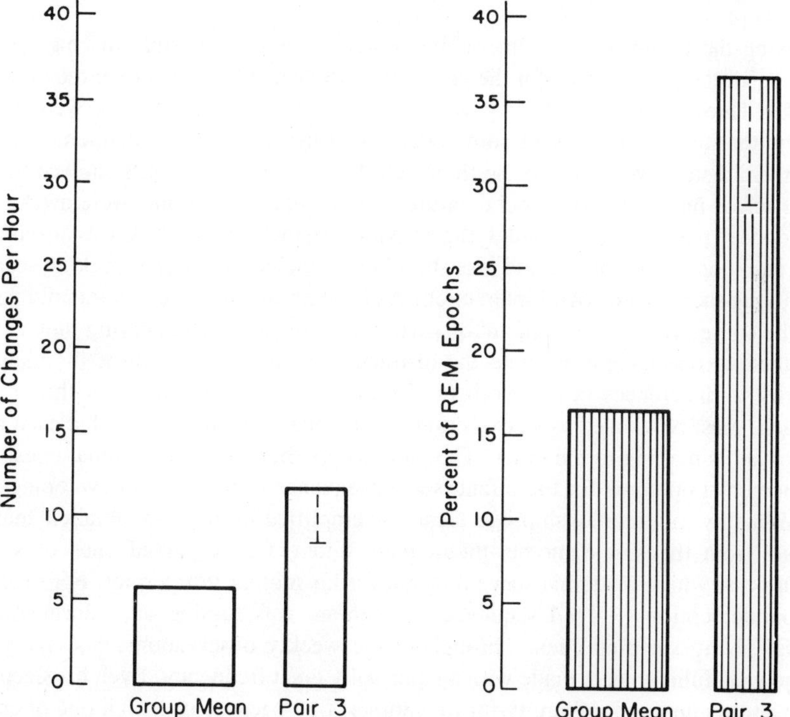

Figure 4. Mean number of state changes per hr and mean percentage of REM epochs spent in open-eyed REM: Group mean (20 infants) and mother-infant pair 3. Dashed lines show 95% confidence limit.

tions, the frequency of change in behavioral states was recorded across active sleep, quiet sleep, drowse, and uncertain. The frequency data, converted to rate-of-change per hr of sleep, are shown in Figure 4 for infant 3 compared with that for the total group over the 4 weeks. Infant 3 had the second highest rate of state change, significantly higher than the mean for the entire group.

Finally, a characteristic that was expected to differentiate infant 3 from the other infants was the amount of open-eyed REM during active sleep. The percentage of REM periods in which open-eyed REM occurred was determined for each infant on each week. Figure 4 shows infant 3 compared with the total group. On this measure, infant 3 was higher than any other infant in the study.

DISCUSSION

The extensive behavior sampling undertaken in this study resulted in measures that are highly stable across the infants' first 5 weeks of life. This stability is quite important for long term prediction of behavior. When the principles of reliability theory are applied, it seems unlikely that observations markedly reduced in number or duration would yield measures with sufficient stability to be useful in long term prediction of behavior. For the study of individual infants and mother-infant pairs, such assessment of measures is a critical step.

Using the highly reliable interactive variables, it was possible to characterize the frequency of their occurrence for the group of 20 mother-infant pairs over the infants' first 5 weeks. Three infants who later gave evidence of developmental delay were compared with the total group, to present commonalities in the nature of their interactions which made them distinctive. Each of the three selected mother-infant pairs showed much less mother-infant interaction of a social nature, that is, when the infants were awake and the mothers were not engaged in caregiving activities. In these pairs, there was also much less visual attention to the infants and less stimulation, including patting, rocking, caressing, and moving them, with social interaction. As a subgroup, the three infants did not differ from the entire group in the amount of wakefulness or fussing and crying they exhibited. Nevertheless, one cannot attribute the distinctive qualities of the three individual pairs primarily to differences in the mothers. Behavior patterns of a dyad, within a systems approach, must be viewed as an expression of the ongoing adjustments that each member of the dyad is making to the other. The patterns are therefore truly mutual ones, and the developmental outcome for the infant is a consequence of the earlier developing system.

Mutuality in a relationship was clearly exemplified in the more detailed analyses of the data from the single mother-infant pair. Infant 3 gave mixed cues of sleep and wakefulness, which made his states difficult for his mother to interpret. For example, in the nonintervention → feed sequences, the infant was fussing and, during the same periods, giving sleeping cues. Throughout the weekly observations, his changes from sleep to wakefulness were made with an unusually great frequency. Even his sleeping was erratic and a source of ambiguity for the mother: first because of a high rate of change in state within sleep periods, and second because of the frequent episodes of open-eyed REMs during active sleep, which the mother interpreted as wakefulness. Her uncertainty was expressed verbally and behaviorally, in terms of frequent but brief episodes of holding and feeding her infant.

From these detailed analyses, it appears that there was a lack of modulation in this mother-infant pair, like a positive feedback system in which each individual accentuated the volatility of the other. The pattern that emerged was one in which both partners made changes abruptly: the mother from one activity to another, and the infant from one state to another. The abruptness of the changes presumably required rapid adjustments by both mother and infant.

Results from the follow-up assessments implicated volatility as a continuing characteristic of infant 3. Neither the neurological examination nor the developmental assessment could be completed, and the professionals who attempted to administer the tests independently commented on the infant's lack of cooperation. We do not have detailed information about the course of the neurological examination. However, on the developmental assessment at 33 months, the child cooperated well on some items, performing within normal limits on a few. On other items, he simply refused to respond. There was no consistent pattern of types of tasks accepted or refused; the examiner's impression was that the child was just very changeable.

A variety of relatively simple data analyses have been used to illustrate that systems-type variables can be derived and used to describe mother-infant pairs, and that the characteristics of a dyad when the infant is very young may be related to later behavior. The results and interpretations of the data in this report have been made without any inferences as to direction of influence between mother and infant. Most important, the results presented are consistent with the notion that the continuities in development are not in the infant, nor in the environment, but in the infant-environment system.

ACKNOWLEDGMENTS

This project was carried out with invaluable assistance from Emelia DeMusis, Linda Abramson, Leslie Gerber, and Margaret Becker.

REFERENCES

Ainsworth, M. D. S., Bell, S., and Stayton, D. 1972. Individual differences in the development of some attachment behaviors. Merrill-Palmer Q. 18:123–143.

Bayley, N. 1969. Bayley Scales of Infant Development. The Psychological Corp., New York.

Bertalanffy, L. V. 1968. General System Theory, Revised Ed. George Braziller Inc., New York.

Brazelton, T. B., Tronick, E., Adamson, L., Als, H., and Wise, S. 1975. Early mother-infant reciprocity. In: Parent-Infant Interaction. Associated Scientific Publishers, New York.

Brody, S. 1956. Patterns of Mothering. International Universities Press Inc., New York.

Burns, P., Sander, L., Stechler, G., and Julia, H. 1972. Distress in feeding: short-term effects of caretaker environment of the first ten days. J. Am. Acad. Child Psychiatry 11:427–439.

Clarke-Stewart, K. A. 1973. Interactions between mothers and their young children: characteristics and consequences. Monogr. Soc. Res. Child Dev. 38:Sections 6–7 (Serial No. 153).

Cohen, S., and Beckwith, L. 1975. Caregiving behaviors and early cognitive development as related to ordinal position in preterm infants. Paper presented at meetings of the Society for Research in Child Development, April, Denver, Colorado.

Eckerman, C. O., and Rheingold, H. 1974. Infant's exploratory responses to toys and people. Dev. Psychol. 10:255–259.

Escalona, S., and Corman, H. 1971. Impact of mother's presence upon behavior: the first year. Human Dev. 14:2–15.

Freese, M. P. 1975. Assessment of maternal attitudes and analysis of their role in early mother-infant interactions. Unpublished doctoral dissertation, Purdue University, Lafayette, Indiana.

Gewirtz, H. B., and Gewirtz, J. L. 1969. Caretaking settings, background events and behavioral differences in 4 Israeli child-rearing environments: some preliminary trends. In: B. M. Foss (ed.), Determinants of Infant Behavior, Vol. IV. Methuen & Co. Ltd., London.

Korner, A. F., and Thoman, E. B. 1970. Visual alertness in neonates as evoked by maternal care. J. Exp. Child Psychol. 10:67–78.

Korner, A. F., and Thoman, E. B. 1972. Relative efficacy of contact and vestibular stimulation in soothing neonates. Child Dev. 43:443–453.

Lewis, M. M., and Goldberg, S. 1969. Perceptual-cognitive development in infancy: a generalized expectancy model as a function of the mother-infant interaction. Merrill-Palmer Q. 15:81–100.

Lewis, M. M., and Lee-Painter, S. 1974. An interactional approach to the mother-infant dyad. In: M. Lewis and L. A. Rosenblum (eds.), The Effect of the Infant on Its Caregiver. John Wiley & Sons Inc., New York.

McCarthy, D. 1972. McCarthy Scales of Children's Abilities. The Psychological Corp., New York.

Moss, H. A., and Robson, K. S. 1968. Maternal influences in early social visual behavior. Child Dev. 39:401–408.

Papousek, H., and Papousek, M. 1975. Cognitive aspects of preverbal social infant-adult interaction. In: Parent-Infant Interaction. Associated Scientific Publishers, New York.

Richards, M. P. M., and Bernal, J. F. 1971. Social interaction in the first days of life. In: H. R. Schaffer (ed.), Origins of Human Social Relations. Academic Press, New York.

Rosenthal, M. K. 1973. Study of infant-environment interaction: some comments on trends and methodologies. J. Child Psychol. Psychiatry 14:301–317.

Sander, L. 1964. Adaptive relationships in early mother-child interaction. J. Am. Acad. Child Psychiatry 3:231–264.

Sander, L., Stechler, G., Burns, P., and Julia, H. 1970. Early mother-infant interaction and 24-hour patterns of activity and sleep. J. Am. Acad. Child Psychiatry 9:103–123.

Schroedinger, E. 1935. Science Theory and Man. Allen & Unwin Ltd., London.

Stern, D. N. 1971. A micro-analysis of mother-infant interaction: behavior regulating social contact between a mother and her 3½-month-old twins. J. Am. Acad. Child Psychiatry 10:501–517.

Stern, D. N. 1974. Mother and infant at play: the dyadic interaction involving facial, vocal and gaze behaviors. In: M. Lewis and L. Rosenblum (eds.), The Effect of the Infant on Its Caregiver. John Wiley & Sons Inc., New York.

Tulkin, S. R., and Kagan, J. 1972. Mother-child interaction in the first year of life. Child Dev. 43:31–41.

Uzgiris, I. C., and Hunt, J. McV. 1975. Assessment in Infancy: Ordinal Scales of Psychological Development. University of Illinois Press, Urbana, Illinois.

Weiss, P. 1971. The basic concept of hierarchical systems. In: P. Weiss (ed.), Hierarchically Organized Systems in Theory and Practice. Hafner Publishing Company Inc., New York.

Wohlwill, J. F. 1973. The Study of Behavioral Development. Academic Press, New York.

Yarrow, L. J., Rubenstein, J. L., and Pedersen, F. A. 1975. Infant and Environment: Early Cognitive and Motivational Development. John Wiley & Sons, Inc., New York.

chapter 5

Contingent Interaction Between Mothers and Their Developmentally Delayed Infants

Peter M. Vietze, Steven R. Abernathy, Mary Lou Ashe, and Gretchen Faulstich

In the past seven years, the focus of understanding infant development in the context of interaction between infant and caregiver has shifted from an emphasis on the parent's role in shaping the infant to interest in the infant's contribution to such transactions. Some attempts to illustrate this have centered on demonstrations that the arousal state, sex, and age of the infant have differential effects on the kinds of behavior in which the caregiver engages with the infant. In one such study, Moss (1967) concludes that the infant initially controls maternal behavior and, if the mother responds to the infant contingent on the infant's behavior, the mother will acquire value as a reinforcing agent which enhances her ability to control the infant's behavior. This conclusion that the infant contributes to the interaction with its caregiver is representative of what R. Q. Bell (1971) and others call "the effect of the infant on the caregiver." In a recent volume edited by Lewis and Rosenblum (1974), several perspectives are presented illustrating this "infant effects" phenomenon.

There are may ways to study how the infant can affect the caregiver and contribute to interactions in which it is a member. A number of studies have focused on differential responses of caregivers to atypical infants. However, the immediate effect of the infant's behavior on that of the parent has been neglected as a topic of study in both the experimental setting and the naturalistic context. Although there is experimental evidence of some ways in which adults can have direct effects on the level of infant responding (e.g., Bloom and Esposito, 1975; Weisberg, 1963), there is not much direct evidence of the immediate effect of the infant's behavior on that of the parent. However, recent experiments by Gewirtz and Boyd (1977) have demonstrated that infant headturns and vocalizations were

---

This research was supported in part by Grants 00973, HD-07054, and HD-00043 from the National Institute of Child Health and Human Development, and by Biomedical Science Support Grant FR-RR07087 from the General Support Branch, Division of Research Resource, Bureau of Health Professions, Education, and Manpower Training, National Institutes of Health. In addition, support was received from research contract NE-C-00-3-0260 from the National Institute of Education.

effective reinforcers in conditioning mothers' communicative responses. Furthermore, there is little evidence that the infant or the parent in interaction show effects that can be detected in one another when the infant is older. This is the case even though there is a widely accepted view that the parent-child interaction system is the arena of early learning.

The view of the infant's behavioral contribution to its own development has evolved in the present century from discoveries that stimulation, especially that originating with the human caregiving environment, is essential for normal, healthy development. Early studies of infants raised in institutional environments devoid of adequate stimulation by consistent caregivers indicated that maternal deprivation accounted in part for the emotional, physical, and intellectual retardation so prevalent among institutionalized children. These findings contributed to the great interest already shown by many psychologists in the role of early experience on later development.

Experimental studies with infrahuman organisms revealed a plethora of effects that could be attributed to varying amounts and varieties of early stimulation. In applying these results to research with human infants on early experience, the emphasis was placed on whether there was sufficient stimulation. Casler (1968) and Yarrow (1961, 1963), however, pointed out the need to differentiate the kinds of early stimulation that might account for varying developmental outcomes in infants. These views have led some investigators to examine various aspects of caregiving environments in order to better understand how the developing organism interacts with its surroundings.

At least one formulation of the environment's influence on development has been concerned with a number of dimensions, each of which has been derived from theoretical writings. Yarrow, Rubenstein, and Pedersen (1975) report the results of an extensive investigation in which they attempted to characterize environmental variables in terms of the variety, complexity, and responsiveness of the inanimate as well as the social environment. In their book they emphasize the importance of developing methodologies to define more precisely the responsiveness of the animate environment. They acknowledge that both psychoanalytic and behavioral persuasions emphasize the salience of a responsive environment for early development. The psychoanalytic school sees responsiveness of caregivers as a reflection of their sensitivity to the infant's needs. For behaviorists, the salient feature of a stimulus is its responsiveness or contingency. The present research illustrates how one methodology, developed for studying the responsiveness of the caregiver and infant to one another, was adapted to the study of developmentally delayed infants.

The observational methodology described in the present chapter was designed to study mother-infant interaction in the natural environment, allowing for the sequencing and duration of mother and infant behaviors (Strain, 1975, Anderson and Vietze, 1977; Anderson, Vietze, and Dokecki, 1977). In addition, it was our intention to record behaviors believed to have communicative value in the context in which they occurred. The observational system is described more fully below, although the data presented focus on vocal interactions between mothers and their infants as illustrative examples. This provides comparisons with other studies that have emphasized vocal responding of mothers and infants to one another.

MOTHER-INFANT VOCAL INTERACTION

The significance of vocal behavior in the mother-infant interactional system has been emphasized by several writers. Bowlby (1969), in his presentation of attachment theory, has pointed out that infant vocal behavior serves to elicit and maintain proximity which is important for the development of attachment. Maternal vocal responses in turn stimulate additional infant vocalization, which enhances the value of interaction and proximity. Other investigators who have suggested the importance of the reciprocal nature of mother-infant vocal responding include Bateson (1975) and Brazelton, Koslowski, and Main (1974). The former has underlined the fact that vocal interchange, as opposed to its content, solidifies the bond between infant and adult.

Several different methods for studying vocal interchange in the context of mother-infant interaction have been reported. Some have used time-sampling (Lewis, 1972; Yarrow, Rubenstein, and Pedersen, 1975), others have video-taped or filmed interactions (Brazelton et al., 1974; Condon and Sander, 1974; Stern, 1974), whereas still others have continuously recorded mother and infant behaviors (Jones and Moss, 1971; Brown et al., 1975; Strain, 1975; Vietze, Strain, and Falsey, 1975). Results of these investigations have suggested that, for infants between the ages of 3 and 6 months, maternal vocalization contingent on the vocal responding of the infant was positively related to the overall infant vocalization, although measures of total maternal vocal responding were not related to infant vocalization (Jones and Moss, 1971; Yarrow et al., 1975).

Most recently, investigators have begun to look more closely at the structure of vocal interaction between mothers and infants. Anderson and Vietze (1977) and Stern et al., (1975) have reported that 3-month-old infants show signs of approximating dialog interactions with their mothers, alternating vocal responding with them. (Both of these reports are based on a model suggested by Jaffe and Feldstein, 1970.) Furthermore, Vietze et al. (1975), in a longitudinal study of 51 mother-infant pairs, found that from 2 to 6 months of age, the infant seems to become a more active participant in the reciprocal "conversations" with the mother. The low variability across different mother-infant dyads reported in these investigations suggests that the conversational model might be one of the characteristics of social interaction that is relatively unaffected by individual differences. Data reported in the present chapter examine this proposition as it might apply to children whose development is delayed.

INTERACTION BETWEEN ATYPICAL CHILDREN AND THEIR MOTHERS

Research examining parent-child interaction in which the children were atypical has been limited. Among these, several studies have appeared in which premature infants and their mothers were observed (Barnett, Leiderman, Grobstein, and Klaus, 1970; Klaus et al., 1970); interaction between blind infants and their mothers have been studied (Fraiberg, 1971); observations of mothers and their cerebral palsied children have been reported (Shere and Kastenbaum, 1966; Kogan and Tyler, 1973); mother-child interactions in families with mentally retarded young children have been observed using a variety of techniques (Kogan, Wimberger, and Bobbitt, 1969; Marshall, Hegrenes, and Goldstein, 1973); and atypical infants and their mothers were filmed during structured interaction sequences (Greenberg, 1971). These studies have indicated that the parents of atypical infants display interaction patterns that often differ from those exhibited by mothers whose young children and infants are not atypical.

Shere and Kastenbaum (1966), in referring to their own sample of children with cerebral palsy, point out that "the development of these children thus appeared to be in double jeopardy—jeopardized by . . . the affliction and jeopardized potentially by the emergence of an interaction pattern that might inhibit rather than foster psychological growth" (p. 257). Kogan, Wimberger, and Bobbitt (1969), in comparing their two groups of mother-child pairs, found that mothers of the retarded children showed much lower levels of submissiveness to their children than did comparison mothers. There was a higher level of neutral co-acting between the retarded children and their mothers than there was in the comparison group, such that "retardates and their mothers 'did nothing together' more often than other things, while comparison children and their mothers 'took turns'" (p. 807). The retarded children had mothers who showed less sensitivity or responsiveness to them than did the comparison children. In another study comparing retarded, physically handicapped and normal children interacting with their mothers, Kogan and Tyler (1973) found that the mothers of both groups of atypical children were more overprotective than were the mothers of the nonhandicapped children. Similarly, Marshall et al. (1973), studying the verbal interactions of retarded children and their mothers, found higher rates of assertive verbal behavior among these mothers than among mothers of nonretarded children. This took the form of a significantly higher number of *mands* (verbal operants which include commands, demands, and requests) used by mothers in playing with their retarded children. The conclusion that can be drawn from this limited number of studies is quite general: there is some disturbance in the mother-child interactional system when the child is atypical in some way. However, in none of these studies investigating mother-child interaction have there been any attempts to examine contingent relationships between the two dyad members.

The purpose of the present research was to examine the interactional system of mothers and their retarded children in order to understand the contingencies that operate between them. Among the previous research efforts that have attempted to study contingent interaction between mothers and infants, some (Lewis, 1972; Yarrow et al., 1975) have done so by designating a behavior as either "stimulus" or "response" during data collection. The present authors believe that this imposition is not conducive to the study of the natural contingencies that might exist between infant and mother. Condon and Ogston (1967) discussed this issue in their presentation of a general model that can be applied to the study of dyadic interaction:

> The fundamental problem involves finding an empirical, decisional basis for the analysis of an ongoing process across the multiple and interlocking levels of that process as it occurs naturally. . . . Behavior, to re-emphasize, occurs as patterns of "whiles," a person speaks connecting segments of sound, "while" eyes and brows move, "while" arms, hands and fingers move, "while" the other person or persons move. Behavior *is* what they all are "while" they occur. . . . We are seeking to illustrate that the components of behavior are not discrete and isolated events which are then combined to form behavior, but are regular and predictable patterns of change within an ongoing process (pp. 222, 225).

Recently, investigators in several laboratories have developed observational methods consistent with the model of the reciprocal, bidirectional nature of mother-infant (and perhaps other) interactional relationships (e.g., Bakeman and Brown, 1977; Brazelton et al., 1974; Stern et al., 1975; Anderson and Vietze, 1977). These methods allow for the continuous recording of sequential interactions between individuals and the subsequent analysis of the behavior stream to determine the contingent relationships. The remainder of this chapter describes the use of such an observational system and how the data are analyzed to compare groups of mother-infant dyads that include developmentally delayed children with respect to the contingent nature of their interactions.

METHODS

Subjects

Families with Developmentally Delayed Children Subjects in this sample consisted of 28 children (17 boys, 11 girls) and their mothers. The families were enrolled in a home-based intervention program for developmentally delayed infants. Three additional children and their mothers were observed but were dropped from the present analyses because their Bayley scores could not be obtained. Within 4 months prior to data collection, the children had been administered the Bayley Scales of Infant Development as part of the regular assessment procedures of the program. In order to determine whether the interactional measures were related to developmental level, the sample was divided equally into two groups of 14 children. The high developmental level group had Bayley MDI scores between 50 and 74, while the low developmental level group had Bayley MDI scores below 50. Thus, all of the children in this sample showed a wide range of developmental delays. (Although the age range in this sample includes children above what is typically considered infancy, they all functioned at levels within the infancy period; therefore, they will be referred to as infants hereafter.) Descriptively, the sample consisted of children with various handicaps, including retardation resulting from prenatal-perinatal trauma, Down's syndrome, various motor handicaps, and visual impairments. Although it was expected at the outset of the study that balanced selection for chronological and developmental age might be made, it was later discovered that self-selection by families and the nature of the population prevented this. Thus, the two groups differed in chronological age with the low MDI group having a mean age of 28.82 months and the high MDI group having a mean age of 18.36 months. Observations were carried out in the subjects' homes and lasted about 40 min.

Potential subjects were selected from the total number of cases served by the Infants Program. The two observers, in consultation with home visitors who had responsibility for the cases, contacted the families by mail, phone, and in person to recruit them for inclusion in the study. Of 38 families who were asked to participate, seven refused.

Families with Nondevelopmentally Delayed Infants This sample consisted of 48 mothers and their normal infants, 22 males and 26 females. These mother-infant pairs were recruited for participation in a longitudinal study in which data were taken when the infants were 2½, 6½, and 12½ months of age. Infants were administered the Bayley scales at these ages. Mean MDI scores were 110.7, 111.9, and 115.33 at 2, 6, and 12 months, respectively. Although this study included laboratory assessments of infant learning and perception, the results to be reported here are from observations of mother-infant interaction carried out in the subjects' homes at the three ages. The observations at each age lasted between 70 and 90 min.

Procedure

Observations were carried out by two observers who had extensive training in the use of the recording equipment and the observational instrument. They arranged to arrive at each subject's home just before the child was expected to awaken from a nap. Parents had previously been informed that we wished to observe the child in a variety of situations, including a feeding, a bath, and a play period. However, it was emphasized that the mother should maintain her normal routine as much as possible.

Apparatus

Data were collected using an electronic digital recording device (Datamyte, Model DAK-8, Electro-General Corporation, Minnetonka, Minnesota), consisting of a 12-button keyboard and a cassette tape recorder. The keyboard contains buttons representing the digits 0 through 9, an asterisk button to flag errors, and a button that enters the codes pressed since the previous entry. An internal clock records the time, in seconds, each time the "enter" button is pushed. Once an observation has been made, the cassette tape is played through a decoder and entered directly onto a computer disk. This raw data file can then be edited for errors and prepared for data reduction and analysis.

Observational System

The observational system (Anderson, Faulstich, Ashe, and Vietze, 1975) consists of a set of numerical codes representing patterns of infant and mother behavior. The ongoing behaviors of the mother and infant are coded continuously as onsets of one of the set of mutually exclusive and exhaustive patterns. Each behavior pattern is defined as a composite of one or more behavior categories as depicted in Table 1. For infants there are five behavior categories: a) visual attention to mother, b) nondistress vocalization, c) smile, d) distress vocalization, and e) no signalling behavior present. There are, likewise, five behavioral categories recorded for the mother: a) visual attention to the infant, b) vocalization directed to the infant, c) smile, d) tactile play stimulation, and e) no behavior directed to the infant. Each behavior pattern consists of one or more of these categories and is entered as a unique 2-digit code. Finally, context codes for infant arousal state, maternal proximity to the infant, and maternal caregiving activities are entered at the beginning of the observation and whenever changes in context occur, these three contexts are also comprised of mutually exclusive categories and each of the three contexts is monitored separately from each other and separate from the behavior patterns. In the present report, only vocalizations that occurred while the mother and child were in each other's presence are considered.

Table 1. Outline of observation categories

Infant behavior patterns
Vocalize
Look at mother
Look/smile
Vocalize/look
Vocalize/look/smile
Vocalize/smile
Smile
Cry
Cry/look
No signalling behavior
Maternal behavior patterns
Vocalize to infant
Look at infant
Look/smile
Vocalize/look
Vocalize/look/smile
Vocalize/tactile-play
Look/smile/tactile-play
Vocalize/look/smile/tactile-play
Tactile-play
No behavior to infant
Caregiving
Feed
Bathe-diaper/dress
Put to sleep
No caregiving
Infant state
Active-awake
Quiet-awake
Drowsy
Asleep
Maternal proximity
Holds infant
Within 3 feet
Greater than 3 feet
Out of room

Observers

The observers were trained initially by viewing video tapes of mother-infant interaction and coding from these tapes until the level of inter-observer agreement for both frequency and duration of each category reached at least 0.80. Following this training period before the TV monitor, 90-min observations of pilot families were carried out until interobserver agreement in homes also reached 0.80. Reliability on pilot homes and periodic reliability checks during the studies yielded acceptable interobserver agreements ranging from 0.82 to 0.94 for durations, and 0.87 and 0.98 frequencies for the vocalization data being presented here.

Reduction of Observational Data

In this report, vocalizations of mother and infant are reported as they were subjected to a time series analysis. The purpose of this analysis was to evaluate the second-by-second alternation of vocal activity between mother and infant through a conditional probability analysis of the vocal interactions. To prepare the data for this analysis, each observational record was divided into consecutive fixed time intervals of 1 sec. The choice of 1-sec units was made as this was the smallest time unit for which the behavior was coded and for which the Datamyte could have timed a behavior. For the relevant portions of the record, one of the following four mutually exclusive dyadic vocal states was assigned to each 1-sec unit: a) simultaneous vocalization (both mother and infant vocalizing), b) mother vocalizing alone, c) infant vocalizing alone, and d) neither mother nor infant vocalizing (distress vocalizations were not included for the infant). The sequence of states formed from this reduction fit the assumptions of a finite Markov process: a) the number of steps in the sequence is finite, b) the sequential transitions are discrete, and c) the probability of a given event depends only on the last preceding event.

A first order transition matrix was constructed for each dyad. This matrix gave the frequency with which a vocal state at time "*t*" moved in the next 1-sec interval time (t + 1) to any vocal state including itself. From this matrix of transition frequencies, transition probabilities for each cell were derived by dividing a cell frequency by its corresponding row total. Thus, the outcome of this data reduction was the conditional or transition probabilities represented in the cells of the matrix constructed for each of the infant-mother dyads. These conditional probabilities are the dependent variables that were used in the present analysis of the interaction observations.

RESULTS

The transition probabilities derived from the transition matrices constructed for each mother-child dyad were treated as scores representing the various changes in vocal interaction. The mean probabilities for the dyads with nondevelopmentally delayed infants may be found in Table 2, while those for the dyads with developmentally delayed children are shown in Table 3. In both tables, the transition probabilities are listed below the simple probabilities for each of the four vocal states.

It should be noted that the transition for mother vocalizing alone followed by infant vocalizing alone (MV→IV) and its converse, and the transition for both vocalizing followed by neither vocalizing (BV→NV) and its converse, are not given. The observation procedure does not allow the possibility for coding simultaneous initiations, terminations, or alternations of mother and infant without 1 sec elapsing, because a single observer is coding both dyad members' behavior. Thus, these transitions are coded sequentially. (In examining transitions lagged by 2 sec where these four transitions are possible, we have found that such simultaneous transitions are rare.) Another noteworthy phenomenon relates to the transition where any state follows itself. The entries for these transitions are quite high: BV → BV = 0.815; MV → MV = 0.925, etc. This is an indication that the ongoing behavior of the members of the dyads continues through time; the smaller the fixed time

Table 2. Probabilities of behavior patterns for the 49 mother-infant dyads with nondevelopmentally delayed infants

Behavior patterns	Two months		Six months		Twelve months	
	Mean	s.d.	Mean	s.d.	Mean	s.d.
Both vocalizing	0.083	0.058	0.121	0.045	0.167	0.084
BV-BV	0.815	0.059	0.838	0.034	0.772	0.237
BV-MV	0.149	0.057	0.111	0.023	0.086	0.035
BV-IV	0.036	0.023	0.051	0.021	0.079	0.141
Mother vocalizing	0.454	0.154	0.377	0.133	0.291	0.107
MV-MV	0.925	0.028	0.906	0.032	0.794	0.255
MV-BV	0.023	0.012	0.035	0.016	0.049	0.021
MV-NV	0.051	0.025	0.058	0.021	0.095	0.167
Infant vocalizing	0.049	0.046	0.121	0.083	0.142	0.067
IV-IV	0.771	0.126	0.838	0.051	0.744	0.239
IV-BV	0.098	0.101	0.072	0.037	0.108	0.158
IV-NV	0.128	0.057	0.091	0.023	0.093	0.035
Neither vocalizing	0.414	0.146	0.381	0.112	0.345	0.156
NV-NV	0.932	0.028	0.915	0.026	0.834	0.240
NV-MV	0.055	0.029	0.055	0.024	0.084	0.167
NV-IV	0.013	0.009	0.030	0.014	0.040	0.023

interval used, 1 sec in the present case, the higher these same state transition probabilities tend to be.

Before making specific comparisons between transition probabilities, a number of general features of the data are described. The strategy for presenting results is to describe first the findings for the nondevelopmentally delayed infants and mothers and then to present the comparable data for the developmentally delayed children-mother dyads. It can be seen in Table 2 that for the nondelayed sample the mothers tended to dominate the dialogues (summing both vocalizing and mother alone vocalizing) at all three ages. However, although the infants vocalized a little more than 10% of the time at 2 months (summing both vocalizing and infant alone vocalizing), by the time they were a year old, the infants had increased their rate of vocalization. In addition, the amount of time neither partner vocalized decreased over the 10-month period indicating the effect of the infant's increasing competence on the interactional system. Examination of the delayed sample (see Table 3) reveals that for these mothers there is slightly more mother vocalization in the low MDI group than in the high MDI group, although the infants in the two groups do not show much difference. However, the mothers clearly show considerably more vocal activity than do the infants at both developmental levels. If the ratio of vocal activities from the two samples are compared, it is found that the developmentally delayed infants resemble the nondevelopmentally delayed infants at 12 months whereas the mothers of the developmentally delayed children vocalize at a rate comparable to the mothers of the

Table 3. Probabilities of behavior patterns for the 28 mother-infant dyads with developmentally delayed infants

Behavior patterns	Low MDI		High MDI		Total sample	
	Mean	s.d.	Mean	s.d.	Mean	s.d.
Both vocalizing	0.204	0.101	0.172	0.100	0.188	0.098
BV-BV	0.829	0.047	0.834	0.055	0.832	0.049
BV-MV	0.116	0.036	0.114	0.048	0.115	0.041
BV-IV	0.054	0.021	0.051	0.030	0.053	0.025
Mother alone vocalizing	0.388	0.121	0.347	0.152	0.368	0.134
MV-MV	0.881	0.043	0.882	0.046	0.882	0.043
MV-BV	0.054	0.026	0.051	0.024	0.053	0.024
MV-NV	0.065	0.029	0.069	0.032	0.066	0.030
Infant alone vocalizing	0.116	0.006	0.118	0.075	0.117	0.068
IV-IV	0.769	0.070	0.804	0.082	0.786	0.076
IV-BV	0.129	0.045	0.094	0.056	0.112	0.052
IV-NV	0.101	0.040	0.102	0.039	0.102	0.038
Neither vocalizing	0.292	0.116	0.363	0.147	0.327	0.132
NV-NV	0.864	0.064	0.905	0.043	0.884	0.056
NV-MV	0.084	0.042	0.060	0.034	0.072	0.039
NV-IV	0.052	0.034	0.040	0.016	0.044	0.027

normal infants at 2 months. This may be a reflection of the way in which mothers of developmentally delayed children respond to the atypicality of their children. It might also be the result of their participation in the program in which they were enrolled and may reflect their efforts to stimulate language in their children.

To evaluate the relative probabilities of the dyadic system being in any one of the four vocalization states, the data for the nondevelopmentally delayed children were analyzed using a mixed design analysis of variance (sex × vocal state × age). Results of this analysis indicated a significant main effect for vocal state, F (3, 138) = 125.5, $p < 0.001$, and a significant vocal state by age interaction, F (6, 276) = 22.9, $p < 0.0001$. No sex differences were found for this or for any of the other analyses to be presented here. Figure 1 indicates that as the infants became older, the probability of both vocalizing simultaneously increased at each age while that for mothers decreased. Infants vocalizing alone increased significantly from 2 to 6 months, but not from 6 to 12 months. There was no significant difference at 2 months between infant vocalizing and both vocalizing.

A mixed design analysis of variance (developmental level × vocal state) was also conducted for the delayed sample with the simple probabilities as the dependent variables yielding only a significant main effect for vocal state, F (3, 78) = 22.56, $p < 0.0001$. This is also represented in Figure 1. Although the main effect suggests that the four vocal states were different for both developmental levels, and the interaction was not significant ($p <$

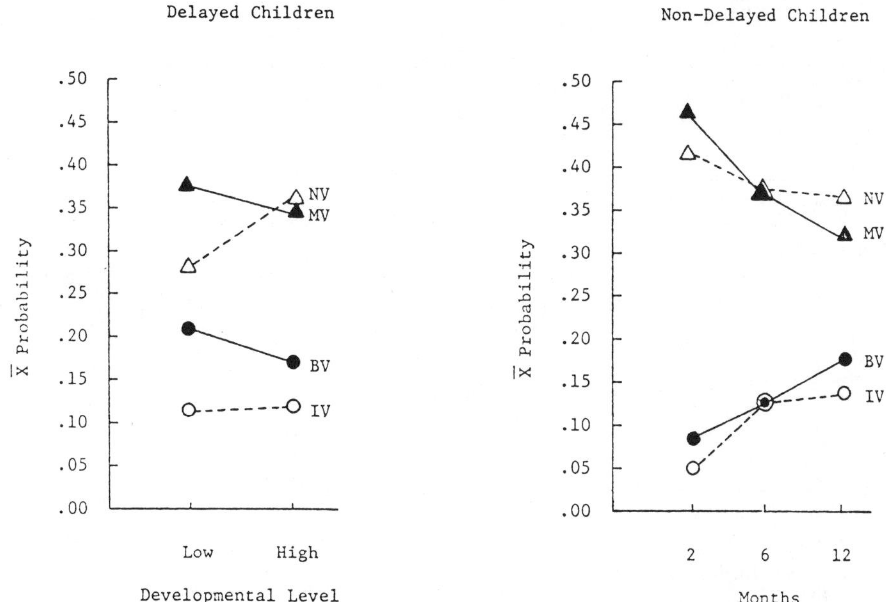

Figure 1. Mean probability for dyadic vocal states in nondevelopmentally delayed and delayed children.

0.37), inspection of the means indicates that for the high developmental level there was no difference between neither person vocalizing and mother vocalizing. Comparison of the two samples by inspection reveals that, as indicated above, the probabilities for the delayed sample most resemble the nondelayed sample at 12 months of age.

Effect of Infant Vocalizing on Parent Vocal Onset

In order to evaluate the contingent nature of the mother's vocalization(s) in relation to the infant's vocalization(s), the transition from infant vocalizing alone to both vocalizing (mother vocalization onset contingent on the infant's vocalizing) was compared to the transition from neither vocalizing to mother vocalizing alone. Figure 2 illustrates these comparisons. A sex × transition × age analysis of variance was computed for the dyads with nondevelopmentally delayed infants with transition probabilities for IV → BV and NV → MV as dependent variables. The analysis revealed a significant main effect for transition probability, $F(1, 47) = 34.32, p < 0.0001$, and a significant age × transition interaction, $F(2, 94) = 3.16, p < 0.05$. No effects were found for sex of infants. Subsequent analyses (Newman-Keuls Multiple Comparison, $p < 0.05$) indicated that the rate of IV → BV decreased from 2 to 6 months but did not change significantly between 6 and 12 months. The rate of NV → MV did not change as the infants grew older. It is apparent from Figure 2 that mothers are more likely to vocalize if the infant is already vocalizing. However, it seems that as the infant increases in age, the mother's tendency to respond to the infant decreases.

In order to examine the contingency relationship for the delayed children and their

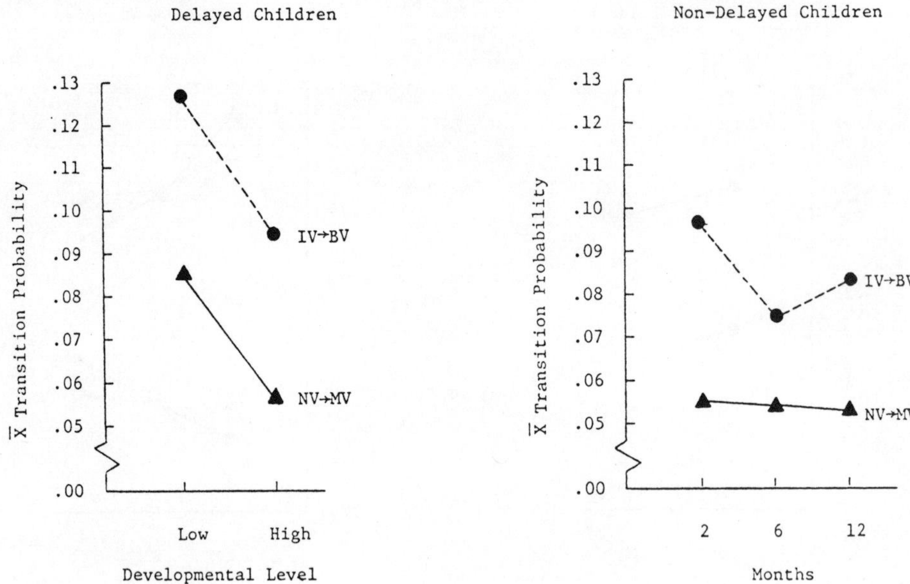

Figure 2. Mean transition probabilities indicating the effect of infant vocalization on contingent mother vocalization for nondevelopmentally delayed and delayed children.

mothers, the transition probabilities IV → BV and NV → BV were subjected to a transition × developmental level analysis of variance. A main effect for transition was found, $F(1, 26) = 17.61, p < 0.001$, indicating that IV → BV was greater than NV → BV. It seems from this comparison that mothers of developmentally delayed young children respond more contingently than they do "noncontingently" with respect to vocal interactions. It seems, moreover, from inspection of the data for the developmentally delayed children, that mothers of lower functioning children show a higher probability of responding whether the children are responding or not, than do the mothers of the higher functioning children. This must be considered, however, in light of the fact that there were generally no differences in maternal vocalizations between the two groups of delayed children.

Effect of Mother Vocalizing on Infant Vocal Onset

In order to consider the interactional system as a reciprocal system, the effect of the mother's vocalization on infant vocal onset was also considered. This effect is assessed by comparing the transition probabilities MV → BV and NV → IV. It will thus be possible to determine whether the infant is more likely to initiate vocalization when the mother is already vocalizing than when neither of them is vocalizing.

Comparisons of these two transition probabilities for the two samples of children and their mothers are represented in Figure 3. To evaluate the change in the effect of mother vocalizing on infant vocal onset as the infant increases in age, a sex × transition × age analysis of variance was computed for the nondevelopmentally delayed children. The

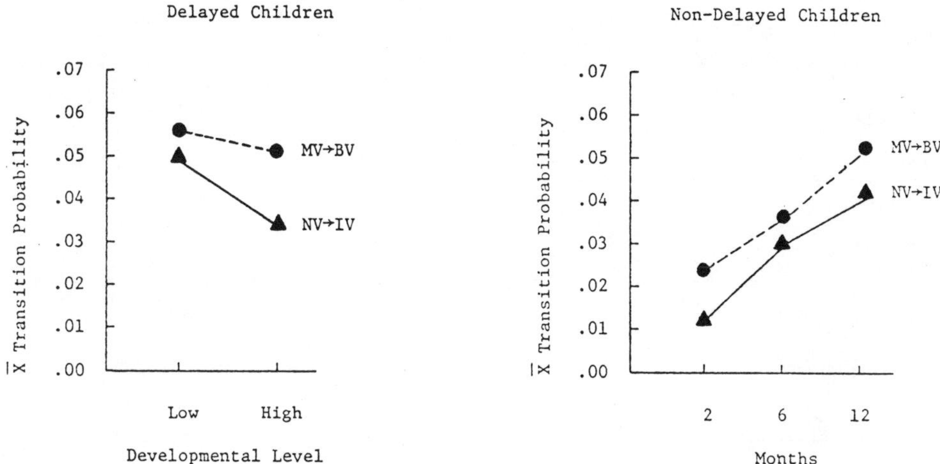

Figure 3. Mean transition probabilities indicating the effect of maternal vocalization on contingent infant vocalization for nondevelopmentally delayed and delayed children.

analysis revealed only a significant main effect for transition probability, F (1, 47) = 48.13 $p < 0.001$, indicating that infants were more likely to initiate a vocal response contingent on mother vocalization than not contingent on mother vocalization. The two groups of developmentally delayed children and their mothers were compared to see if there were any differences between developmental levels in contingent infant vocalizations. The transition × developmental level analysis of variance indicated a significant main effect for transition, F (1, 26) = 7.65; $p < 0.01$, and a significant group × transition interaction, F (1, 26) = 4.83, $p < 0.03$. One explanation for this interaction is that the children in the lower developmental group showed no difference in vocal onset whether the mother was vocalizing or not vocalizing, whereas the higher developmental level children did manifest vocalization contingent on maternal vocal responding.

Suppression Effects

Several investigators have suggested that maternal vocal behavior may inhibit infant vocalizations (Brazelton et al., 1974; Webster, 1969). Such a phenomenon might be considered as a type of contingent behavior although in this case, the contingency is a negative one. Basically, the effect of one person's behavior on the termination of another's behavior might be seen as interfering with continued social interaction.

The suppression of infant vocalization contingent on mother vocalization was tested by comparing the transition probabilities BV → MV and IV → NV. A sex × transition × age analysis of variance carried out on these two transition probabilities for the non-delayed sample revealed a significant main effect for transition, F (1, 47) = 19.82, $p < 0.0002$, and a significant interaction between age and transition, F (1, 94) = 7.34, $p < 0.001$. The means illustrating this comparison are shown in Figure 4. It can be seen that, at the two younger ages, the mothers did seem to inhibit infant vocal behavior. However,

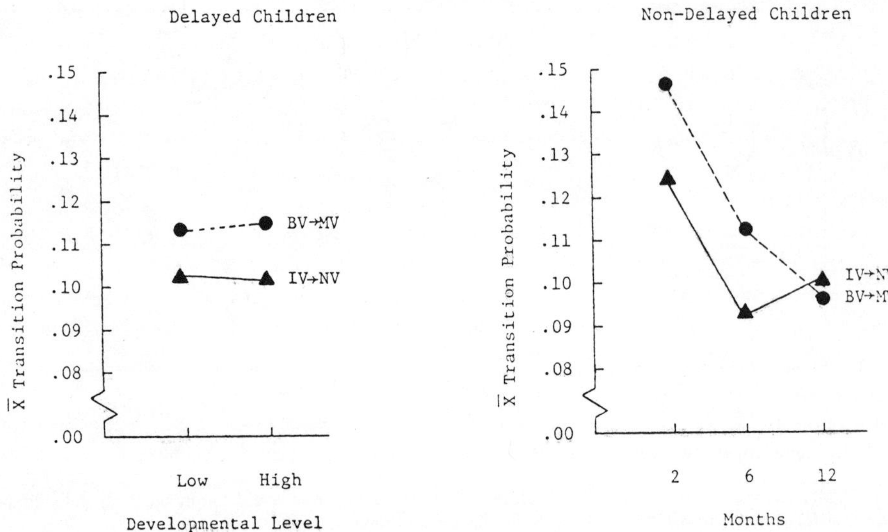

Figure 4. Mean transition probabilities indicating the effect of maternal vocalization on termination of infant vocalization for nondevelopmentally delayed and delayed children.

at one year, this effect was no longer evident and the change seems to be due to a decrease in the infant's tendency to terminate its vocal behavior.

The suppression effect was analyzed for the developmentally delayed sample using analysis of variance (transition × developmental level). The analysis indicated no significant effects, suggesting that there was no suppression of child vocalization by mothers for the delayed population. Thus, the children cease their vocalizations whether the mother is already engaged in vocal responding or not. Taken by itself, this might be an indication that the developmentally delayed children do not differentiate between the two circumstances. However, given that the 12-month-old infants in the normal sample also show no suppression effects, this would not seem to be a reasonable explanation.

DISCUSSION

The present investigation examined observational data of mother-infant interactions collected continuously and sequentially. Vocal interactions were subjected to a transitional probability analysis for each mother-infant dyad, and these probabilities were used to define contingency relationships between the dyad members. Two samples of mothers and children, one including young children judged to be developmentally delayed, the other, children judged to be nondelayed, were compared.

Results indicated that, for the nondelayed infant-mother pairs, both infants and mothers exhibited contingent vocal responsiveness in relation to one another. This suggests that the mother-infant vocal interactional system is a reciprocal one with each dyad member taking the other's behavior into account in vocal responding. It was also evident that examination of either mother or infant behavior, without taking into account the sequential nature of the transactions, might give a biased view of the effects of the two on one another. For instance, the presentation of simple probabilities for the four dyadic states indicated that mothers' vocalizations to their infants decreases as a function of the infants' increasing age. However, consideration of the transition probabilities separates the changes in maternal vocal responding according to the antecedent events and shows that, as the infants grow older, there is no change in maternal initiation of vocalization from a state in which neither person is vocalizing.

Another result from the analysis of vocal state transitions was that although the mothers seemed to dominate the vocal transactions when the infants were 2 months, the nondevelopmentally delayed infants became more active participants with increasing age. The change that took place seems to have been a function of the mothers' withdrawing from their dominant position in the interchanges concurrent with the infants' increased participation. This is especially evident in the increasing probability of infant vocalizing contingent on the mother's vocalization. Thus, there seems to be an increasing tendency for the dyadic vocal system to become more reciprocal as the infants increase in age from 2 to 12 months. The change in the balance of vocal interactions was also manifested by decreasing maternal suppression of infant vocalization as the infants increased in age. Taken collectively, the results for the nondevelopmentally delayed infants and their mothers suggest a reciprocal interactive system for vocal responding which, although showing its basic nature as early as the second month of the infant's life, tends to become more balanced and reciprocal as the first year progresses.

The results for the mothers and their developmentally delayed children are strikingly similar to those for the nondelayed sample at 1 year. Basically, there is strong evidence that these children and mothers also demonstrate reciprocal vocal interactions. The similarity between dyads with low functioning and higher functioning developmentally delayed children suggests that the children's level of mental development may not affect the mother's interactive style of vocal behavior. However, it should be pointed out that the difference found between low and high functioning infants in contingent responding to the mother's vocalizations eventually affects the interactive style of the mothers. Failure of the children to differentiate between presence and absence of maternal vocalization may lead to the mothers' responding less contingently.

Outcomes of the present analysis for the nondelayed infant-mother pairs can be compared with those reported by Anderson and Vietze (1977) for a similar population of 3-month-olds. In the Anderson and Vietze study, both mothers and infants initiated vocalization with a higher probability when the other was vocalizing than if the other person was not vocalizing. In addition, no sex differences were found for any of the transition probability scores, as was true in the present sample. This was interpreted as indicating the strength of the conversational model suggested by Stern et al. (1975) to describe early mother-infant vocal interaction. The relative similarity of the transition matrices for individual mother-infant dyads in these previously reported studies was replicated in the present sample of nondevelopmentally delayed infants and mothers. In addition, results from the nondelayed infants and their mothers indicate that the structure of vocal interaction continues to approximate the adult model reported by Jaffe and Feldstein (1970) as the infants increase in age. Thus, the initial maternal domination of the dialogues decreases as the infants become more vocal with age.

The findings for the delayed children and their mothers are largely in agreement with the basic model of reciprocal vocal interaction found to exist for nondelayed infants and their mothers in the first year. However, the lower functioning, developmentally delayed children seem to show less differentiation between their mothers' vocalizing and not vocalizing than the higher functioning children; the mothers in these two groups do not differ. Thus, the hypothesis that children delayed at different developmental levels would differ in their interactions with the mothers was not substantiated with respect to their level of contingent responsiveness.

The present results differ somewhat from those reported by Anderson and Vietze (1977) with respect to the mother's suppression of infant vocalization. Anderson and Vietze found no evidence of suppression effects, whereas the present study with the nondevelopmentally delayed infants showed evidence of these effects at 2 and 6 months—the ages most comparable to the previous study—and no suppression at 12 months. In addition, there were no significant suppression effects for the delayed sample. The only possible explanation that can be offered at this time for the conflicting findings is that our sample is larger. Further analysis of the two samples may reveal an alternative explanation for the difference.

Comparisons between the present results for the sample of developmentally delayed children and previous studies are difficult to make since the focus of this study was on molecular aspects of the interactions whereas previous studies have examined more molar features of mother-child interaction. Further investigation of the molecular aspects of mother-child interaction with developmentally delayed children is needed, controlling for age and developmental level.

ACKNOWLEDGMENTS

We would like to express our sincere appreciation to the directors, home trainers, nurses, social workers, and secretaries of the Infants Program at Western Carolina Center, Morgantown, North Carolina, for their friendly, helpful cooperation and patience in facilitating the data collection for this study. In addition, we are very thankful to the parents and children who served willingly as subjects in the study reported. Special thanks go to Gloria Gannon Mason and Wanda Stocks for preparing the manuscript, and to Diane Sandler for her help with data analysis. To Susan Falsey, who wrote the computer programs for the transition probability analyses, we are humbly indebted.

REFERENCES

Anderson, B. J., Faulstich, G., Ashe, M. L., and Vietze, P. M. 1975. Observation manual for assessment of behavioral sequences between infants and mothers: newborn to 24 months. DARCEE, George Peabody College, Nashville, Tennessee.

Anderson, B. J., and Vietze, P. M. 1977. Early dialogues: the structure of reciprocal infant-mother vocalization. In: S. Cohen and T. Comiskey (eds.), Child Development: Contemporary Perspectives. F. T. Peacock Publisher, Itasca, Illinois.

Anderson, B. J., Vietze, P. M., and Dokecki, P. R. 1977. Reciprocity in vocal interactions of mothers and infants. Child Dev.

Bakeman, R., and Brown, J. V. 1977. Behavioral dialogues: an approach to the assessment of mother-infant interaction. Child Dev. 48:195–203.

Barnett, C. R., Leiderman, P. H., Grobstein, R., and Klaus, M. H. 1970. Neonatal separation: the maternal side of interactional deprivation. Pediatrics. 45:197-205.

Bateson, M. C. 1975. Mother-infant exchanges: the epigenesis of conversational interaction. Ann. N.Y. Acad. Sci. 263:101-113.

Bell, R. Q. 1971. Stimulus control of parent or caretaker behavior of offspring. Dev. Psychol. 4:63-72.

Bloom, K., and Esposito, A. 1975. Social conditioning and its proper control procedures. J. Exp. Child Psychol. 9:209-222.

Bowlby, J. 1969. Attachment and Loss, Vol. 1. Hogarth Press Ltd., London.

Brazelton, T. B., Koslowski, B., and Main, M. 1974. The origins of reciprocity: the early mother-infant interaction. In: M. Lewis and L. A. Rosenblum (eds.), The Origins of Behavior. pp. 49-76. Vol. 1. The Effect of the Infant on Its Caretaker. John Wiley & Sons Inc., New York.

Brown, J. V., Bakeman, R., Snyder, P. A., Fredrickson, W. T., Morgan, S. T., and Helper, R. 1975. Interactions of black inner-city mothers with their newborn infants. Child Dev. 46:677-686.

Casler, L. 1968. Perceptual deprivation in institutional settings. In: G. Newton and S. Levine (eds.), Early Experience and Behavior: The Psychobiology of Development. pp. 573-626. Charles C. Thomas Publishers, Springfield, Ill.

Condon, W. S., and Ogston, W. D. 1967. A segmentation of behavior. J. Psychiatr. Res. 5:221-235.

Condon, W. S., and Sander, L. W. 1974. Neonate movement is synchronized with adult speech: interactional participation and language acquisition. Science 183:99-101.

Fraiberg, S. 1971. Intervention in infancy: a program for blind infants. J. Am. Acad. Child Psychiatry 10:381-405.

Gewirtz, J. L., and Boyd, E. F. 1977. Experiments on mother-infant interaction underlying mutual attachment acquisition: the infant conditions the mother. In: T. Alloway, P. Pliner, and L. Krames (eds.), Attachment Behavior. Plenum Press, New York.

Greenberg, N. H. 1971. A comparison of infant-mother interactional behavior in infants with atypical behavior and normal infants. In: J. Hellmuth (ed.), Exceptional Infant: Studies in Abnormalities, Vol. 2. Bruner/Mazel, New York.

Jaffe, J., and Feldstein, S. 1970. Rhythms of Dialogue. Academic Press, New York.

Jones, S. J., and Moss, H. A. 1971. Age, state, and maternal behavior associated with infant vocalizations. Child Dev. 42:1039-1051.

Klaus, M. H., Kennell, J. H., Plumb, N., and Zuehlke, S. 1970. Human maternal behavior at the first contact with her young. Pediatrics 46:187-192.

Kogan, K. L., and Tyler, N. 1973. Mother-child interaction in young physically handicapped children. Am. J. Ment. Defic., 77(5):492-497.

Kogan, K. L., Wimberger, H. C., and Bobbitt, R. A. 1969. Analysis of mother-child interaction in young mental retardates. Child Dev. 40:799-812.

Lewis, M. 1972. State as an infant-environment interaction: an analysis of mother-infant interaction as a function of sex. Merrill-Palmer Q. 18:95-121.

Lewis, M., and Rosenblum, L. A. (eds.). 1974. The Effect of the Infant on its Caregiver, Vol. 1: The Origins of Behavior Series. John Wiley & Sons Inc., New York.

Marshall, N. R., Hegrenes, J. R., and Goldstein, S. 1973. Verbal interaction: mothers and their retarded children vs. mothers and their nonretarded children. Am. J. Ment. Defic., 77(4):415-419.

Moss, H. A. 1967. Sex, age, and state as determinants of mother-infant interaction. Merrill-Palmer Q. 13:19-36.

Shere, E., and Kastenbaum, R. 1966. Mother-child interaction in cerebral palsy: environmental and psychosocial obstacles to cognitive development. Genet. Psychol. Monogr. 73:255.

Stern, D. N. 1974. Mother and infant at play: the dyadic interaction involving facial, vocal, and gaze behaviors. In: M. Lewis and L. A. Rosenblum (eds.), The Effects of the Infant on Its Caregiver. John Wiley & Sons Inc., New York.

Stern, D. April 1975. Infant regulation of maternal play behavior and/or maternal regulation of infant play behavior. Paper presented at the meetings of the Society for Research in Child Development, Denver.

Stern, D. N., Jaffe, J., Beebe, B., and Bennett, S. L. 1975. Vocalizing in unison and in alternation: two modes of communication within the mother-infant dyad. Ann. N.Y. Acad. Sci. 263:89–100.

Strain, B. A. 1975. Early dialogues: a naturalistic study of vocal behavior in mothers and three-month-old infants. Doctoral dissertation, George Peabody College, Dissertation Abstracts International, University Microfilms, No. 75-14168B, Ann Arbor, Michigan.

Vietze, P. M., Strain, B., and Falsey, S. March 1975. Contingent responsiveness between mother and infant: who's reinforcing whom? Paper presented at the annual meetings of the Southeastern Psychological Association, Atlanta.

Webster, R. L. 1969. Selective suppression of infants' vocal responses by classes of phonemic stimulation. Dev. Psychol. 1:410–414.

Weisberg, P. 1963. Social and nonsocial conditioning of infant vocalizations. Child Dev. 34:377–388.

Yarrow, L. J. 1961. Maternal deprivation: toward an empirical and conceptual re-evaluation. Psychol. Bull. 58:459–490.

Yarrow, L. J. 1963. Research in dimensions of early maternal care. Merrill-Palmer Q. 9:101–114.

Yarrow, L. J., Rubenstein, J. L., and Pedersen, F. A. 1975. Infant and Environment: Early Cognitive and Motivational Development. John Wiley & Sons Inc., New York.

OBSERVATIONAL METHODS IN THE STUDY OF COGNITIVE DEVELOPMENT

Introduction

Bruce A. Grellong

The study of cognitive development in American psychology has traditionally been a laboratory endeavor. Yet some of the major contemporary theoretical descriptions of cognitive function come directly from the observational methods utilized by researchers such as Piaget. These uses of observational methods in both laboratory and natural settings have been challenged for both lack of rigor and lack of insight into basic cognitive processes. Butterfield's analysis in chapter 6 calls for a new look at the potential interaction of observational and experimental methods for studying cognition.

Butterfield describes the contribution that each method may make to what is known about processes underlying cognitive development, the malleability of cognitive performance, and the implications of research for interpreting and altering the performance of persons labeled mentally retarded. Both Charlesworth in chapter 1 and Butterfield suggest the strategy of looking for problems by observing in the real world, establishing a sense of the importance of these problems by measurement during unstructured behavior, and then going to the laboratory. For the experimentalist, this process may maximize the chances that something of actual importance will be studied. For the theorist using observational methods, this process may yield an explanation of the naturalistic observations. Because the experimentalist's basic task is understanding how to control behavior, the laboratory research tradition has attempted to eliminate individual differences whenever possible. However, even the crudest observations of real world behavior underscore the fact of individual differences as a basic phenomenon in cognitive functioning. Butterfield's analysis suggests that attention to such observational ''facts'' should lead the laboratory investigator toward multivariate studies that can actually account for individual differences, rather than simply averaging out these clearly nonrandom sources of variability.

Butterfield's discussion proposes a carefully outlined set of procedures for identifying and validating explanations of deficient cognitive performance in terms of basic underlying processes. This analysis leads to Butterfield's conclusion that it is not sufficient to simply attribute failures of training or instruction with retarded persons to structural limitations. Rather, a theory-guided instruction or training procedure proceeds by testing each presumed cognitive process under varied conditions until performance is modified to its limit in either laboratory or natural settings. Structural defects can be validly inferred only when performance fails to reveal the existence of a proposed process after testing under a variety of conditions known to utilize that process. Thus, the complementary relationship between natural observation and laboratory experiment involves identifying the uses of knowledge in everyday life that can be assessed in the laboratory to yield an explanation of performance.

The two chapters of data that follow Butterfield's theoretical analysis raise specific issues concerning the application of both observational and experimental methodology to cognitive problems. Chapter 7 by Price-Williams and Ciborowski offers an example of cross cultural anthropological field research. This study concerns the development of the concept of animism within the cultural and linguistic context of a rural Hawaiian population. The study illustrates how a concept serves as a "weltanschauung" or response set in determining performance on a particular type of cognitive task within a particular culture. The work is an instructive example of one major source of variation that might underlie apparently deviant cognitive development and performance by retarded people. To the extent that such people grow up in a culture markedly different from societal norms, such as an institution, the organization of their experiences may be at least as responsible for cognitive failures as any structural or organic processes.

Chapter 8 by Uzgiris and Lucas presents an example of the integration of observational with experimental methodology. Observational data from studying object permanence behaviors were used to identify patterns used by infants while searching for toys in near and far space. Subsequent experimental manipulations were designed to explain the influence of different variables on these search behaviors. These research examples illustrate how observations can highlight the links between specific cognitive functions and the infant's broader experience in the world. For example, Uzgiris found that the ability to locomote in space was an important variable related to object permanence development. Uzgiris suggests that the development of such links can be profitably studied among groups of deviant or at risk infants. They provide an "experiment of nature" in which the contribution of specific limitations on experience (e.g., sensory handicaps, delayed locomotion) can be observed for effects on the acquisition of specific cognitive abilities (e.g., concepts concerning spatial relations and object permanence). This approach seems to have instructive implications for designing research comparing normal and deviant development and for planning intervention programs with infants at risk for mental retardation.

chapter 6

On Studying Cognitive Development

Earl C. Butterfield

The recent history of developmental cognitive psychology is a complex saga whose theme seems to be that the experimental means of researchers have evolved far less rapidly than their theoretical goals (Kuhn, 1974; Belmont and Butterfield, 1977). The time is ripe to ask whether *any* identifiable methods can bridge the gap between the richness and subtlety of contemporary cognitive theory and the poverty and coarseness of current methods (Chase, 1973; Newell, 1973; Weimer, 1974). This conference provides the occasion to ask more particularly whether observational methods can fill the tactical needs of developmental cognitive researchers.

If by observational research is meant the characterization of behavior in ecologically typical settings, then the easiest answer is that the study of cognitive development cannot be pursued observationally. The study of cognition focuses upon processes and capacities that underlie behavior. Clarifying the unobservable underpinnings of behavior requires careful engineering of environmental arrangements and precise measurement of behavior. Therefore, developmental cognitive psychology must be a laboratory undertaking.

The purpose of this paper is to explore the limits of the conclusion that observational methods cannot be used to study cognitive development. The senses in which the conclusion is invalid are shown, and the ways in which observational and experimental methods might complement one another in the study of cognitive development are highlighted. To anticipate, observational data have already importantly oriented the study of cognitive development. This can be seen in Piaget's reliance on observational methods and his profound influence on laboratory scientists. It can also be seen in the minor revolution that linguists have helped introduce into cognitive science with arguments based on exceptionally informal observations of children's language. It is also true that innovative methods are being pioneered by scientists who study cognition of children and mentally retarded persons. These innovations have to do with isolating individual differences (Ghatala, Levin, and Subkoviak, 1975; Underwood, 1975; Butterfield and Dickerson, 1977) and with instructing normal and retarded children to think maturely (Brainard and Allen, 1971). The use of these tools is providing new empirical foundations for cognitive theory,

The preparation of this chapter was supported by United States Public Health Service Grants HD-00870, HD-08911, HD-02528, and HD-04756.

but it is also pinpointing the need for additional procedures, particularly to establish the significance of processes isolated by laboratory research (Kuhn, 1974; Belmont and Butterfield, 1977). Observational methods seem appropriate to this goal, since part of the significance question is whether typical behavior depends on mechanisms isolated in the laboratory (Brown, 1974).

HISTORIC ORIENTATION

The study of the cognitive characteristics of mentally retarded people is so tightly interwoven with the study of normal cognitive development that nothing is lost by considering the two efforts as one. This is partly a sociologic observation. Most scientists who study the cognitive aspects of mental retardation also study normal children. All who study the retarded rely heavily on methods and theories that are used in the study of normal development. These methods and theories come, in turn, either from pure developmentalists, mostly of the Genevan school, or from basic experimental laboratories that focus on normal adults. Contemporary developmental cognitive psychology has taken neither its methods nor its theoretical issues from other scientific traditions that might have influenced it, and seeing why gives definition and perspective to the argument that observational methods can play no role in the study of human mentality.

Maturational Metrics

Looking back, one developmental tradition stands out as depending heavily upon observation of typical behavior in typical settings. It is exemplified best by Gesell's (Gesell et al., 1940) remarkably thorough codification of the things babies and children do and the ages at which they typically do them. Gesell's norms are still used as clinical metrics of children's general developmental progress, but few, if any, students of cognitive development cite Gesell's work or even consider using his approach. If the reasons for this rejection were conscious and deliberate, they would probably have been put this way: Gesell focused on motor behavior, so his descriptions say very little about cognition, and the maturational theory which his descriptions imply does not clarify underlying mechanisms. Moreover, maturational accounts of development militate against ever obtaining analytic understandings of psychological mechanisms, because they assume that the causes of development lie deep in the biology of the organism. This leaves the psychologist with too slight a purchase on analytic tools.

Psychometry

Psychometric traditions are also represented only weakly in recent investigations of mental development (Horowitz and Dunn, 1976). The probable reasons are the following. Intelligence tests are meant to rank people according to their intellectual performance. Cognitive scientists (e.g., Hunt, Frost, and Lunneborg, 1973) have concluded that performance rankings do not elucidate underlying processes, similar to the presumptive shortcomings of the maturational and descriptive tradition of Gesell. The reason IQ tests are mute about process is not that they attribute development to biological maturation. Quite the contrary, intelligence tests are based squarely on the assumption that intellectual development requires congenial experience. This assumption might have formed the basis for a concerted attack on the determinants of cognitive performance, but viewing the IQ as a measure of the *trait* called intelligence eliminated this possibility. In order to represent the IQ as an estimate of a stable trait, it is necessary to assume that everyone has equivalent experiences, and that assumption is as unsupportive of psychological analysis of process as the assumption that maturation determines development. Efforts to build culture-free intelligence tests provided no more support for those who would analyze cognition. These efforts also accepted the goal of performance ranking, and they tried to avoid an examination of environmental determinants by selecting test items that might be uninfluenced by experience. Like Gesell, the psychometricians provided no effective purchase on tools with which to analyze cognition. From the viewpoint of developmental cognitive psychology, the maturational and psychometric approaches survive largely as relicts whose ecological niches are the clinic and the school, not the arena of mental science.

One way to construe an intelligence test is as an elicited sample of behavior. It is a substitute for observing naturally occurring intellective behaviors. By failing to adopt the methods of the psychometric or the maturational approaches, developmental cognitive psychology has suggested that neither direct observation nor comprehensive sampling of spontaneous behavior help one to understand cognitive development. However, it seems that it is not their observational nor sampling techniques per se that led to the neglect of these two traditions. Rather, the critical factors seem to have been these approaches' theoretical nihilism and analytic barbarism. Consider now the methodological consequences of borrowing from Piaget and from adult experimentalists.

METAMORPHOSIS OF THE GENEVAN APPROACH

As practiced in Geneva, the Piagetian approach depends absolutely on naturalistic observation. Currently, that is not true of American Piagetian research, and seeing why is crucial to defining the role of observation in the study of cognitive development.

When theorizing about a cognitive development, Piaget first noted the order in which behaviors enter the repertoire of infants and children. His observations on the emergence of different varieties of imitation provide a suitable example (Piaget, 1951).

The earliest sort of imitation with which Piaget credits the infant has this form: infant does A; adult imitates A as a model for infant; infant does A again. This is called pseudo-imitation, and it occurs during the first 3 or 4 months of life. The next development is imitation of gestures which the infant can see himself perform. Piaget credits the infant with imitation of visible gestures when he does something that he has not recently done with a visible portion of his body shortly after a model performs that act. Imitation of acts that the infant cannot see himself perform comes later. It refers to the infant doing something with an invisible portion of his body (e.g., his face) shortly after seeing a model do that thing. Finally, there is deferred imitation, which typically occurs at 18 months of age or later. Instead of imitating only while the model is present, the infant sometimes imitates after the model's departure.

The next step in the Genevan approach is to interpret observed sequences. The interpretation always assumes that invariant orders of behavioral emergence result from invariant sequences of underlying cognitive developments. These prerequisite cognitive sequences, not their behavioral manifestations, are the object of Piagetian theory. For example, here is one aspect of Piaget's account of the cognitive accomplishments that underlie the transition from visible to invisible imitation.

> An important new phase begins with the imitation of facial movements. . . . The difficulty is then that the child's own face is known to him only by touch and the face of the other person by sight, except for a few rare tactile explorations of the other person's face. Such explorations are very interesting to note at this level, when the child is forming correspondences between the visual and tactilo-kinesthetic sensations in order to extend imitation to the non-visible parts of the body. Until these correspondences are elaborated, imitation of facial movements remains impossible, or is accidental (Piaget and Inhelder, 1969, p. 55).

This quotation exposes Piaget's view that development is the increasing coordination of previously unrelated internal states, or as he and Inhelder say here, the development of correspondences between different sensory inputs. The reason the infant does not imitate invisible gestures before he imitates visible ones is that substantial experience is required to build up internal correspondence between the visual and the tactilo-kinesthetic modes. The infant *cannot* translate his visual experience of what someone else does into kinesthetic terms upon which he might act until those correspondences have been established. The infant imitates things that he can see himself do before he imitates things he cannot see himself do, because the former depends only upon visual guidance and does not require cross modal correspondences. The quote also shows Piaget's belief that cognitive development results from experience. Correspondences between visual and tactile sensations are the result of such experiences as the tactile exploration of another's (visible) face. Moreover, the quote shows that it is the *order* of cognitive developments that matters to Piaget, not the age at which any particular behavior occurs.

Above all, Piaget's account of cognitive development is hierarchical. Each mental accomplishment is constructed out of the accomplishments that preceded it. Since internal reorganization results from experience, and since experiences can vary widely, any particular child or children in any particular culture can progress at different rates, achieving any developmental stage at different ages. However, no child can bypass any prerequisite stage, because each stage builds upon and incorporates its predecessors.

To invalidate any aspect of Piaget's theory, one must show that the order of behavioral manifestations upon which it is built is not invariant. That is why American Piagetian researchers have turned away from strictly observational methods. They have turned to automated and standardized techniques for recording behavior, and they have turned to giving children specially engineered experiences. The questions have been whether the sequences which Piaget and others have observed naturalistically lose their invariant order when other measurement procedures are used or when exceptional experiences are provided. If they do, then Piagetian assertions about the necessity of passing through an invariant order of cognitive stages might be invalid.

One Small Step: Instrumented Observation

The smallest of the several steps that American researchers have taken away from naturalistic observations in order to test Piagetian theory is to instrument their observational procedures. Research on imitation shows how large the implications of that step can be (Meltzoff and Moore, 1977).

Several considerations prompted Meltzoff and Moore to doubt Piaget's interpretation of the development of imitation, but we need consider only one, which is that several investigators, including Piaget himself, had reported observing what appeared to be invisible imitation by infants who were so young that they could not have passed through the stages of pseudo and visible imitation (Guillaume, 1926; Valentine, 1930; Piaget, 1951, Zazzo, 1957). Meltzoff and Moore concluded that they could not take these observations as definitive refutations of the invariant sequence upon which Piaget built his account of imitation, because of the way the observations were taken. In each case, the observers were the models for the young infants' imitative behavior, and they were also the judges of whether imitation had occurred. It seemed necessary to separate the modeling and judging functions, and to provide for reliability determinations of the judgments. Moreover, since there is now good evidence that neonates can be instrumentally conditioned (Papousek, 1967; Butterfield and Siperstein, 1972), it seemed essential to rule out the possibility that the model had inadvertently reinforced spontaneous occurrences of the to-be-imitated responses. The critical question for Piaget's interpretation is not whether very young infants can be taught to make particular responses, but whether they will make them in response to a model without benefit of reinforcement. Finally, spontaneous behaviors. In short, Meltzoff and Moore pointed out that naturalistic observations are incapable of supporting strong inferences about the existence of *imitative* responses. They were willing to believe that very young infants had made responses which they could not see themselves produce, but determining that the responses resulted from imitation required more stringent procedures than the observation of naturally occurring behavior.

The key to solving all of these problems was to automate the recording of imitative behavior. To do this, Meltzoff and Moore used two cameras. One filmed only their neonate subjects and the other recorded only their experimenter model. The model performed four acts. One could have been imitated visibly: sequential finger movements. Three could only be imitiated invisibly: lip protrusion, mouth opening, and tongue protrusion. Six independent raters viewed film segments of the infants' behavior following each modeled act. The judgments showed that the response which had been modeled immediately before the film segments occurred far more frequently than any of the other three responses. Moreover, observations of films of the models showed hardly any behavior that could have reinforced the infants. The babies observed were only 2 weeks old, so these results are strong evidence that invisible imitation does not occur according to the invariant sequence that Piaget thought he had established. Theoretically, the conclusion is that the infant does not need to go through a sequence of stages during which experience provides a prerequisite cognitive basis for invisible imitation.

Meltzoff and Moore's reasons for moving away from naturalistic observations to study imitation illustrate a larger movement among American Piagetians. The objects of their interest are unobservable cognitive structures, and to improve the quality of their inferences about those structures they have moved from unaided observation to instrumented observation. Another trend is illustrated by the way in which Kahn (1975) tested Piaget's account of the developments that permit language use.

Another Small Step: Standardized Testing of Developmental Deviants

According to Piaget, the occurrence of deferred imitation signals the development of the ability to act upon representations of events. That ability, in turn, is required for the development of productive language. Accordingly, children should not speak until they make deferred limitations. Kahn (1975) provided a particularly strong test of this prediction by studying profoundly retarded children, who begin to speak much later than normal children.

Kahn (1975) used naturalistic observations to identify eight profoundly retarded children who spoke 10 or more words, and eight who did not speak at all. Those with spoken language averaged 71 months of age, and those without averaged 67 months, a trivial difference. He administered a standardized scale (Uzgiris and Hunt, 1966) to assess whether the children had achieved Piaget's stage VI of sensorimotor development. One of the subtests of the Uzgiris and Hunt scale measures imitation, and for our purposes we need focus only on it. (Kahn gives reasons for looking at the other subscales.)

Kahn found that none of the eight nonspeaking retarded children passed the test for deferred imitation, but seven of the eight speaking ones did pass. This finding is compelling support for Piaget's analysis, because it shows that deferred imitation is an imposingly accurate predictor of language use even among a group with marked language delays. By studying severely retarded persons, Kahn importantly reduced the chance that unknown age-related processes mediate the correlation between deferred imitation and speaking, thereby strengthening Piaget's theoretical analysis. According to Piaget's analysis, the age at which cognitive accomplishments occur is unimportant; the important thing is their sequencing. Kahn's data show that the sequence of deferred imitation followed by spoken language is invariant across widely varying ages. His findings also suggest that it may be useful to determine where retarded people fall in relation to Piaget's cognitive stages before undertaking to teach language to them.

Methodologically, Kahn's approach illustrates another sort of movement away from simple observation. Investigators need to choose where they will place their effort. Experimenters can let environmental conditions vary freely, after the fashion of ethologists, and put their primary effort into data collation and analysis. Or, they can put their effort into developing ways to constrain behavior during data collection, and spend far less time manipulating their data. When someone else has spent the time developing ways to constrain data collection, investigators can seemingly have the easiest of possible worlds. Standardized tests permit this easy existence, and enough of them have been developed for assessing Piagetian cognitive development that American investigators are now using them in place of natural observations. Thus, Kahn's work illustrates the movement by many students of cognitive development away from observational methods toward the use of standardized tests. A price that they are paying for this easier style of research is that they less often study uncharted behaviors and processes, but to many the price has seemed small.

A Large Step: Cognitive Instruction

The largest departure from the standard observational procedure of the Genevan School is the use of instructions and special experiences to induce forms of thinking before they emerge spontaneously. Various reasons have been given for the rise of this instructional approach to developmental cognitive psychology (cf. Kuhn, 1974; Belmont and Butterfield, 1977). Observing that the instructional movement is confined largely to the United States, Deanna Kuhn raised the ignoble possibility that it was simply a manifestation of that uniquely American fetish for speed, according to which faster is better. There may be some truth to the view that the experimental effort to accelerate cognitive development is driven by the impatient chafing of a pony express mentality against the bridle of Piaget's succession of cognitive stages. But the more illuminating view is that Piaget has laid down theoretical challenges that seem uniquely testable by active manipulations of children's cognition, and he has set a congenial climate for those tests. The shootout between observation and instruction seems to have been provoked by Piaget, not by any uniquely American craziness.

The stimulus for instructional experiments is the standard Genevan tenet that development proceeds sequentially. It is the frequent Piagetian assertion that such and such cognitive accomplishment cannot occur until some other mental milestone has been passed. However, if there is any lesson in the plethora of modern studies on cognitive development, it is that infants and children can do far more, far earlier than anyone would suspect from watching their everyday business. According to Piaget, it is the assimilation of and accommodation to experience that prompts cognitive progress, so it seems inevitable that his assertions of immutable sequencing would be pitted against the test of special experience. That has happened for the various conservations (Brainard and Allen, 1971; Kuhn, 1974) and for headier thought too, like scientific inference (Siegler, Liebert, and Liebert, 1973; Siegler and Liebert, 1975). The approach is well illustrated by the attack of Siegler et al. on the pendulum problem.

The question posed for the child by the pendulum problem is: what determines how long it takes a metal object swinging by a string to move between the tops of its arc? Is it the force of the push that starts the swinging? Is it the weight of the metal object? . . . the length of the string? Inhelder and Piaget (1958) observed that 10, 11, and 12-year-old children almost always conclude that the weight of the object influences the speed with which the object travels. Providing such preadolescents with swinging examples of various string lengths and object weights did not lead them to conclude that string length alone matters. Inhelder and Piaget concluded that sorting out the effects of push force, string length, and object weight requires formal reasoning skills that do not develop until adolescence, and that these formal reasoning skills underlie scientific problem solving. Siegler et al. (1973) saw this conclusion as a challenge to induce scientific thinking. Their question was whether 10 and 11-year-olds lacked formal reasoning abilities or whether they needed simple guidance in how to approach a problem like the swinging pendulum. As it turned out, they needed guidance.

Without any instruction, the 10 and 11-year-olds of Siegler et al., like those of Inhelder and Piaget, failed the pendulum problem. With instruction, they solved it. The instructions concerned how to use a stop watch to measure (*M*) the speed of swinging objects, an explanation of the conceptual framework (*C*) of dimensions and levels of variables and the logic of interpreting main and interactive effects, and practice in solving two problems analogous (*A*) to the pendulum that did not involve motion. None of the three instructions by itself induced correct solutions, but the *AM* and *CM*, as well as the *CAM* combinations did provoke correct solutions. Preadolescents are clearly *able* to solve the pendulum problem. All they need is appropriate instructions. Furthermore, they can quickly be induced to use other sorts of formal reasoning (Siegler and Liebert, 1975). Their problem seems not to be the Piagetian one of having failed to progress to mature stages of conceptual readiness.

Faced with findings of the foregoing sort, champions of the Piagetian school raise an interesting issue, whose resolution of at least one may require a return to heavier reliance upon observational methods. The issue concerns how to distinguish the induction of a particular performance from the promotion of underlying cognitive growth. For Piaget, this is a critical distinction.

Accelerating Cognitive Development versus Improving Task Performance

According to Piaget, cognitive development is a reorganization of cognitive structures. It is not the acquisition of any specific information nor of any particular mental skill. With development, various cognitive operations become amalgamated into new and different wholes or systems, and it is Piaget's contention that development concerns these underlying reorganizations. Therefore, it is not a satisfactory demonstration of departure from invariant sequencing to show that a particular task performance can be taught to children long before they naturally perform it. The argument is a straightforward extension of the deceptively simple assertion that the subject matters of cognitive developmentalists are internal states and processes, not external behaviors.

There is no direct window to cognition. There are only behaviors from which cognition can be inferred. That inferential process is easily corrupted, and one major corruption can occur when experimenters use induced changes in performance to infer induced changes in cognitive development. The corruption comes from the narrowness of the trained behaviors. Inducing mature performance on any particular task is not the same as showing a general cognitive reorganization. Piagetians find it satisfactory to infer general change from the spontaneous emergence of particular behaviors, partly because they can often account for many emerging behaviors by infering a single underlying cognitive reorganization. Instructional experiments almost always show increased performance on one task only, leaving the possibility that the instructions have not created any general cognitive reorganization. One way to see whether particular instructions produce general effects would be to observe uninstructed, naturally occurring cognitive behaviors outside of the laboratory while training a particular task in the laboratory. If theoretically related, naturally occurring behaviors were to emerge along with increased performance on the trained laboratory task, then Piagetians would be more inclined to accept the conclusion that the instruction had accelerated cognitive development (cf. Kuhn, 1974). The need to provide additional bases for interpreting cognitive instructional effects thus might be satisfied by ethological and observational methods. Can it be satisfied that way?

The Problem of Specifying Process

Another way to judge the significance of cognitive instruction is to ask whether it has influenced theoretically important cognitive mechanisms. If not, then one might doubt that the instructions have told us anything important, no matter how impressive the behavioral gains effected and no matter how widely those gains manifest themselves. From this viewpoint, Piagetian instructional experiments have been uninformative. They have not been based on analyses of the mechanisms underlying the behaviors they changed, because Genevan theory does not specify underlying processes that might be trained (Kuhn, 1974). Thus, Siegler et al. (1973) could not design their conceptual, analogue, and measurement instructions to influence particular mechanisms of formal operational thought. They had to base their instructions on the loose observations that 1) modern science is characterized by a reliance on quantitative techniques, experimental analogues, and integrative theoretical principles and 2) solving the pendulum problem requires a scientific sort of approach. Although these authors explicitly questioned Piaget's notion that scientific thinking requires prerequisite cognitive developments that occur after age 10, they could find no adequate specification in Piagetian theory of the specific cognitive mechanisms that they might train to promote earlier scientific thinking. The best they could do was to inculcate special knowledge and procedures that seemed consistent with the way scientists work, and this they did to elicit a particular problem solution from children whose uninstructed performance implied that they had not passed through (unspecified) cognitive stages necessary to solve the problem.

Because Genevans have not specified underlying cognitive mechanisms, comparisons between Piagetian theory and the results of instructional experiments have been very crude. For the same reason, instructional experimenters have had to become a functional bunch. Their functionalism can be seen in the following quote, in which Hall et al. grouse at cognitive theorists and advise cognitive researchers all at once.

> When capacity limitations are implied or stages hypothesized, . . . (one) must investigate and rule out alternative explanations. A more plausible solution to employ when a task proves too difficult for a group of subjects is to continue searching for other possible training conditions rather than using labels (such as maturation) as explanations. One strategy for looking at these other possibilities is to employ a detailed analysis of the criterion task (Hall, Salvi, Seggev, and Caldwell, 1970, p. 427).

A fair paraphrase of this passage is as follows. Do not look to cognitive theory for a specification of why particular behavioral developments occur when they do. Look instead to functional analyses of particular tasks, and try various ways to improve performance of children who normally do those tasks poorly. Because analysis of processes that underlie task performance is largely a laboratory effort, following this advice seems to lead away from observational methods, which is precisely the opposite direction suggested by the Piagetian reaction to the instructional approach (see "The Problem of Specifying Process" above or Kuhn, 1974). The route of task analysis is being pursued vigorously by cognitively oriented experimental child psychologists. After seeing why, it will be possible to judge better the possible contributions of both observational and laboratory approaches to cognitive development.

TRENDS WITHIN EXPERIMENTAL CHILD PSYCHOLOGY

Experimental child psychology can be distinguished by its sources from developmental psychology of the Piagetian sort. It grows from basic science laboratory efforts to understand human adult functioning, rather than from observational efforts to understand children's behavior. Observational methods have never been particularly important to experimental child psychology. Like Piagetians, experimental child psychologists have been concerned with behavior's underpinnings, but they have not depended on establishing invariant sequences to justify their inferences.

Use of Interactions to Define Processes

Before the mid-1960's, correlations of age or intelligence with performance on single tasks were often attributed to process differences among children of different ages or IQ's. Then, experimental child psychologists were introduced to the alternative of showing interactions between experimentally manipulated variables and age (Gollin, 1965) or intelligence (Baumeister, 1967). The notion was that simple age and IQ effects implicate no process, but interactions with manipulated variables do allow inferences about particular processes that distinguish age and IQ groups. The argument simply extends the idea that processes themselves are defined by experimental interactions. This latter idea is illustrated by the way experimental adult psychologists came to distinguish primary from secondary memory.

Experimentalists of the verbal learning persuasion had long studied adults' recall of serially presented lists of digits, letters, nonsense syllables, words, etc. They knew that the bowed serial learning curve was one of the most reliable laboratory phenomena in psychology. Many experiments had shown that adults recall least accurately from the middle serial positions of lists, more accurately from the initial serial positions than from the middle ones, and most accurately from the terminal positions. For years, adult experimentalists tried to account for this main effect of serial position by invoking variants of the notion of conditioned associations between adjacent items. But even sophisticated mathematized versions of such single process ideas failed to account for variations in the basic bowing of the serial position curve that result from changing presentation conditions and recall requirements. For example, changing the rate at which the lists' items were presented changed recall accuracy primarily at the early and middle serial positions. Slower presentation rates gave higher recall at these serial positions, but changes in rate had little effect on recall at terminal positions. Interpolating attention-consuming activities between list presentation and recall produced another sort of interaction with serial position; recall accuracy was decreased by interpolated activities, but almost exclusively at the terminal positions.

The effects of presentation rate and interpolated activity illustrate that the initial and terminal portions of the serial learning curve are influenced differently by many experimental variables. Interactions of experimental variables and serial position eventually drove adult experimentalists to advance multiprocess accounts of the bowed serial learning curve. Performance on the terminal portions of serial lists was attributed to primary memory, which is short-lived and depends upon relatively passive input operations. Performance on the early portions of serial lists was attributed to secondary memory, which is long-lived and depends upon active input operations generally referred to as rehearsal. The distinction between primary and secondary memory seems roughly equivalent to the long-standing distinction between short and long term memory, but it is based on interactive evidence of a discontinuity in underlying process rather than on the simple operational distinction between experiments that use short retention intervals and experiments that use long ones. Experimental adult psychologists conclude these days that distinct underlying mechanisms are at work when experimental manipulations interact with one another, and experimental child psychologists have adapted this interactive strategy to isolate developmental changes in underlying psychological mechanisms.

Isolating Processes that Develop

Ellis's (1970) research on the relationship between intelligence and memory performance illustrates the approach. He administered a sort of serial recall task to average and retarded people, and he varied the items' presentation rate. He observed an interaction between intellectual level, presentation rate, and serial position, and from this interaction he inferred process differences between people of different intellectual levels. Figure 1 shows his findings.

Ellis used lists containing 9 digits, each of which was presented for 0.5 seconds. There was no interval between digits in the massed condition, whereas 2.0 seconds intervened between each digit under the spaced condition. These presentation rates made a marked difference for the normal people, whose recall was much more accurate at the early and middle positions under the spaced condition. No such difference was observed for the retarded people, who recalled inaccurately under both massed and spaced presentation. Normal and retarded people both recalled highly accurately at the terminal serial positions under both presentation rates. From this pattern of results, Ellis inferred that average and retarded people differ hardly at all with respect to primary memory, but that they differ markedly with respect to secondary memory. Since adults' secondary memory presumably depends upon rehearsal, he concluded that retarded people have a rehearsal deficit that might account for poor performance in a variety of behavioral domains.

Ellis's approach is entirely representative of child psychology experiments. It is a large advance over simply correlating age and task performances. Still, it is highly inferential, that is, indirect. The indirectness can be seen in the fact that the explanatory process invoked concerns mechanisms that operate during list learning, but the dependent measures were taken well after that learning was completed. Measures taken during learning would be more direct, and they would be less subject to distortions introduced by mechanisms of forgetting and information retrieval.

Beyond Interactions: Direct Measurement

Belmont and Butterfield (1969, 1971a, b) are among the investigators who have advocated more direct measurement procedures to study cognitive development. This may be

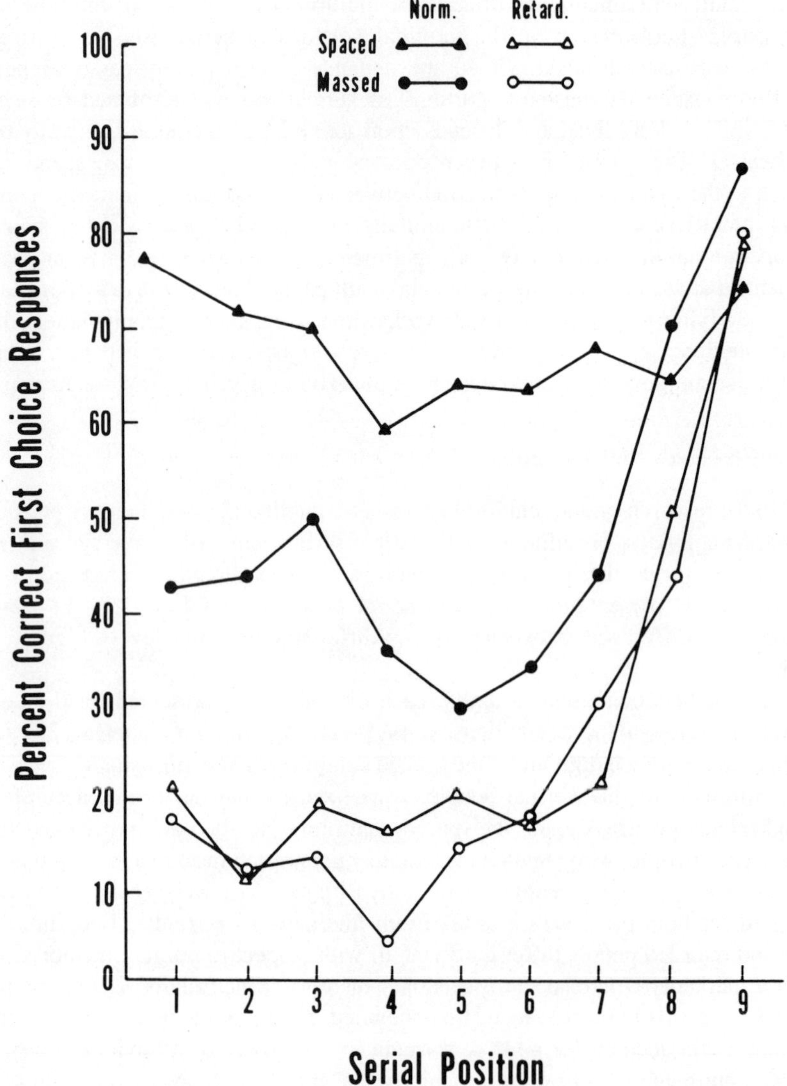

Figure 1. Recall of normal and retarded people following massed or spaced input. (Ellis, 1970.)

seen in the following quotation, in which the term *primacy* refers to recall from early and middle positions.

> . . . primacy performance depends at least partially upon the rate at which *E* presents the items of a serial list. The faster the stimuli appear, the weaker the primacy. The consensus is that slow presentation rates permit more rehearsal than fast presentation rates, and it is the greater rehearsal permitted under slow rates that results in greater primacy. Following this line of reasoning, Ellis (1970) has concluded that mentally retardeds, who exhibit equally poor primacy under fast or slow presentation, must simply not be rehearsing even when given

> sufficient time. The deficiency in recall accuracy thus translates into a hypothetical rehearsal deficiency, and what is now required is to collect hard data support for this hypothesis. One ought to be able, after all, to document the deficiency by directly measuring the retardeds' learning strategies and comparing them with learning strategies produced by normals who are given the same task (Belmont and Butterfield, 1971a, pp. 411, 412).

In order to measure rehearsal strategies more directly, Belmont and Butterfield gave retarded and normal people control over the presentation of items in a serial list. The items themselves appeared briefly, and only the time spent between them was measured. The total such time for a list was taken as an index of the amount of learning activity expended by the subjects. Belmont and Butterfield (1969, 1971a, b) found that normal people spend more time than retarded ones, which is a relatively direct confirmation of the proposition that normal people rehearse more. Moreover, normal adults spent more time than normal children, and within all age and IQ groups, people who spent more time recalled more accurately. Furthermore, plotting time spent between items against their serial positions indicated that active learners used their time to study the early and middle items in the lists, not the terminal ones. This is precisely what they should do according to the theoretical distinction between primary and secondary memory, but it could not have been seen with less direct methods.

Relatively direct measurement has been used in enough child psychology experiments (e.g., Flavell, Beach, and Chinsky, 1966; Milgram, 1968; Taylor, Josberger, and Knowlton, 1972; Turnure, Buium, and Thurlow, 1975) to prompt the conclusion that it is a premier technique in developmental child psychology (Belmont and Butterfield, 1977). But the significance of direct measurement is not that focusing as precisely as possible upon one's object of study is inevitably more informative than more inferential methods. Its main significance is that direct measurement has fostered a peculiarly fecund combination of process analysis and instructional experimentation. This can be seen in the long line of research into normal children's use of verbal mediators. The line began before 1940 with Vygotsky's and Luria's notions about the verbal control of behavior, which it took more than 20 years to bring to the test of direct measurement (Flavell et al., 1966). Thereafter, it took only 10 years for the results to send experimental child psychologists far down entirely new research highways using radically different signposts to judge their progress (Brown, 1974; Butterfield and Belmont, 1977; Flavell and Wellman, 1977). Where before the benchmark was a statistically significant interaction, now various standards are being used, including proportion of variance accounted and the magnitude, durability, or transfer of instructional effect achieved.

Mediation and Production Deficiencies

The mediational issue was introduced into American experimental literature by Kuenne (1946). Like many experimental child psychologists, she fashioned her dependent measures after those of laboratory scientists who had never studied children. Her question concerned the relation of age to size transposition. Children were first rewarded for selecting one of two squares that differed in size. Once they consistently selected the rewarded square, for instance the smaller one, they were given a transposition test, in which the children were rewarded for selecting the smaller of another two squares. Older children solved the second problem more rapidly than the first, but the younger ones did not. Kuenne attributed the older children's performance gain to their use of verbal mediation. But since she did not measure verbal behavior, there was an essential ambiguity about Kuenne's conclusion that the young child "is able to make differential verbal responses . . . but this does not control or influence his . . . behavior." She knew that even her youngest subjects could say which square was smaller. But failing to measure whether they did so during the experiment left pertinent questions unanswered. Could it be that younger and older children make precisely the same covert verbal responses, which are only effective mediators for the older children because of the greater development of some mechanism in their central nervous system? Or perhaps the system is developed, but the responses of the younger children are not appropriate. Or perhaps the younger children's responses to size cues are appropriate, but they fail to make them in the experimental situation.

Twenty more years of research clarified the issue only a little. The Kendlers used discrimination procedures similar to those of Kuenne, and although their transfer tests were more sophisticated than Kuenne's transposition tests, they too failed to measure verbal behavior (Kendler, Kendler, and Wells, 1960). A substantial literature on paired associates learning managed no more direct a look at the mechanism responsible for older children's quicker learning (cf. Reese, 1962). Young children still seemed mediationally deficient, but no one knew precisely what that meant. By 1964, the issue of whether and how children mediate verbally must surely have become tedious, but Maccoby reviewed the voluminous literature and suggested that young children possess mediators which they do not produce unless "experimental situations are arranged so the relevant verbalizations will be elicited." The sticking point was that practically no one had any idea what constituted a relevant verbalization for any laboratory task. Before the production deficiency hypothesis could be tested by eliciting relevant verbalizations, someone needed to determine what they were for some experimental task.

Flavell et al. (1966) arranged to observe children's lips during a developmental memory experiment. Lip reading neither interfered with nor even required knowledge of children's recall, but it showed what children with accurate recall said to themselves as they prepared for memory tests. Armed with this knowledge, Flavell and his colleagues elicited verbalizations from children who did not recall accurately, thereby effecting marked increases in their memory performances (cf. Flavell, 1970). This strategy has been generalized widely: having measured or otherwise determined what produces good task performance, poor performers are instructed. Although not always successful, cognitive instruction has worked well enough, often enough to convince experimental child psychologists that children suffer few if any mediation deficiencies. Theirs are deficiencies of production. They possess cognitive subroutines that they fail to call up and combine. Resnick and Glaser (1975) put it this way:

> In each of the studies . . . the subjects demonstrated unequivocally that they could competently perform each of the routines necessary for solving the presented problems. Not only did they pass pretests on the component routines; but in every instance, direct prompting of the transformation routine was sufficient to promote full solution of the task if the child had not "invented" the solution himself. Yet many did not invent. The routines were available but not accessible when needed.

Independently, we made the same argument:

> Clearly, the retarded subjects' passive (primary) memory capacity is not greatly impaired, for if it were they could not have rehearsed the 3 letters accurately. Clearly, too, they can rehearse, and having rehearsed, they can recall accurately even after doing an interfering task that seems at least as disruptive as attending passively to 3 letters. Yet, . . . they recalled accurately only when they were also instructed to use a retrieval strategy appropriate to the instructed learning strategy. These retarded subjects did not lack the memory processes. . . . What they did lack was spontaneous access to the processes and coordination among them (Butterfield, Wambold, and Belmont, 1973, p. 688).

Rohwer (1973, p. 9) generalized the conclusion across people:

> . . . the underlying elaboration process is . . . common to virtually all people (except infants); what varies across persons is the type of prompt necessary to activate the process.

Similarly, Morrison, Holmes, and Haith (1974, p. 424) concluded:

> . . . to use a computer metaphor, the basic "hardware" of visual memory seemed to exist at all age levels.

Butterfield and Belmont (1977) generalized across tasks:

> . . . if a task solution plan is given to the child, he will perform as if he had invented the strategy himself.

These quotes are marvelous in view of the Piagetian demurrers on cognitive training (see "The Problem of Specifying Process"). Unlike Piagetians, experimental child psychologists see little reason to question the importance of instructional effects. This is partly because the experimentalists' tradition gives them no theoretical commitment to the view that development is limited by the rate of underlying cognitive reorganization. Probably more important, direct measurement and process analyses give experimentalists reason to believe that they have specified the underlying mechanisms that they instruct, and the effects of instruction strengthen that view. Instead of questioning their instructional effects, experimentalists have asked why young children so often fail to use processes that work so well for them. To find out, experimental child psychologists have gone off in quest of metamemory (Flavell and Wellman, 1977), the executive functions of cognition (Butterfield and Belmont, 1977) and the development of knowing about knowing (Brown, 1975). The hunt has bagged impressive game, but there are indications too that grave problems of method have been flushed into the open along with the quarries. Consider the catch and then the problems.

Beyond Production Deficiencies: Metamemory

Having seen how easily children can be induced to use effective memory mechanisms, Flavell (1971) suggested that their problem was partly one of metamemory. Since they could do mnemonically effective things when instructed, their failure to do so when invited only by the presentation of problems and arrangements of materials might mean that they lack knowledge about 1) their own capabilities, 2) the mnemonic requirements of different tasks, and 3) potential strategies for meeting task demands and for capitalizing on one's own capabilities (Flavell and Wellman, 1977). The hypothesis is that children may not rise to the challenges of memory tasks until they understand when and why they should intentionally store and retrieve information, and this metamemoric understanding may develop slowly. Many intriguing questions arise from this view.

When do children first sense the objective need for efforts to retrieve information from memory and the need to actively prepare for future retrieval? What sorts of memory mechanisms do they use before they sense the need for deliberate mnemonic behavior? When do children realize that what they do not remember easily may come to mind if they concentrate or think more about it? When do they distinguish things they do not remember from things they did not know in the first place, and when do they use this distinction to decide whether to continue trying to recall something? What standards do people use to decide to stop trying to remember something they know they know, and when do children apply those standards? When can children accurately estimate how well they will remember, and how do they decide that they have prepared sufficiently for later recall? When does a child understand that parental injunctions to remember such and such later are requests to have intellectual commerce with such and such now? When do children appreciate the distinction between veridical memory for events and inferential memory with which unexperienced events are constructed from memories of experienced ones? Do children appreciate the need to prepare for future recall long before they make such preparations? Do children appreciate the utility of providing themselves with external memory aids (e.g., putting completed homework next to the front door to guarantee seeing it and taking it to class) before they appreciate the utility of internal memory aids (e.g., visualizing a completed homework assignment tied with a bright bow to the front door knob)?

Research questions like these might be approached experimentally in the laboratory, by interview or, in some cases, observationally. In fact, interview and experimental techniques dominate the metamemory literature. Interview techniques have seldom been used by experimental child psychologists, but questions of metamemory concern what people know more than what people do, so interviews are reasonable tools, and they are being used more often. Their use is well illustrated in the monograph by Kreutzer, Leonard, and Flavell (1976).

Kreutzer et al. interviewed 20 children from each of four ages: 6, 7, 9, and 11 years. The interview concerned five sorts of metamemory: 1) knowledge about the temporary and enduring attributes and states of people that influence their retrieval of information; 2) knowledge about the properties of information which influences its retrievability; 3) knowledge of what to do with information to influence its subsequent retrieval; 4) knowledge of what to do in order to retrieve information previously stored in memory; and 5) knowledge of the effects of different sorts of retrieval tests (e.g., recall versus recognition). The richness and extent of the findings by Kreutzer et al. defy succinct description. Here are a few of their conclusions: Even 6-year-olds have substantial knowledge in all five metamemory categories. They have some appreciation that information is lost rapidly from short term memory; that previously learned but forgotten information can be relearned more easily than it was originally acquired; that the amount of past preparation influences the amount of present recall; and that the familiarity and number of items to be studied affects how well they will later be recalled. As for developmental trends, older children were more aware that accurate recall often depends upon the use of deliberate and systematic input and retrieval efforts, and they were considerably more aware that relationships among pieces of information affect their recall. Like so many of Flavell's undertakings, this study will have great impact upon students of cognitive development, and the reader who is interested beyond seeing that interviews are now used in experimental child psychology should see the full report (Kreutzer, Leonard, and Flavell, 1976).

Interview approaches have the disadvantage that one never knows how fully children understand the premises of the questions posed. Younger children especially might not grasp hypothetical situations, and if they do not, then their answers are misleading (Flavell and Wellman, 1977). Yussen and Levy (1975) combined an experimental and interview procedure in a way that should have minimized this problem. Their 5, 9, and 20-year-old subjects were shown sequences of pictures at the rate of one picture per sec. The sequences varied from one to ten pictures. Having seen a sequence, the subjects were asked to predict if they could recall the names of the pictures they had just seen. The dependent measure was the length of the longest sequence the subject predicted he could recall. Predicted recall length *decreased* with age. The younger children believed they could recall longer sequences than the older children. The next step was to test recall. The length of the sequences actually recalled *increased* with age. The average sequence length that the youngest children recalled correctly was 3.29. Their predicted recall length was 8.12. Moreover, following recall, during which it should have been clear that they had not recalled sequences as long as 8, 9, or 10, several of the youngest subjects nevertheless asserted that they could recall 9 or 10 items if they were given another chance. Under the conditions of this experiment, the average sequence length recalled correctly by the 20-year-olds was 5.9. Clearly, the youngest subjects were not in touch with their own memory functioning nor with the difficulty of the task they had just experienced. Data like these are compelling evidence that metamemory develops, but they do not say whether that development has anything to do with age-related increases in recall accuracy. Are metamemorics post hoc epiphenomena, or do they influence performance?

To see whether metamemory is epiphenomenal, one must collect recall and metamemory measures from each experimental subject. The epiphenomenon question is tested by correlating the measures. Calculating the correlation is essential. Appel et al. (1972) observed study behaviors that index children's awareness that memory requires deliberate activity, which seems a matter of metamemory. Study behavior and the children's recall accuracy both increased with age, suggesting that metamemory and recall are correlated, which in fact they were not. So far as the data from Appel et al. can say, metamemory is an epiphenomenon; it is unrelated to accuracy.

A chief advantage of the laboratory approach is that it permits special arrangements to increase power of measurement. Regarding metamemory, this advantage was not well realized in the study by Appel et al. as they made no special provision to measure study behavior. They simply watched for spontaneous overt evidence of study. All covert study went undetected, and that might account for the failure to observe a relationship between recall and metamemory as indexed by study behavior. Belmont and Butterfield have employed measures that do capture covert study behaviors (Belmont and Butterfield, 1969; 1971a, b; Butterfield and Belmont, 1972; 1977).

Beyond Production Deficiencies: Executive Functions

In an effort to come to grips with why children do not use cognitive tactics that work for them, Belmont and Butterfield eschewed reference to knowledge about cognition in favor of looking at behavioral indices of executive functions of cognition. Contemporary theorists (Atkinson and Shiffrin, 1968; Greeno and Bjork, 1973; Reitman, 1970) distinguish control processes, by which they mean something like cognitive tactics, from the executive functions, which are responsible for organizing the control processes into strategies. The control processes with which Belmont and Butterfield have been concerned are 1) attention to and 2) rehearsal of material to be recalled later. By measuring how long people spend following their own exposure of serially occurring items, it has been shown that they combine attention and rehearsal into distinctive strategies, the character of which varies with memory requirement and age (Belmont and Butterfield, 1971b). Because the executive functions are responsible for combining tactics into strategies, the measurement procedures that reflect strategic behavior have been used to index the executive. The executive function has been examined by changing the requirements of memory tasks and measuring how people change their strategies. We consider that the executive function is exhibited when a person spontaneously changes a control process or sequence of control processes in reasonable response to an objective change in an information processing task (Butterfield and Belmont, 1977). With this approach, the epiphenomenon question can be answered without measuring what the subject knows. The test is to determine whether indices of executive functions that are operationally independent of recall accuracy, nevertheless predict accuracy. The results of such a test have never been reported, but the data which enable one have been collected (Butterfield and Belmont, 1977). The pertinent experiment can be appreciated by referring to Figure 2.

The experiment had 37 trials, during each of which an eight-word list was studied for subsequent recall. Each of the first nine trials, data from which are shown in the top panel of Figure 2, was composed of a unique list, as none of their words appeared in any other list. On each of the next nine trials, shown in the second panel from the top, a single list was presented over and over again. For the next seven trials, shown in the third panel from the top (Figure 2), seven new unique lists were presented. For the final 12 trials, another list was presented repeatedly, except that on trials 31 and 37 new words were introduced at two positions in the otherwise familiar list. Thus, on trial 37, the first two words had not been seen in this experiment, but the remaining six words were the same as those used on trials 26 through 30. On trial 31, the fourth and fifth words were new to the otherwise familiar list.

Extensive analysis of this memory task (Belmont and Butterfield, 1969; 1971a, b; Butterfield and Belmont, 1972; Butterfield, Peltzman, and Belmont, 1971; Butterfield, Belmont, and Peltzman, 1971; Kellas and Butterfield, 1971; Butterfield, Wambold, and Belmont, 1973) led us to require recall in a circular order, beginning with the sixth serial position and proceeding in the order 6-7-8-1-2-3-4-5. (The numbers designate the order in which the words appeared during study.) Our task analyses told us that this recall requirement is best satisfied by cumulative rehearsal of the first five words and simple attention to the last three words. On each trial with a novel list, subjects who correctly diagnose the processing demands of the circular recall requirement should pause increas-

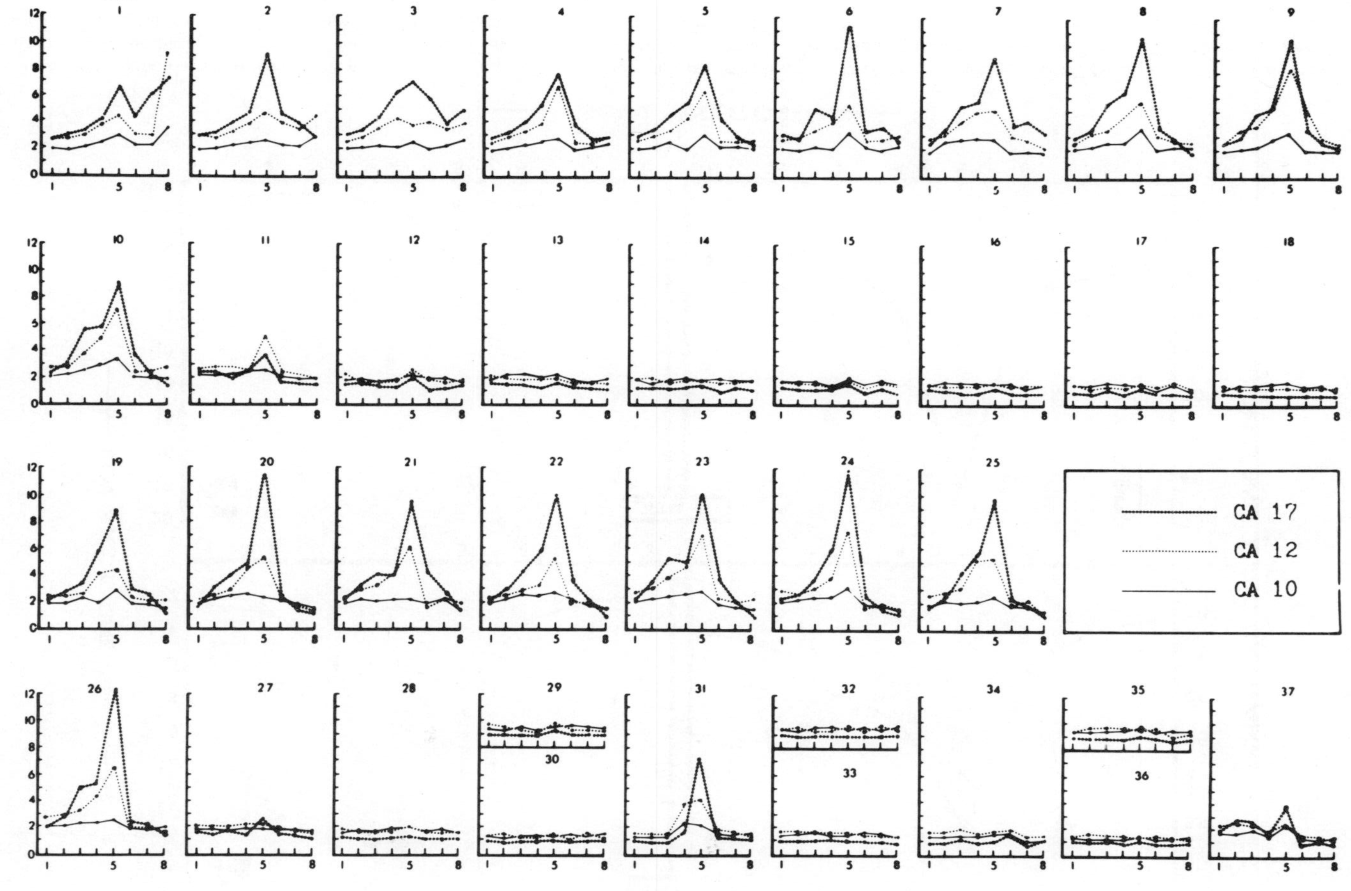

Figure 2. Input pause times for 10, 12, and 17-year-olds. (Adapted from Butterfield and Belmont, 1977.

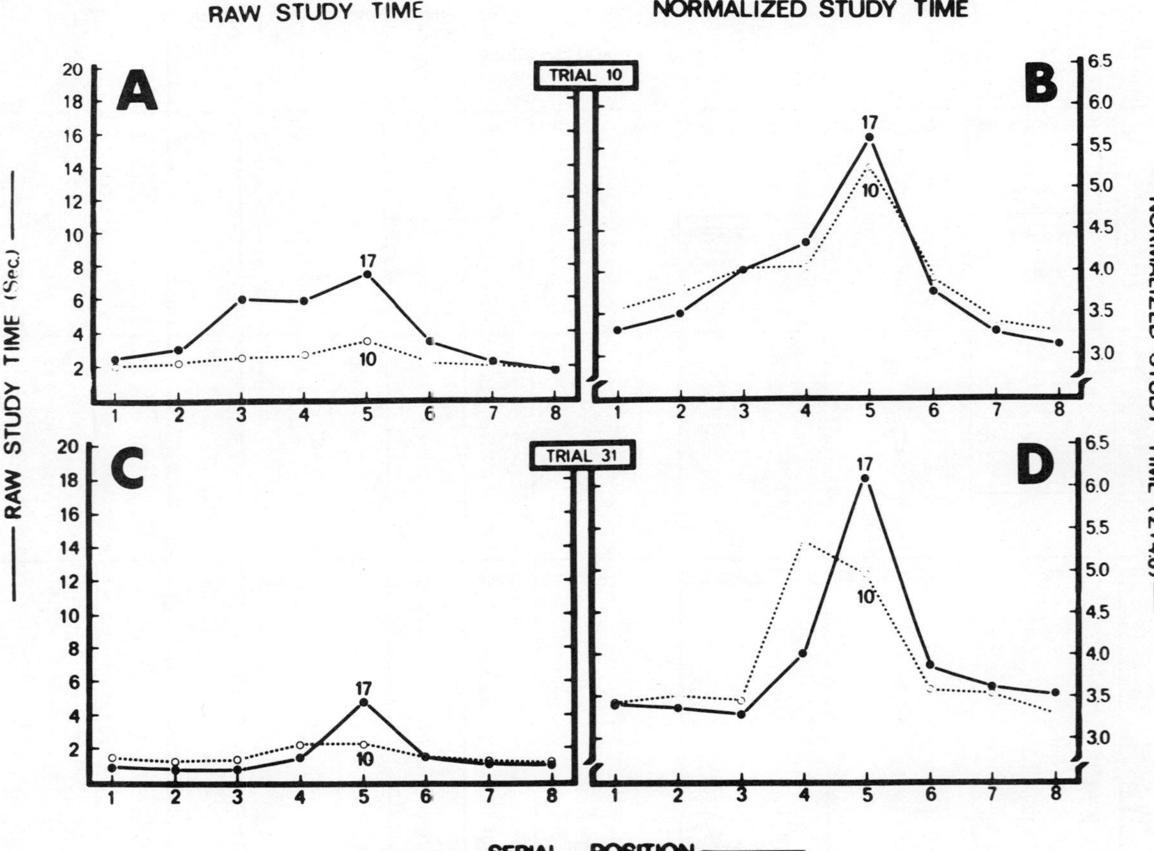

Figure 3. A: trial 10 median ad lib study-time patterns for children (10) and youth (17) under instructions to recall last three words of list followed by first five; B: same data normalized to show similarity of forms independent of level; C: study-time patterns later on (trial 31) for a highly overlearned list in which novel words unexpectedly appear at positions 4 and 5; D: same data normalized to show dissimilarity of children's and youth's responses to novel words.

ingly from serial positions 1 through 5, but at positions 6 through 8, they should pause only long enough to attend to the items. Since lists that have already been learned need not be rehearsed, mature processors should abandon their pausing during the repeated lists (e.g., trials 11 to 18).

There were 80 subjects, 20 each at ages 10, 11, 12, and 17. They paced themselves through the lists, and they were free to pause as long as they chose at any serial position. Figure 2 shows the average pause patterns for the 10, 12, and 17-year-olds. The first thing to notice is that total study time for the unique lists (trials 1 to 10 and 19 to 25) increased with age. Averaging across trials 6 to 10, the mean number of seconds per trial was 22.2, 32.5, 35.6, and 43.0 for the 10, 11, 12, and 17-year-olds, respectively. For the 80 subjects as a group, average study time for these trials ranged from 12.7 to 104.6 seconds. Because all subjects decreased their study time to nil for the repeated lists, it can be inferred that time spent is an index of the subjects' assessment of the amount of effort required by the task, and it is a reflection of executive functions. The second thing to notice is that the shape of the pause patterns changes systematically across the first several trials of the experiment, and the shape gradually approximates the form predicted as a result of task analyses. The number of trials required for that approximation decreases with age, but by trial 10, all age groups paused increasingly long up to position 5, and then went rapidly through the remainder of the lists. In Figure 2, this is clearest for the 17-year-olds, who spent more time overall. Eliminating total time differences by converting each subject's trial 10 pause times to standard scores, and plotting the averages of these against serial position, shows that all age groups distribute their time according to the expected pattern (see Figure 3, A and B). The third piece of pertinent background concerns trials 9, 18, and 19. On trial 18, no group showed any differential pausing, since they had already learned the list. On trial 19, the groups showed patterns of pausing that are more or less similar to the patterns of trial 9. The similarity was greater for the older group. The similarity between the pattern on trial 19 and the one on trial 9 reflects the executive function called strategy reinstatement. Finally, note that the groups departed from their low flat pause patterns on trials 31 and 37, showing what can be called strategy modification. It is a modification in the sense that the pause pattern is different from the patterns used both for entirely unique lists (e.g., trials 6 through 10) and for well learned lists (e.g., trials 30, 32, and 36). Moreover, the form of the modification depends upon where in the familiar list the two new items were inserted. The form of the modification also varied with age, and a closer look at that fact is given in Figure 3, C and D.

The data shown in Figure 2 and 3 illustrate four sorts of executive functions, each of which shows development: 1) effort selection, indexed by total study time; 2) strategy selection, indexed by the distribution of times across serial position during the first ten trials; 3) strategy reinstatement, seen in the similarity between the initially selected strategy and the one used on trial 19; and 4) strategy modification, indexed by the pause patterns on the partly new lists of trials 31 and 37. Accuracy also increases with age. For example, the average number of words correctly recalled on trials 6 through 10 was 22, 24, 28, and 32 for the 10, 11, 12, and 17-year-olds, respectively (the maximum possible correct was 40). The correlations between age and accuracy and between age and executive functions suggest that executive functioning and accuracy are related, but to answer the epiphenomenon question directly, indices of accuracy and executive functions must be correlated directly. To do that, multiple correlations were calculated in which recall accuracy was the criterion measure and four executive functions were the predictors.

The total number of words recalled correctly on trials 6 to 10 was the dependent measure. The maximum possible score was thus 40, and the observed scores ranged from 12 to 40. Indices of two of the executive functions were derived directly from the data summarized in Figure 2. The measure called effort selection was the mean total pause time on trials 6 through 10. The measure called reinstatement was derived by calculating omega square (w^2) between the normalized pause pattern of trial 19 and the normalized patterns on each of trials 7, 8, 9, and 10. The w^2 expresses the similarity between two pause patterns as a variance ratio that can range from 0 to 10. The larger the ratio, the moresimilar the patterns. Our predictor was the highest w^2 of the four calculated between trials 7:19, 8:19, 9:19, and 10:19. The use of normalized scores in these calculations assured that variability in total time did not influence the w^2 computations. Indices of the other two executive functions were derived from w^2 comparisons of data summarized in Figure 2 with what we call ideal standards. The strategy selection index was a measure of how closely each subject approximated the theoretically ideal strategy for the circular recall requirement of this experiment. The modification index was a measure of how closely the subject's pause pattern on trials 31 and 37 approximated the modification of a mature information processor who had used the theoretically ideal strategy on all of the unique lists in the experiment. To quantify the selection and modification ideals, the experiment summarized in Figure 2 was repeated with 20 adults who were instructed to use cumulative rehearsal for the first five words and simple attention for the last three. The average pause pattern produced by these instructed adults on trials 25, the last unique list in the experiment, was converted to standard scores. Then w^2 values were calculated between these values and each subject's standardized pause patterns on trials 8, 9, and 10. The sum of these three values was taken as an index of the extent to which each subject selected the ideal circular strategy. A similar procedure was used for trials 31 and 37, yielding an index of the extent to which each subject selected ideal modifications of his basic strategy. Notice that each of the predictor variables is derived from data that is operationally independent of recall accuracy.

Multiple correlations were calculated separately for each age group, leaving no possibility that unknown age-related factors might mediate any observed correlation. Also, the computations within each group stand as replication tests for the other groups. For the 17-year-old subjects, $R = 0.75$, indicating that 57% of the variance in recall accuracy is accountable in terms of the four executive functions. Executive functions are not epiphenomena. The variance accounted among the 12, 11, and 10-year groups was 42%, 47%, and 25%, respectively. Only the 10-year-old correlation was unreliable ($p > 0.05$). Since the 10-year-olds were the youngest subjects tested, the interpretation is that they had not yet developed effective executive functions. This interpretation is bolstered by the data in Figure 2 (cf. Butterfield and Belmont, 1977).

Reprise

Like experimental psychologists who study adults, child experimentalists have adopted the idea that unobservable processes are defined empirically by interactions among experimental variables. To determine whether development can be characterized as changes in underlying processes, experimental child psychologists have sought interactions between experimental variables and either age or IQ. Their selection of experimental variables has frequently been based on the results of process anlyses of adult cognition. The question has been whether processes isolated in adult performance emerge during development. The approach of adult experimentalists has been highly inferential, and that has been true of much developmental research too. Lately, however, there has been more effort to measure processes as directly as possible. Although there is no way to look exactly at underlying meachanisms, increasing the directness with which they are measured has provided bases for instructing children who do not spontaneously use mature processes. These instructional efforts have easily effected major increases in children's cognitive performance. The interpretation has been that children do not lack the basic cognitive tactics required for mature performance. Instead, they somehow fail to produce these tactics unless explicitly directed to do so. In order to account for such production deficiencies, many experimental child psychologists have shifted their focus to a higher level of theoretical abstraction. One question has been whether children fail to produce because they lack knowledge of their own cognitive apparatus and of the requirements of problems posed by their environment. To answer this question, experimental child psychologists have focused on knowledge about memory problems and mechanisms, which knowledge is called metamemory. Neither adult nor child psychologists have often focused upon knowledge, and neither the method of seeking interactions with age nor the methods of task analysis and cognitive instruction are well suited to the purpose of exposing metamemory. The methodological response has been to depend increasingly upon interviewing children, taking experimental child psychologists away from their procedural forte. Perhaps as a consequence of this, or perhaps because of a desire to pursue as rapidly as possible fascinating new findings that have emerged from querying children, several loose ends have been left dangling. One of these concerns the question of whether metamemory matters as regards children's performance. As if to answer this question, investigators have remarked that knowledge about memory problems and performance on them both increase with age. But there are empirical demonstrations in the literature of the statistical fact of life that correlating knowledge and performance with age does not justify the inference that knowledge and performance themselves covary. To tie up this loose end, some investigators have turned to the study of executive functions, which they have defined in terms of measurements that are independent of recall accuracy. Securing operational measures of executive functions has required a reliance on detailed analyses of standard laboratory tasks. This has brought experimental psychologists back to their procedural strengths, but it has also kept them away from new substantive areas of investigation, which concern knowledge, meaning, semantic memory, and other complex processes. Nevertheless, the study of executive functions has established that some higher level cognitive processes not only develop, but also importantly account for information processing accuracy, independently of age.

APPRAISAL OF THE EXPERIMENTAL APPROACH TO CHILDREN'S COGNITION

One other set of considerations seems relevant to seeing how experimental and observational methods might be combined to study cognitive development. These concern limits on the experimental study of thinking by children and mentally retarded people. Since recent developments in experimental child psychology have stemmed from the apparent success of cognitive instructional experiments, we may as well begin with a problem of interpreting instructional effects.

The Unrealized Logic of Instructional Experiments

Huttenlocker and Burke (1976) recently reported an experiment with which they attempted to clarify the development of memory input mechanisms by looking instead at recall output. As Newell (1973) and Allport (1975) have shown, it frequently happens in the report of such influential experiments that the discussion of results is tortuously reasoned and nearly interminable, because indirect methods leave enormous room for undisciplined speculation about what might account for the results obtained. So it was with Huttenlocker and Burke, but they nevertheless made one telling argument, the general form of which should sober any investigator who would use cognitive instruction. Concerning the use of training to clarify memory differences between groups of people differing in age or intelligence, these authors say:

> The hypothesis that differences in rehearsal account for differences in recall in different population groups is more directly tested through the training approach. That is, it would be support for the hypothesis if one found greater effects of forced rehearsal for groups whose recall is poor. On the other hand, if forced rehearsal helps all population groups equally, the hypothesis would be disconfirmed. Most forced rehearsal studies have not reported such differential effects of training, nor has the issue been explicitly considered in interpretations of data. (Huttenlocker and Burke, 1976, p. 19)

The general argument is that instructed processes can be invoked as explanations of age or other group differences only if identical instructions are applied to various groups, and then only if the instructions leave the groups performing at identical levels. The effect of the instructions can be to lower the performance of the more accurate group or to raise the performance of the less accurate group. However, if after instruction there remain reliable differences between the groups, then the processes affected by the instructions may not be responsible for the differences between the groups under uninstructed conditions. In the case where instructions are intended to improve poor performance, the notion is that groups who naturally perform better are already using the instructed processes, but the groups who perform poorly are not. Therefore, the more accurate group should benefit little or none from the instructions, but the less accurate group should benefit greatly. Conversely, in the case where the instructions are intended to eliminate the processing thought to account for accurate performance, the inaccurate performers should be impaired relatively little, since they are presumably not using the target processes anyway. If the goal is to account for why young children or retarded people perform inaccurately, then the instructional approach requires that older or normal people be instructed along with the younger or retarded ones.

Most instructional experiments have not included older or more normal groups (e.g., Butterfield et al., 1973). Even those experiments that have included appropriate comparison groups have usually failed to eliminate differences between or even to affect differentially the accurate and inaccurate processors (e.g., Belmont and Butterfield, 1971).

This implies that children may be no more production deficient than adults. No evidence refutes this implication completely, although there is reason to doubt its strong form, which is that experimental child psychology has made no progress in accounting for memory development.

Consider further the data described above to show that executive functions predict recall accuracy. Eighty people contributed data, and they ranged in age from 127 to 232 months. The correlation between age and accuracy on trials 6 through 10 was 0.51. That value seems small, but it is probably representative of experimental studies of memory development, which invariably report their effects as means of groups leveled on age, rather than as correlations. The mean age effects in our data (see p.157) seem every bit as large as those in the literature. This problem of nomothetics is discussed next. However, the current question is can the size of this correlation be importantly reduced by partialling out of it the measures of executive functioning that were shown above to account for performance within age groups?

The answer is that the variance shared by age and accuracy is more than halved by partialling out the four executive functions defined above (p.157). The square of the correlation between age and accuracy is reduced from 0.27 to 0.13. Despite the fact that this latter value is nor reliably greater than zero, we are not inclined to claim that we have completely accounted for the development of memory as measured by the circular recall task. In the first place, the four executive functions that reduce the correlation account for only half of the variance in adults' circular recall. Also, all of these functions are derived from measures of input activity. It is known that output processes also have substantial effects upon recall in very similar memory tasks (Butterfield and Belmont, 1971) and that instructing output causes further improvements in mentally retarded people's recall beyond instructing input alone (Butterfield et al., 1973). The challenge is to account for *all* of the variance in recall both between and within age and IQ groups. No process analysis of any sort of memoty can be regarded as adequately valid until it does that. The role of the instructional experiment is to test the analytic accounts of between-group differences, the instructional experiment is to test analytic accounts of between-group differences, and the problem remains: no instructional experiment has met the criteria required to establ-matter of within-group differences.

Neglect of Individual Differences

A prominent feature of experimental adult psychology is its nomothetic approach, according to which all individual differences are error variance. Until recently, few prominent voices were raised against this absurdity. Now, Allen Newell (1973), William Battig (1975), Benton Underwood (1975), and others (Hunt, Frost, and Lunneborg, 1973; Simon, 1975) have argued that individual differences can no longer be neglected. Their argument is important, because it suggests that the nomothetic approach could never bring the experimental enterprise to its goal, which is valid theory.

Battig (1975) examined data from the most thoroughly analyzed procedures yet employed by psychologists: serial learning, paired associates learning, verbal discrimination learning, and free recall. By capitalizing on the accumulated understanding of processes underlying performance on these tasks, he was able to show not only that different people use different processes on the same task, but that each individual uses different processes on different trials and even on different items within single trials. To quote Battig (p. 225):

> we have to date been able to identify no task or conditions whatever where the typical individual subject will use only one type of processing consistently for different items of a particular type either within or across successive trials. We find . . . (within-individual differences) . . . whether we assess them at the time the individual is actually studying the materials, immediately after they have been responded to correctly, or through some type of post-experimental inquiry.

His conclusion is that

> no matter where or how it is evaluated, any theory or model may well be both entirely correct or totally wrong, depending upon what type(s) of processing the particular subject happens to be using for a given item within a particular task.

The point is that individual differences and variability from time to time within individuals must be directly measured, manipulated, and given theoretical status. Failing to do these things simply damns psychological theory to eternal imprecision and irrelevance, because the existence of *systematic* variability between and within people precludes valid discovery by averaging. To work, averaging requires random variability, but whenever psychologists have worked with the most direct available methods and with thoroughly analyzed tasks they have found that random variability among people is the exception, not the rule. Skipping from task to task, without completely analyzing any of them, is no solution (cf. Newell, 1973), although it does mask the problem.

Until recently, experimental child psychology was hardly less nomothetic than experimental adult psychology. By individual differences, child experimentalists usually meant differences between groups leveled on age or IQ. All within-age differences were viewed as random, which they are not. This not only caused substantial imprecision, as in adult psychology, it excluded an important test from the developmentalist's arsenal. There is always question about any correlate of age: Is it due to some unknown developmental process? To answer the question negatively, which is always the goal, requires that the age-correlated process account for significant variance within narrowly constituted age groups. If it does not, then the demonstration that something varies with age only highlights our ignorance about what its development signifies.

Developmentalists seek to account for changes in behavior with age. To give compelling bite to their explanations of age effects, they must show that their theoretical notions have explanatory status independent of age. This requires analysis of within-age differences. That analysis can take the form of correlations between measures within ages, as in our demonstrations that executive functions predict accuracy for 11, 12, and 17-year-olds (see p. 158). The analysis can show that particular developmental sequences obtain even when the age at which they occur varies widely, as in Kahn's (1975) demonstration that deferred imitation precedes language regardless of the age at which imitation first occurs (see p. 142). Or, the within-age analysis can take a more instructional form in which some processes are regularized by training in order to clarify others (cf. Butterfield and Dickerson, 1977). Regardless of the form of the test used to study individual differences, the theoretical treatment they are given will remain inadequate until it accounts for all variability on at least one experimental task to which the theory addresses itself. The need to account completely for performance variability arises because there is no direct way to measure any cognitive process.

Incomplete Process Analyses

Because their theories focus on unobservables, experimental psychologists have devised tactics to increase their confidence that their behavior measures tap particular mechanisms. One tactic has achieved special importance. It is called convergent validation, which is the use of two or more operationally distinct performance measures of each mechanism. The idea is that worthy processes should reveal themselves in more than one measurement setting. If a theoretical mechanism does not show itself in at least two experimental ways, then the scientist may be studying an idiosyncrasy of performance on a single experimental paradigm. Convergent validation has bolstered the postulation of several cognitive processes, such as iconic memory (Sperling, 1960; Averbach and Coriell, 1961). But neither convergent validation nor any other experimental tactic has yet permitted satisfying cumulation of theoretical understanding of cognition (cf. Chase, 1973; Newell, 1973). There are forever unresolved disputes about alternative hypothetical processes that might account for each performance phenomenon. Eventually the disputants tire and go on to other phenomena, leaving a clutter of unresolved issues and no cumulated knowledge. The problem is to find empirical tactics that can lend priority to one or another process account of behavioral performances.

As long as any appreciable performance variability remains unaccounted in any measurement paradigm, an indefinite number of process accounts of behavior in that paradigm can be entertained. The solution is to exhaustively explain variability. One exhaustive account of performance can be challenged seriously only by another, and given two theories that explain all behavioral variability in the same situations, the choice between them reduces to matters of elegance, parsimony, and generality.

Although the matter of incomplete analysis has been treated here as a problem for experimental adult psychologists, it plagues experimental child psychologists too. Since age cannot be accelerated, reversed, or otherwise manipulated, the processes that are invoked to explain development can gain experimental veracity only through within-age analysis. Lacking within-age explanations, questions always remain as to whether an unknown process correlated with age explains development. Within-age process analyses, in turn, require the explanation of all performance variability. The reality of a process hinges not only on demonstrations that it can be measured in various ways, but on an explanation of how it combines with other processes to account entirely for particular behaviors. The experimental child psychologist can provide no compelling account of behavioral developments unless he can also account compellingly and independently of age for the behaviors whose development he seeks to explain.

A Laboratory Strategy

This appraisal of experimental child psychology has identified three problems that need solution: the logic of instructional experimentation has never been satisfied experimen-

Table 1. How to validate a process explanation of deficient performance

Step 1. Perform a process analysis of performance on your task, within deficient and proficient groups.
- A. Make process measurements that correlate with performance.
- B. Show correlations between independent measures of each process.
- C. Manipulate each process.
- D. Show that each process manipulation changes performance.

Step 2. Differentiate between groups with measures of processes that undrelie performance within groups
- A. Demonstrate correlations between each process measure and subject characteristics (e.g., CA, MA, IQ) that differentiate deficient and proficient groups.
- B. Using performance measures, show interactions between subject characteristics and process manipulatoins. Collect concurrent process measurements.

Step 3. Teach deficient people to process as proficient ones, thereby raising their performance to the level of similarly instructed proficient performers.
If the instructed deficients' performance falls short of the instructed proficients', check concurrently collected process measures to see that instructions actually induced the deficient to process as the proficient:
- A. If instructions failed to induce proficient processing, revise them and instruct other groups.
- B. If instructions did induce proficient processing, retreat to steps 1 and 2 for further process analysis.
- C. If the instructed groups' performances are equal, but the instructions raised the proficient group's performance, use concurrently collected process measure to see that the proficient group members who contributed to the increase were using deficient processes prior to instruction.

Step 4. Teach proficient people to process as deficient ones, thereby lowering their performance to the level of similarly instructed deficient performers.
If the instructed proficients' performance lies above the instructed deficients', use concurrently collected process measures to see that instructions actually induced the proficient to process as the deficient.
- A. If instructions failed to induce deficient processing, revise them and instruct other groups.
- B. If instructions did induce deficient processing, retreat to steps 1 and 2 for further process analysis.
- C. If the instructed groups' performances are equal, but the instructions lowered the deficient group's performance, use concurrently collected process measurements to see that the deficient who contributed to the decrease were using relatively proficient processing prior to instruction.

tally, systematic individual differences have been ignored, and no process analysis has been completed. In principle, all of these problems can be solved in the laboratory. Before proceeding to other problems, for whose cures extra-laboratory procedures seem required, a possible solution to the foregoing three should be examined.

The solution begins after the selection of an experimental task, and it is confined to experimentation with that task. It has four interactive and recursive components, called steps in Table 1. Step 1 calls for a process analysis of performance on the experimental task. The goal is to account for all between-subject and all within-subject variance in task performance, but that goal need not be reached before the other steps are taken, because there are criteria for reverting to further process analysis depending upon where the other steps lead.

Table 1 sketches some of the tactics required by each of the four steps. Thus, step 1A calls for the use of process measures that correlate with performance measures. The process-performance distinction is basic to developmental cognitive psychology, and it must be reflected in experimental operations. Performance measures are indices of the outcome of cognition. In a memory task, the performance measure is generally an index of recall or recognition accuracy. Process measures are supposed to be more direct reflections of what people do to produce the performance outcome. Examples are temporal measures taken during preparation for recall (Ellis and Dugas, 1968; Belmont and Butterfield, 1969; Wilkes and Kennedy, 1969), quantification of forced overt rehearsal (Rundus and Atkinson, 1970; Kellas, McCauley, and McFarland, 1975), timing of inter-item intervals of tape-recorded overt recall efforts (Pollio, Richards, and Lucas, 1969; Ashcraft and Kellas, 1974), and trial-by-trial structured introspections (Anders, 1973). The purpose of establishing correlations between the process and performance measures is to insure that the processes are not epiphenomenal concomitants of performance. When the process measures are taken prior to criterion performance, the correlations can rule out this possibility with substantial certainty. Step 1B calls for convergent validation of each process through the use of more than one measurement procedure, and in addition it incorporates an individual-differences test. The idea is that it is insufficient to show that two separate measures lead to the same conclusion about processing. In addition, the two measures must be taken from the same people and be shown to covary significantly, to provide evidence that the measures tap at least one shared process (cf. Underwood, 1975; Butterfield and Dickerson, 1977). Step 1C asks the investigator to cause theoretically comprehensible changes in his process measures. This will usually require the demonstration of interactions among manipulated variables, as outlined above (pp.146–147). The investigator should also show that manipulations which influence his process measures change task performance. This is a variation on the test in step 1A, where correlations were established between process and performance. All parts of step 1 should be performed within narrowly defined age groups, optimally within more than one.

The purpose of step 2 is to show in the usual fashion of experimental child psychologists that process and performance measures relate to age or some other variable on which subjects are leveled (see p. 147).

Steps 3 and 4 apply the instructional criterion outlined above (pp.160–161). In addition, they specify what to do when differences remain between proficient and deficient groups following training. If concurrent process measures do not account for all instructed increases or decreases in behavior, the investigator should return to steps 1 and 2 for further process analysis.

This laboratory strategy incorporates the criterion that cognitive instruction must produce equivalent performance by groups which differ substantially before instruction. It provides explicitly for examining within-age individual differences. It allows reasonable hope of accounting for all variance in task performance. Applied successfully, it would account for age-related changes in performance on one task. It would specify processes that change with development, and it would show how to mimic development by manipulating those processes in the laboratory. Like every research strategy with which I am familiar, it would leave untouched the matter of what prompts the normal development of the processes it specifies. The *how* of normal development is still beyond the reach of developmentalists' scientific and conceptual tools.

Four problems with which this strategy does not cope are discussed next. Three of these highlight ways in which the laboratory study of cognition might be combined with observational techniques.

Structural Limits on Development?

The foregoing research strategy embodies the hypothesis that all individual differences in cognition can be eliminated by theory-guided instruction. Otherwise, the experimental child psychologist could not aspire to raise the most deficient thinker to the level of the most proficient, similarly instructed thinker. According to Zeaman (1973), that hypothesis must be wrong, because there are structural limits on cognitive development. His argument merits consideration.

Atkinson and Shiffrin (1968) distinguished control processes from structural features, and that distinction remains fundamental to contemporary theories of cognition. The notion is that certain invariant aspects of the human's cognitive apparatus cannot be changed by any amount of training. These invariants they called structural features. The control processes of cognition are indefinitely flexible. Atkinson and Shiffrin did not speak of individual differences between people, nor did they speak of cognitive development. From what they did say about control processes, it is easy to infer that many transient differences among people result from the use of different control processes to solve the same cognitive problems. It seems less clear whether they would attribute to differential control processing, or to varying structural features, the sort of enduring cognitive differences that separate idiocy from genius. Their arguments seem moot on this matter; the structural features of cognition may be identical for all people, or they may account for all cognitive differences between people.

Zeaman (1973) sees it differently. He argues that mental retardation must be a matter of structural features. He notes that although individual IQ's may not be constant, rate of mental growth is, and on this matter the data are compelling (Fisher and Zeaman, 1970). Mental growth rate does remain stable and it does distinguish normal from retarded people. From this fact, Zeaman infers that intellectual differences among people must be the result of structural features, and he views his research as an effort to identify the structural limits that account for mental differences. He points out that his research has, from time to time, identified differences between normal and retarded people that might have been structural. But in practically every case, those differences were easily eliminated by experimental intervention. When that has happened, the conclusion has been that the identified difference was not a structural feature. According to Zeaman, a difference that can be trained away is not a structural matter, but it is inconsequential as regards intelligence. Like Piaget, Zeaman believes that genuine intellectual change cannot be achieved by instruction.

Then how should we view the research strategy outlined here? Does it trivialize experimental child research by making instructability the key test of theory? On the contrary, it is the only approach to the problem of cognitive differences that might conceivably justify the structural position. To see how it might do that, consider Brown's (1974, p. 61) argument against Zeaman's position.

> There appears to be a problem with establishing a valid distinction between fixed-capacity restrictions and trainable control processes in that this would require that the effectiveness of a training procedure be independently evaluated. The problem is not acute if a particular training procedure is successful since it would then be possible to conclude that a trainable control process was involved and had responded to training. However, difficulty arises when training does not alter performance. Is this due to the presence of a structural capacity limitation or due to the inadequacy of the training technique itself? It would be necessary to exhaust all possible training techniques before concluding that an untrainable structural feature had been discovered, surely a logical impossibility.

Strictly speaking, Brown is correct. Zeaman's position is logically indefensible. A structural feature cannot be established by failing to change behavior. A better training technique may be just around the corner. But science is a practical business that does not require logical certainty, only estimated probability. The trick is to reduce the probability that a more effective training procedure will be found. When the probability is sufficiently attenuated, reasonable people will infer structural features.

The purpose of the first two steps in the foregoing laboratory strategy is to provide a theoretical basis for cognitive instruction. Completing the first two steps produces a full theory of the behavior to be changed. Given such a theory, the number of appropriate training procedures would be finite and small, and away would go Brown's argument, the force of whose "all possible training techniques" is the spectre of an infinity of unknown procedures. The argument gives too little credit to the possibility of a theoretical basis for reducing the matter from one of all possible training techniques to one of all appropriate training techniques.

In practice and for some time to come, there may be no complete process accounts of any behavioral domain. The strategy outlined above is only a promissory note against the future. Therefore, the number of training procedures that might be tried before inferring a structural feature may remain indefinitely large. This does not vindicate Brown's argument. It means simply that the inference of structural features will be based on other considerations, such as the effort required to produce a complete account of the variance in particular behaviors. The strategy calls for recursive retreats from the instructional steps (3 and 4) to the analytic steps (1 and 2). When instruction does not result in identical performance by proficient and deficient groups, more process analysis is indicated. However, if further process analysis fails to account for more performance variance, there will come a time when the investigator judges that there are no more processes to capture. If the investigator has applied the strategy diligently, that judgment may suffice for inferring a structural feature. The point of the strategy is to guarantee an assiduous test of the belief that cognitive growth cannot be promoted. It is to guarantee that experimental child psychology has no more 20-year periods during which it believes in mediation deficiencies because it did not bother to observe mediational processes so that it might instruct them. Notice the similarity between the notions of mediational deficiency and structural feature (cf. Brown, 1974).

It should also be noted that not all memory performances develop, but those that do may all depend upon the strategic use of control processes (Brown, 1975). If so, then the working hypothesis of instructability may serve centrally in the validation of developmental accounts of mnemonic cognition.

Durability and Transfer of Instructional Effects

When Zeaman (1973) invoked instructability to discount the possibility that performance depends on a structural feature, he also observed that instructing theoretically important processes has not eliminated mental retardation. It is not modifiability alone that makes a process seem incapable of accounting for individual differences in intelligence; it is also the failure to eliminate intellectual differences. The idea is that instructing a truly important cognitive process would create generalized effects. This is very much like the Piagetian notion that instruction does not accelerate development unless it creates generalized effects (see p. 145). The fact is, instructional effects so far achieved by experimental child psychologists have failed to transfer out of the training environment. Moreover, they have seldom endured from one time to another within the training environment. These matters of durability and transfer go to the heart of the instructional movement within experimental child psychology, and how the field views them will importantly determine the fate of the instructional approach.

What does it mean that children who have been trained to use effective strategies quickly revert to their immature strategies when free to do so (Flavell, 1970; Butterfield and Belmont, 1972; Hagen, Hargrave, and Ross, 1973; Borkowski and Wanschura, 1974; Brown et al., 1974)? It seems that it tells more about durability tests than about children and their cognition. Three examples make this point.

Brown et al. (1974) retested a group of retarded adolescents 6 months after training half of them to use a rehearsal strategy for a keeping track task. By observing overt rehearsal of the trained subjects during the follow-up test, Brown et al. defined two subgroups: those who did and those who did not rehearse. The rehearsers recalled very accurately, whereas the nonrehearsers performed identically to the untrained control group. Had the follow-up data from the rehearsing and nonrehearsing trained subjects been averaged together, the comparison of trained and untrained subjects could have been uninterpretable.

Brown et al. did not look back to see if the trained subjects who later abandoned the strategy were in any way separable before or during original training. Borkowski and Wanschura (1974) and Butterfield and Belmont (1972) did look back at pretest and training data for their retarded subjects who later maintained the trained strategy and for those who did not. Borkowski and Wanschura's training procedures were so good relative to the task difficulty that all of their subjects were very near the ceiling during training, leaving too little variability to predict strategy maintenance from the training data. Butterfield and Belmont were more fortunate. We divided our subjects according to whether their post-test pause-time curves showed strategy maintenance. Looking back at the training data, it was clear that all subjects had followed rehearsal instructions during training, but only those who maintained the strategy at post-test actually improved their criterion performance during training. Their improvement was nearly maximal. evidently, training in this study resulted in all-or-none benefits, and it is not surprising that strategy maintenance was seen only in children who originally enjoyed those benefits. This implies that durability is a useful measure of instructional effects only when measures of instructed processes that are independent of criterion performance are used to expose and classify individual differences in response to training. Since durability tests have seldom conformed to these injunctions of the instructional approach (cf. Belmont and Butterfield, 1977), it is simply premature to conclude that failures to achieve enduring instructional effects reveal anything about children's or retarded people's cognition.

Borkowski and Wanschura (1974) addressed the matter of transfer as it concerns mental retardation, Kuhn (1974) did likewise for Piagetians, and Denny (1973) examined it in the areas of cognitive style, cognitive tempo, and cognitive strategy (constraint seeking versus hypothesis testing). These people wrote from very different perspectives, yet they struck the same theme: unless a child exhibits activity akin to the training activity in some situation other than the training task, he has done nothing but parrot the instructor. Borkowski and Wanschura called this parroting "rote mediation," Denny called it "task-specific response set," and Kuhn called it "specific rote-learning responses." All agreed that even when parroting is seen long after the instructions, durability does not mean that the child has grasped what the instruction was all about. He has not necessarily exhibited what Kellas, Ashcraft, Johnson, and Needham (1973) called "cognitive understanding," or Denny's "comprehension of the essential nature of the behaviors being trained." Only transfer can show Kuhn's "genuine structural change," or Denny's "true changes along an information processing dimension," or "real acquisition of generalized cognitive functions." Words like *genuine, true,* and *real* always signal problems for behavioral research. Their use to rationalize failures of transfer signals a failure to appreciate sufficiently the role of process analysis of experimental tasks.

It would be lovely if informed guessing or loose reasoning could provide the process analysis required for tests of transfer. Unfortunately, the task analytic requirements are much too specific and detailed. The investigator who would demonstrate transfer must thoroughly understand both his training and his transfer tasks. By definition, training and transfer tasks are similar; both require processes taught during training. However, they are not identical. Performing the transfer task must also require processes not taught during training. If it did not, the test would be for durability rather than for transfer. Since the tasks are not identical, both must be analyzed to demonstrate that they require the instructed processes. But certain knowledge that the two tasks require shared processes does not guarantee that failing the transfer task results from not transfering the trained processes. The child might well understand that the transfer task requires use of his newly learned processes, and he may use them, but fail the transfer test for not engaging the untrained processes it requires. Without knowing precisely where each subject's performance breaks down, an investigator cannot interpret a failure to obtain transfer. No investigator has known these things about his transfer test. All should have, and here is another reason, advanced by Belmont and Butterfield (1977).

> Transfer tests are given only to people who require instruction on the training task. The fact that training is successful, which it must be before the investigator tests for transfer, says that the people who are tested never did lack the appropriate control processes. They simply failed to invoke them without training. Assuming that they were suitably motivated it seems the subjects' failure on the original task was in the business of assessing its cognitive requirements. This we identify as an executive shortcoming. Observing that training and transfer tasks come from the same class of cognitive problem, and assuming that the executive is no

less important on the second task than on the first, the most reasonable prediction is that the instructed child would not transfer, unless he were trained in matters of executive decision making. We have seen no reports of attempts to do so.

From the experimentalist's vantage all the shortcomings of previous durability and transfer tests might be resolved in the laboratory. The laboratory strategy outlined above incorporates the features needed for adequate durability tests, because it provides for process measures to assess individual differences in response to training. That same strategy can be generalized to solve the major problem with previous transfer tests, which is that investigators have not had adequate process analyses of either their training or transfer tasks. As outlined, the strategy provides for analysis of training tasks, and the requisite generalization simply requires applying the strategy to transfer tasks as well.

The analytic view required to make informative durability and transfer tests seems more congenial to laboratory than to ethological approaches. But laboratory research by itself cannot answer the transfer question raised by Kuhn (1974): Do laboratory-based instructions produce changes in children's everyday cognitive behavior? Ethological observations might answer this question, and until it is answered affirmatively, important doubt will remain about the wisdom of expending the experimental effort required to generate process measures and complete analyses of a few experimental tasks. Naturalistic observation can be no substitute for durability and transfer tests, but it may importantly supplement them.

Artificiality of Procedure

Laboratory arrangements seem artificial compared to people's typical surroundings. Some have argued that laboratories' artificiality trivializes much experimentation (Jenkins, 1971), particularly with children and retarded poeple (Brooks, 1976), but it remains uncertain whether laboratories are damagingly artificial. Damage would result only if experimental arrangements elicited idiosyncratic forms of cognition that serve no extra-laboratory function. It seems unlikely that people suspend their everyday ways of thinking when they enter the laboratory. Still, it would be reassuring to know that children's failures of executive functioning, which have been observed in the laboratory (Butterfield and Belmont, 1977), also occur in the outside world. Determining whether they do might require simply looking at how often children act deliberately to solve environmental problems. Observational methods might bring data to the question of whether laboratory research is trivial, or whether it clarifies everyday functioning.

The more pertinent question about the laboratory artificiality is whether it interferes with data collection. It is worth noting that some of the methodological wrinkles that gave rise to current emphases in experimental child psychology look like accommodations to ecological considerations. For example, in order to observe children's lip movements, Flavell et al. (1966) turned their memory experiment into a game involving a space helmet. Lowering the helmet's visor during the experiment's retention interval may have encouraged overt mouthing. Or perhaps it put the children in the swing of things so that they did more nearly what they typically do to remember exactly. In either case, making it into a game contributed to the success of this seminal experiment. Another example is provided by the measurement procedures of Belmont and Butterfield. The typical laboratory practice has been for memory experimenters to tightly control the timing of stimulus presentation. Giving over control to the children (Belmont and Butterfield, 1969) may have made the task more like their usual learning experiences.

The atypicality of laboratory arrangements may affect young children more than older ones. Standard laboratory memory tasks have yielded data suggesting that active efforts to memorize do not occur much before 8 years of age (Butterfield and Belmont, 1972). But Shackelton (1974) showed that the lowest age of rehearsal varies with the recall requirement of the memory test. Free recall tasks elicit rehearsal 2 years before position probe tasks. The position probe task is considerably less like any recall situation a child might normally encounter than the free recall task. Wellman, Ritter, and Flavell (1975) carried the implication further when they found evidence for active memorization in 3-year-olds by using a memory task tailored after things young children were observed doing in their regular environments. The implication is that experimental arrangements would give a different view of children if they were tailored after knowledge of the children's typical activities and if the laboratory arrangements were like the children's typical behavioral settings. Put another way, naturalistic observations might reveal environmental factors that control the quality of children's cognition.

Sterility of Investigative Domains

Question has also been raised about the richness of the processes revealed by laboratory procedures currently used in experimental child psychology. The idea is that children think differently in different settings, and that experimental laboratories constrain the quality of thinking. Thus, list learning experiments dominate the literature on children's memory, but they reveal nothing about the quality of semantic inference that even young children make when dealing with narrative material (Paris and Carter, 1973). Most developmental cognitive experiments study deliberate, time-consuming thinking, and leave unexamined the rapid and seemingly automatic processing that goes on, for example, when a child listens to and comprehends what his mother says to him. Might the experimentalist capture a richer view of children's thought if he patterned his procedures after what children do rather than patterning them after the ways in which adult's verbal learning is studied? Does the analytic power gained from well analyzed procedures satisfactorily compensate for the possible loss of relevance their use entails? The key to disciplined response to these queries is what ethological observations reveal about children. Without detailed observational findings, the benefits of abandoning established laboratory techniques would remain obscure, but the loss of accumulated data and technique would be great.

TOWARD A SYMBIOSIS OF EXPERIMENTING AND OBSERVING

The limits of the currently predominant approaches to cognitive development have been examined in order to identify places where observational methods might become symbionts of experimentation. Tracing trends in American Piagetian research showed three movements *away* from observational methods. The trends were toward instrumented observation, standardized testing, and cognitive instruction. This last trend highlighted the first limit to present approaches. Despite the fact that cognitive instruction has created impressive gains in children's cognitive performance, those gains have not been shown to generalize. A Piagetian response to this limit is to suggest that generalization might be shown by ethological observations made concurrently with cognitive instruction. An extended examination of recent trends within experimental child psychology led to the conclusion that evidence for transfer would more likely be found with a laboratory strategy that combined detailed process analysis of experimental task performance, direct process measurements that focus on individual differences, and cognitive instruction that seeks to eliminate differences between deficient and proficient information processors. The analysis of experimental child psychology also showed that its strengths come to the fore primarily when it uses established laboratory procedures whose processing requirements are well understood. But there is some evidence that the artificiality of established procedures limits the view experimentalists gain of children's cognition. One way observational procedures might catalyze the study of cognitive development is by detailing the things children typically do, thereby showing how to approach children so as to obtain a fuller view of their thinking. The use of established procedures also may have restricted the focus of experimental child psychology to cognitive operations that typify little or none of the thinking children do when they solve their everyday problems. Naturalistic observations might test this charge. In the process they might identify fruitful new forms of cognition for laboratory analysis.

Examination of recent trends in experimental child psychology suggested that metamemory and executive functions of cognition may become important topics of investigation, since both promise to explain a major enigma about children's thinking in the laboratory. The enigma is that children do not use cognitive mechanisms which simple instruction shows are effective for them. The metamemoric hypothesis is that children's production deficiencies result from inadequate knowledge about 1) their own cognitive capabilities, 2) the mnemonic requirements of different tasks, and 3) strategies for meeting task demands and capitalizing upon one's cognitive capabilities. Observational techniques might be used to assess children's functional knowledge of the requirements of different tasks, but the success of the approach would depend upon children being less production deficient in their everyday endeavors than they are in cognitive laboratories. Research on executive functions focuses on how children change their problem-solving efforts when the problems themselves change. The future of the laboratory approach to executive functions may hang on what observational work says about how children vary their problem-solving efforts at home and in school.

The symbiosis toward which this chapter points would carry benefits for both experimentalists and naturalistic observers. The yield for experimentalists from a symbiosis of observational and laboratory procedures would be increased confidence that their analyses concern mechanisms required for everyday adaptation. For the ethologist and the ecologist the yield would be analytic understandings of the phenomena they describe.

REFERENCES

Allport, D. A. 1975. Critical notice: the state of cognitive psychology. Q. J. Exp. Psychol. 27:141–152.

Anders, T. R. 1973. A high-speed self-terminating search of short-term memory. J. Exp. Psychol. 97:34–40.

Appel, L. F., Cooper, R. G., McCarrell, N., Sime-Knight, J., Yussen, S. R., and Flavell, J. H. 1972. The development of the distinction between perceiving and memorizing. Child Dev. 43:1365–1381.

Ashcraft, M. H., and Kellas, G. 1974. Organization in normal and retarded children: temporal aspects of storage and retrieval. J. Exp. Psychol. 103:502–508.

Atkinson, R. C., and Shiffrin, R. M. 1968. Human memory: a proposed system and its control processes. In: K. Spence and J. Spence (eds.), The Psychology of Learning and Motivation, Vol. 2. Academic Press, New York.

Averbach, E., and Coriell, A. S. 1961. Short-term memory in vision. Bell Systems Technical J. 40:309–328.

Battig, W. F. 1975. Within-individual differences in "cognitive" processes. In: R. L. Solso (ed.), Information Processing and Cognition. Lawrence Erlbaum Associates, Publishers, Hillsdale, New Jersey.

Baumeister, A. A. 1967. Problems in comparative studies of mental retardates and normals. Am. J. Ment. Defic. 71:869–875.

Belmont, J. M., and Butterfield, E. C. 1969. The relations of short-term memory to development and intelligence. In: L. Lipsitt and H. Reese (eds.), Advances in Child Development and Behavior, Vol. 4. Academic Press, New York.

Belmont, J. M., and Butterfield, E. C. 1971a. Learning strategies as determinants of memory deficiencies. Cog. Psychol. 2:411–420.

Belmont, J. M., and Butterfield, E. C. 1971b. What the development of short-term memory is. Hum. Dev. 14:236–248.

Belmont, J. M., and Butterfield, E. C. 1977. The instructional approach to developmental cognitive research. In: R. V. Kail and J. W. Hagan (eds.), Perspectives on the Development of Memory and Cognition. Lawrence Erlbaum Associates, Publishers, Hillsdale, New Jersey.

Borkowski, J., and Wanschura, P. 1974. Mediational processes in the retarded. In: N. R. Ellis (ed.), International Review of Research in Mental Retardation, Vol. 7. Academic Press, New York.

Brainard, C. J., and Allen, T. W. 1971. Experimental inductions of the conservation of "first-order" quantitative variants. Psychol. Bull. 75:128–144.

Brooks, P. 1976. Research in mental retardation: the experimenters' construction of reality. Paper presented at the Gatlinburg Conference on Research in Mental Retardation.

Brown, A. L. 1974. The role of strategic behavior in retardate memory. In: N. R. Ellis (ed.), International Review of Research in Mental Retardation, Vol. 7. Academic Press, New York.

Brown, A. L. 1975. The development of memory: knowing, knowing about knowing, and knowing how to know. In: H. W. Reese (ed.), Advances in Child Development and Behavior, Vol. 10. Academic Press, New York.

Brown, A. L., Campione, J. C., and Murphy, M. D. 1974. Keeping track of changing variables: long-term retention of a trained rehearsal strategy by retarded adolescents. Am. J. Ment. Defic. 78:446–453.

Butterfield, E. C., and Belmont, J. M. 1977. Assessing and improving the cognition of mentally retarded people. In: I. Bailer and M. Sternlicht (eds.), Psychological Issues in Mental Retardation. Psychological Dimensions, New York.

Butterfield, E. C., and Belmont, J. M. Assessing and improving the cognition of mentally retarded people. In: I. Bialer and M. Sternlicht (eds.), Psychological Issues in Mental Retardation. Psychological Dimensions, New York. In press.

Butterfield, E. C., Belmont, J. M., and Peltzman, D. J. 1971. Effects of recall requirement on acquisition strategy. J. Exp. Psychol. 90:347–348.

Butterfield, E. C., and Dickerson, D. J. 1977. Cognitive theory and mental development. In: N. R. Ellis (ed.), International Review of Research in Mental Retardation, Academic Press, New York.

Butterfield, E. C., Peltzman, D. J., and Belmont, J. M. 1971. The effects of practice upon rehearsal in short-term memory. Psychonomic Sci. 23:275–276.

Butterfield, E. C., and Siperstein, G. N. 1972. Influence of contingent auditory stimulation upon non-nutritional suckle. In: J. Bosma (ed.), Oral Sensation and Perception: The Mouth of the Infant. Charles C. Thomas Publisher, Springfield, Illinois.

Butterfield, E. C., Wambold, C., and Belmont, J. M. 1973. On the theory and practice of improving short-term memory. Am. J. Ment. Defic. 77:654–669.

Chase, W. 1973. Visual Information Processing. Academic Press, New York.

Denny, D. R. 1973. Modification of children's information processing behaviors through learning: a review of the literature. Child Study J. Monogr. 3:(Whole No. 1).

Ellis, N. R. 1970. Memory processes in retardates and normals. In: N. R. Ellis (ed.), International Review of Research in Mental Retardation, Vol. 4. Academic Press, New York.

Ellis, N. R., and Dugas, J. 1968. The serial position effect in short-term memory under E- and S-paced conditions. Psychonomic Sci. 12:55–56.

Fisher, M. A., and Zeaman, D. 1970. Growth and decline of retardate intelligence. In: N. R. Ellis (ed.), International Review of Research in Mental Retardation, Vol. 4. Academic Press, New York.

Flavell, J. H. 1970. Developmental studies of mediated memory. In: H. Reese and L. Lipsitt (eds.), Advances in Child Development and Behavior, Vol. 5. Academic Press, New York.

Flavell, J. H. 1971. First discussant's comments: what is memory development the development of? Hum. Dev. 14:272–278.

Flavell, J. H., Beach, D. R., and Chinsky, J. M. 1966. Spontaneous verbal rehearsal in a memory task as a function of age. Child Dev. 37:283–299.

Flavell, J. H., and Wellman, H. M. 1977. Metamemory. In: R. Kail and J. Hagen (eds.), Perspectives on the Development of Memory and Cognition. Lawrence Erlbaum Associates, Publishers, Hillsdale, New Jersey.

Gesell, A., Halverson, H. M., Thompson, H., Ilg, F. L., Castner, B. M., Ames, L. B., and Amatruda, C. S. 1940. The First Five Years of Life. Harper & Brothers, New York.

Ghatala, E. S., Levin, J. R., and Subkoviak, M. J. 1975. Rehearsal strategy effects in children's discrimination learning: confronting the crucible. J. Verb. Learn. Verb. Behav. 14:398–407.

Gollin, E. S. 1965. A developmental approach to learning and cognition. In: L. P. Lipsitt and C. C. Spiker (eds.), Advances in Child Development and Behavior, Vol. 2. Academic Press, New York.

Greeno, J. G., and Bjork, R. A. 1973. Mathematical learning theory and the new "mental forestry." Ann. Rev. Psychol. 24:81–116.

Guillaume, P. 1926. D'imitation Chez L'enfant. Alcan Press, Paris.

Hagen, J. W., Hargrave, S., and Ross, W. 1973. Prompting and rehearsal in short-term memory. Child Dev. 44:201–204.

Hall, V. C., Salvi, R., Seggev, L., and Caldwell, E. 1970. Cognitive synthesis conservation, and task analysis. Dev. Psychol. 2:423–428.

Horowitz, F. D., and Dunn, M. 1976. Infant intelligence testing. Paper presented at the Conference on Early Behavioral Assessment of the Communicative and Cognitive Abilities of the Developmentally Disabled, Orcas Island, Washington.

Hunt, E., Frost, N., and Lunneborg, C. 1973. Individual differences in cognition: a new approach to intelligence. In: G. H. Bower (ed.), The Psychology of Learning and Motivation, Vol. 7. Academic Press, New York.

Huttenlocker, J., and Burke, D. 1976. Why does memory span increase with age? Cog. Psychol. 8:1–31.

Inhelder, B., and Piaget, J. 1958. The Growth of Logical Thinking from Childhood to Adolescence. Routledge & Kegan Paul Ltd., London.

Jenkins, J. J. 1971. Second discussant's comments: what's left to say? Hum. Dev. 14:279–286.

Kahn, J. V. 1975. Relationship of Piaget's sensorimotor period to language acquisition of profoundly retarded children. Am. J. Ment. Defic. 79:640–643.

Kellas, G., Ashcraft, M. H., Johnson, N. S., and Needham, S. 1973. Temporal aspects of storage and retrieval in free recall of categorized lists. J. Verb. Learn. Verb. Behav. 12:499–511.

Kellas, G., and Butterfield, E. C. 1971. The effect of response requirement and type of material on acquisition and retention performance in short-term memory. J. Exp. Psychol. 88:50–56.

Kellas, G., McCauley, C., and McFarland, C. E. 1975. Developmental aspects of storage and retrieval. J. Exp. Child Psychol. 19:51–62.

Kendler, T. S., Kendler, H. H., and Wells, D. 1960. Reversal and nonreversal shifts in nursery school children. J. Comp. Physiol. Psychol. 53:83–88.

Kreutzer, M. A., Leonard, C., and Flavell, J. H. 1975. An interview study of children's knowledge about memory. Monogr. Soc. Res. Child Dev. 40:(1, Serial No. 159).

Kuenne, M. K. 1946. Experimental investigation of the relation of language to transposition behavior in young children. J. Exp. Psychol. 36:471–490.

Kuhn, D. 1974. Inducing development experimentally: comments on a research paradigm. Dev. Psychol. 10:590–600.

Maccoby, E. E. 1964. Developmental psychology. In: Annual Review of Psychology. Annual Reviews Inc., Palo Alto, California.

Milgram, N. A. 1968. The effects of MA and IQ on verbal mediation in paired associate learning. J. Genet. Psychol. 113:129–143.

Meltzoff, A. N., and Moore, M. K. 1977. Imitation of facial and manual gestures by human neonates. Science. 198:75–78.

Morrison, F. J., Holmes, D. L., and Haith, M. M. 1974. A developmental study of the effect of familiarity on short-term visual memory. J. Exp. Child Psychol. 18:412–425.

Newell, A. 1973. You can't play 20 questions with nature and win: projective comments on the papers of this symposium. In: W. Chase (ed.), Visual Information Processing. Academic Press, New York.

Papousek, H. 1967. Conditioning during early postnatal development. In: Y. Brackbill and G. Thompson (eds.), Behavior in Infancy and Early Childhood. Free Press, New York.

Paris, S. G., and Carter, A. Y. 1973. Semantic and constructive aspects of sentence memory in children. Dev. Psychol. 9:109–113.

Piaget, J. 1951. Play, Dreams, and Imitation in Childhood. W. W. Norton & Company Inc., New York.

Piaget, J., and Inhelder, B. 1969. The Psychology of the Child. Basic Books Inc., New York.

Pollio, H. R., Richards, S., and Lucas, R. 1969. Temporal properties of category recall. J. Verb. Learn. Verb. Behav. 8:529–536.

Reese, H. W. 1962. Verbal mediation as a function of age level. Psychol. Bull. 59:502–509.

Reitman, W. 1970. What does it take to remember? In: D. A. Norman (ed.), Models of Human Memory. Academic Press, New York.

Resnick, L. B., and Glaser, R. 1975. Problem-solving and intelligence. In: L. B. Resnick (ed.), The Nature of Intelligence. Lawrence Erlbaum Associates, Publishers, New York.

Rohwer, W. D. 1973. Elaboration and learning in childhood and adolescence. In: H. W. Reese (ed.), Advances in Child Development and Behavior, Vol. 8. Academic Press, New York.

Rundus, D., and Atkinson, R. C. 1970. Rehearsal processes in free recall: a procedure for direct observation. J. Verb. Learn. Verb. Behav. 9:99–105.

Shackleton, P. D. 1974. The effects of age and recall requirement on short-term memory rehearsal strategies. Doctoral dissertation, University of Kansas.

Siegler, R. S., and Liebert, R. M. 1975. Acquisition for formal scientific reasoning by 10- and 13-year-olds: designing a factorial experiment. Dev. Psychol. 11:401–402.

Siegler, R. S., Liebert, D. E., and Liebert, R. M. 1973. Inhelder and Piaget's pendulum problem: teaching preadolescents to act as scientists. Dev. Psychol. 9:97–101.

Simon, H. A. 1975. The functional equivalence of problem solving skills. Cog. Psychol. 7:268–288.

Sperling, G. 1960. The information available in brief visual presentations. Psychol. Monogr. 74, No. 11.

Taylor, A. M., Josberger, M., and Knowlton, J. Q. 1972. Mental elaboration and learning in EMR children. Am. J. Ment. Defic. 77:69–76.

Turnure, J., Buium, N., and Thurlow, M. 1975. The production deficiency model of verbal elaboration: some contrary findings and conceptual complexities. Research Report #82. Research, Development and Demonstration Center in Education of Handicapped Children, University of Minnesota.

Underwood, B. J. 1975. Individual differences as a crucible in theory construction. Am. Psychol. 30:128–134.

Uzgiris, I., and Hunt, J. McV. 1966. An instrument for assessing infant psychological development. Unpublished manuscript, University of Illinois.

Valentine, C. W. 1930. The psychology of imitation with special reference to early childhood. Br. J. Psychol. 21:105–132.

Weimer, W. B. 1974. Overview of cognitive conspiracy: reflections on the volume. In: W. B. Weimer, and D. S. Palermo (eds.), Cognition and the Symbolic Processes. Lawrence Erlbaum Associates, Publishers, Hillsdale, New Jersey.

Wellman, H. M., Ritter, K., and Flavell, J. H. 1975. Deliberate memory in very young children. Dev. Psychol. 11:780–787.

Wilkes, A. L., and Kennedy, R. A. 1969. Relationship between pausing and retrieval latency in sentences of varying grammatical form. J. Exp. Psychol. 70:241–245.

Yussen, S. R., and Levy, V. M. 1975. Developmental changes in predicting one's own span of short-term memory. J. Exp. Child Psychol. 19:502–508.

Zazzo, R. 1957. Le probleme de l'imitation chez le nouveau-né. Enfance 10:135–142.

Zeaman, D. 1973. One programmatic approach to retardation. In: D. K. Routh (ed.), The Experimental Study of Mental Retardation. Aldine Publishing Company, Chicago.

chapter 7

Conceptual and Methodological Factors In the Study of Animism Among Rural Hawaiian Children

Douglass R. Price-Williams, and Thomas J. Ciborowski

Animism has been described as "the belief in the existence of a separable soul-entity, potentially distinct and apart from any concrete embodiment in a living individual or material organism" (Gould and Kolb, 1964, pp. 26–29). Another concept called "animatism," which was originated by anthropologist Marett, refers to the belief that natural objects are animated by some impersonal force, such as the polynesian idea of *mana*. Piaget's definition of animism as "the tendency to regard objects as living and endowed with will" (Piaget, 1972, p. 170) might then apply more to Marett's animatism than to animism itself as defined by anthropologists like Tyler, from whom the idea originated. At any rate, it is clear that special attention should be given to linguistic uses of the fundamental concepts involved in the study of animism, as well as the behavioral context of the people who are thought to hold animistic ideas. This principle applies equally to the study of peoples whose indigenous language is other than English; and it applies to the study of children whose language use might be considered different from that of adults in the same population.

In Piaget's use of the term, the concept of animism is virtually identical with the notion of consciousness (Piaget, 1972). He traces the concept through four stages. In stage I (through chronological ages 6 to 7 years), all things are thought to be conscious. In stage II (through 8 to 9 years), all things that can move are regarded as conscious. In stage III (through 11 to 12 years), only things that can move of their own accord are thought to be conscious. In stage IV (attained at about 12 years of age), only animals are thought to be conscious. Piaget's scheme, therefore, hinges on the differentiation of consciousness,

This research was supported mainly by a grant from the Carnegie Corporation of New York. It was also supported in part by Grant HD 04612 from the National Institute of Child Health and Human Development, Mental Retardation Center, University of California at Los Angeles.

beginning with an all encompassing panpsychic viewpoint, which gradually gets restricted as the child ages. Although ''aliveness'' is thus synonymous with ''consciousness'' in European and presumably most western studies of animism—certainly those that follow the Piagetian model—studies of animism in nonwestern cultures show a cautious heed to possible terminological distinctions made by subjects themselves. Dennis (1943) noted that there was a distinction between the Hopi terms *tavta* and *kayta*. Tavta apparently means ''moving by itself'' but not ''really living,'' whereas kayta means ''really alive.'' Furthermore, tavta expresses the idea that such things as rivers, fire, and the wind are alive, but not in the sense in which people are alive, for which the term kayta is reserved. Jahoda (1958) noted another kind of relevant distinction in West Africa: certain common objects have two different names, one of which is used in ordinary context and the other is used when the object is part of a traditional story or myth. It is this second usage that endows the object with properties characteristic of living things. Margaret Mead (1932) maintained that the ready availability of certain kinds of terms and their precise meaning is crucial for the study of animism, and that the structure of the language itself either encourages or discourages animistic beliefs in children. Although this is a necessary aspect of a culture to know, it is not by itself sufficient, for one has to know when the child assumes the language used by adults. In Mead's studies among the Manus, this point was crucial. The sacred lore of the Manu society was kept from children, with the result that possible animistic notions held by adults were not shared by children. Even the *tchinal* or ''bogeyman'' was not feared by children, although it was greatly respected by adults. Mead noted a necessary distinction in animistic ideas, namely, ''the difference between spontaneous animism and the child's passive acceptance of animistic categories which are explicit or implicit in the linguistic conceptions of the elders'' (Mead, 1932, p. 223).

One might also explore distinctions between metaphor and literalness in a given culture, and ask at what age a child understands the use of metaphor. In the United States, when one talks of ''the sun rising,'' older children and adults understand perfectly that this is only a way of speaking and that no similarity is intended to people rising out of their beds. Also in this culture, metaphors based on similarity (e.g., ''the stars are a thousand eyes'') are comprehended as expertise in concrete operational mechanisms, and metaphors based on proportion (e.g., dreams passed in a parade) are understood as an advance to the formal operational stage (Billow, 1975). We seem to lack such knowledge about other cultures. It thus behooves us to clear the conceptual underbrush before charting a trail for the understanding of animism, and noting what ideas are available in the language and how they are expressed.

With such considerations in mind, we embarked upon a study of animistic concepts among rural Hawaiian children. First, we asked what surface evidence there was for animism in the general population. At the outset, we observed that stories documented in collected myths of the islands (e.g., Westervelt, 1963; Beckwith, 1970; Kalakaua, 1972) were often repeated by the contemporary inhabitants. To get some measure of the contemporary conceptual background the daily field notes of anthropology students who had been working in the area of concern for the last 3 years were searched through for spontaneous remarks by both adults and children. It should be noted that references to such stories are not easily elicited because adult Hawaiians, even in rural areas, are sophisticated enough to harbor their outlook on such matters from the outsider. The field workers lived in the community and engaged in conversations quite freely without inhibiting their respondents.

Their field notes contain numerous instances of what could loosely be called superstitions, but no direct animistic cases in the sense of attributing life or consciousness to inanimate objects, among either adults or children. As a matter of fact, children made hardly any "supernatural" allusions at all.

The references to what we have called superstitions fall into several categories: 1) *obake,* which could be defined as a poltergeist type of ghost; 2) mythological creatures, sometimes regarded as guardian gods, such as the *aumakua,* exemplified in our sample as a shark and as a watersnake; 3) Madame Pele, goddess of the volcano, appearing in certain guises, such as an old woman; 4) appearances of deceased relatives; and 5) *akualele* or fire-balls (thought by some to have animate, sometimes malevolent, attributes). Of all these classes of superstitions, only aumakua and akualele get close to animism in the classical sense, yet even these are recognized as special cases. Not every shark has aumakua properties, and akualele are distinguished from the customary meteor trail. In addition to these five classes, there is a general background of taboolike beliefs, such as putting bamboo sticks around cemeteries to keep obake at bay, or not taking bananas or money with one while fishing. The only example of direct animism that we encountered in these field notes was a mother's warning to her child not to throw stones in the water because the fish would come out and bite him, a cautionary tale that hardly fits the criteria for a true animistic response.

Rather than immediately doing the kind of elaborate experiments in causal thinking that were characteristic of some of Piaget's studies, it was decided to proceed more slowly. The first focused step in studying animism among this Hawaiian population was simply asking the children to name some things that were alive and some things that were dead. Because this paper is concerned with the relationships between the methods used in naturalistic observation and in formal experiment, together with the conceptual and methodological difficulties inherent in such relationships, elaborate quantitative treatment is avoided. A more elaborate treatment is presented elsewhere, in addition to subsequent studies on causality.

An important feature of this investigation is that it was conducted in Pidgin (Hawaiian Islands Dialect). Pidgin is a major dialect of the English language and it shares many of the same features of other Creole variants of English (Carr, 1972). The subjects all had highly competent linguistic skills in Pidgin.

The use of Pidgin, however, led to an unexpected difficulty in experiment I of this study, which we attempted to correct in experiment II. The difficulty revolves around the word "dead." According to the Hawaiian research assistants, an accurate translation of the English word "dead" would be the Hawaiian word *make,* and Pidgin speakers supposedly use the two words interchangeably. This interchangeability was further supported by the most authoritative sources on Hawaiian customs and language (Pukui and Elbert, 1971; Pukui, Haertig and Lee, 1972). Despite these reassurances that the two words are equivalent, difficulties were encountered which are reported in experiment I.

EXPERIMENT I

In the first experiment on animistic thinking among rural Hawaiian children we asked the children to name some things that are alive and some things that are dead (or *make*).

Subjects and Procedures

The subjects were 30 children of predominantly Hawaiian ancestry who live in an isolated fishing village on the south Kona coast of the Big Island of Hawaii. They were divided into five groups of six children each according to age: 4 to 5 years; 6 to 7 years; 8 to 9 years; 10 to 12 years; and 13 to 15 years old. The experimenter was a Hawaiian woman who lives in the village and is highly skilled in Pidgin. She asked each child to tell her some things that are alive, and some things that are *make*. The responses were tape-recorded and transcribed into Standard English by the Hawaiian assistant.

Results

As measures of performance, we calculated the percentage of living and dead things (according to Piagetian definitions) the children reported when asked to name some things that are alive, and the percentage of living and dead things they reported when asked to name some things that are *make*. The percentages proved striking.

In the 4 to 5-year-old group, one child did not respond and another reported no things as living and the category ''boys'' as dead. The remaining children in this age group showed no difference in the things reported as living or dead. When asked to name *make* things the children included chickens, dogs, fish, etc. All the items could be classified as animals! These items all correspond to Piaget's stage IV.

For the 6 to 7-year-olds, over 75% of the reported things that are alive were animals and people, corresponding to Piaget's stage IV. Over 90% of items listed as *make* correspond to Piaget's stage IV. The striking finding is that virtually all the responses to the probe label *make* were names of living things!

For the 8 to 9-year-olds, over 80% of items listed as alive corresponded to stage IV. Over 25% of their responses to the probe word *make* were things that most adults would classify as dead (e.g., dead people, dead battery, etc.). However, a strikingly large proportion of their *make* items were living things corresponding to Piaget's stage IV.

For the 10 to 12-year-olds, 75% of items listed as alive and over 50% of items listed as *make* corresponded to Piaget's stage IV. Just under a third of the responses to *make* were things that most adults would classify as dead.

For the 13 to 15-year-olds, nearly 70% of the ''alive'' items corresponded to stage IV. The responses to the probe word *make* were still somewhat surprising: nearly 25% of the responses correspond to Piaget's stage IV, whereas just over 50% of the responses were things that most adults would classify as dead.

Discussion

This first experiment yielded two major results. First, when asked to name things that were alive (or living), the overwhelming majority of the children responded with things corresponding to Piaget's stage IV. Even children as young as 6 to 7 years old responded at a rate of over 75%, despite the fact that, according to Piaget (1972), this stage is not reached until approximately 11 to 12 years of age. This radically different pattern of responses might be because these methods were completely different than Piaget's, but it is still surprising.

The second major finding, and clearly the most perplexing, is that when asked to name things that are *make* many of the children responded with items that are alive. An interesting developmental pattern emerged in this. As the ages increased, the percentage of stage IV items reported as *make* declined monotonically. Conversely, the overall percentage of items reported as *make* increased monotonically. These striking findings led us to seriously question the basic procedure of the experiment. For example, it was speculated that the children either did not understand the question, or did not understand what was meant by the word *make*. Extensive conversations with a number of Hawaiians in this fishing village unearthed an unexpected outcome.

Apparently, the words dead and *make* are *not* equivalent. In fact, the Hawaiian word *make* does not represent for these children, in any clear way, a permanent state such as death, but rather represents a possibility or potentiality of dying. The word *make* essentially means for this sample something that is (or might be) alive, but will (or may) die at some unspecified time in the future. This seems to be the way the word is currently being used by the Hawaiians in this fishing village, despite the fact that authoritative sources such as Pukui, Haertig, and Lee (1972) define the word *make* as equivalent to the word dead.

EXPERIMENT II

In this experiment, armed with a new understanding of the word *make*, rural Hawaiian children's concept of dead was focused on. This was done in a direct way. First, extensive interviews were conducted with several adult Hawaiians in the village in an effort to obtain a clear and unambiguous set of instructions. The Standard English question we finally arrived at was: "Can you tell me some things that are really dead? Can you tell me some things that have no more life, or never have life?" This was then translated into Pidgin without using the word *make*, and used in the second experiment. The Hawaiian assistants were certain that the new set of instructions would be very clear to the children.

Subjects and Procedures

The subjects were 20 children from the fishing village, not the same children that participated in the first experiment. They were divided into five groups of four children each in the same age ranges used in experiment I. The experimenter was the same Hawaiian assistant who performed experiment I. The key features of the new set of instructions were that the word *make* was not used, and the Hawaiian assistants assured us that the instructions communicated very clearly the concept of dead.

Results

The measure of performance was the percentage of names the children produced that could either be classified by Piaget's four stages, or be classified as items that most adults would consider dead (e.g., rock). As age increased, there was a monotonic decrease in the percentage of stage IV items reported as dead, and a monotonic increase in the percentage of items that most adults would classify as dead. It should also be mentioned that two of the 4 to 5-year-olds and one 6 to 7-year olds did not respond. When pressed they replied that they did not understand the question, even after repetition and coaxing.

General Discussion

Two major findings emerged from these two experiments. First, there is the somewhat perplexing high percentage of stage IV items the children reported when asked to report things that are dead. This pattern of responses decreased sharply for the two older age groups in experiment II. That is, in experiment I the 10 to 12-year-olds responded with 56.8% of stage IV items, and the 13 to 15-year-olds responded with 24.0% of stage IV items. By contrast, these same age groups in experiment II responded with only 17.4% and 7.7% of stage IV items. Thus, the revised set of instructions used in experiment II significantly affected the responses of the two older age groups. However, the change in instructions had practically no effect on the performance of the three younger age groups. This outcome might be interpreted in a variety of ways.

One possible interpretation is that the younger Hawaiian children have a different concept of death (or what is dead) than children in the continental United States. It is not until the Hawaiian children are well over 10 years old, and have had extensive exposure to formal classroom schooling, that they begin to show a "western" understanding of what dead means. By comparison, Nagy (1959) has shown that the concept of dead in the continental United States is thought of as a final state and hence generally understood by about 8 years of age, and by about 10 years of age children have a clear understanding of what dead means. It is therefore possible that the Hawaiian children's understanding of what dead means is a reflection of certain cultural beliefs that we do not understand.

In any event, we feel that it would be too glib an explanation to argue that the Hawaiian children simply didn't understand the questions they were asked. Two factors seem to undercut this interpretation. First, changing the instructions in experiment II substantially altered the pattern of responses. Second, in both experiments I and II we obtained monotonic differences in performance across age levels. The older the child was, the more his performance matched that of children in the continental United States. An argument that the Hawaiian children simply did not understand would have to take into account the growing increase in "understanding" as the children grew older.

The second major finding of these experiments was the very high percentage of things corresponding to Piaget's stage IV when the children named things that were alive. Even the very young children performed at this level much earlier in age than stipulated by Piaget. This result is supported somewhat by Kastenbaum and Aisenberg (1972, p. 27), who concluded that "children abandon their 'animistic' thinking somewhat *earlier* than Piaget reckoned."

As mentioned above, the differences between these results and those of Piaget (1972) could perhaps be attributed to the different procedures. Also, Piaget was primarily interested in causality, whereas this was a preliminary study that sought only to elicit items regarded as alive or dead. However, before coming to any firm conclusions about the differing results, it was decided to do a third experiment, using Standard English, in case the use of Pidgin was influencing the results.

EXPERIMENT III

Subjects and Procedures

The subjects were 30 children of predominantly Hawaiian ancestry who attend the same elementary school located on the south Kona coast of the Big Island of Hawaii. They were assigned, six children to a group, according to grade level: kindergarten, 1, 3, 5, and 8. They were tested individually by a Hawaiian woman who is verbally skilled in Standard English. The approach was to pretend that she was a ''haole'' teacher from the mainland, as stated in the following instructions:

> Let's make believe that I am a haole teacher and that I know nothing about Hawaii, so we can't talk in Pidgin. I am going to ask you two questions. First, I want you to tell me some things that are alive. And remember that we are making believe that I am a haole teacher.
>
> Now I want you to tell me some things that are *dead*. Things that are *not* alive. And remember that we are making believe that I am a haole teacher.

All the children's responses were tape recorded and then transcribed.

Results

As in experiments I and II, the measure of performance was the percentage of living and dead things (according to Piagetian definitions) the Hawaiian children reported when asked to name some things that are living (or alive), and that are dead.

When asked to name things that are alive, the children again responded with an extremely high percentage of stage IV items. In fact, the highest percentages were obtained for the younger children!

When asked to name things that are dead, the children once more named a very high percentage of stage IV items: man, boys, girls, fish, dog, etc. Not until the fifth grade group did we obtain a reasonable percentage of items that most mainland children would classify as dead (e.g., dead battery, sticks, sand, rock, etc.). Comparing these proportions of recognizably dead items with those in the second experiment reveals an increase for the kindergarten and first grades but a considerable decrease for the third, fifth, and eighth grades. It is known from our other investigations of psychological processes in the same population that it is only in the first few grades that performance in Pidgin versus Standard English makes a difference. It is not easy to see, though, how this might relate to the differential proportions noticed here. All that can be stated firmly is that the procedure of experiment II (i.e., using a revised set of Pidgin instructions) was substantially more effective than the procedure of experiment III in producing a set of responses more similar to what would be obtained with mainland children.

It should also be stressed that the important finding of experiment III was the replication of the finding of the Pidgin experiments: when asked to name things that are alive, rural Hawaiian children predominantly name items consistent with Piaget's stage IV.

CONCLUSIONS

Quite apart from specific cultural examples, the literature contains other criticisms of Piaget's notion that the child chronologically progresses from an all-embracing life attribution to the naturalistic phase in which life is attributed only to plants and animals. That children may attribute life to inanimate objects does not of itself suggest a qualitatively different kind of thinking in children than in adults (Huang and Lee, 1945; Klingensmith, 1953; Klingberg, 1957). Although Piaget's main position has its supporters (e.g., Laurendeau and Pinard, 1962), the fact remains that concepts of animism among children are hard to interpret. A study of animism among 7-year-olds in a U.S. midwestern city revealed an incomplete understanding of the concept of "living" (Looft, 1974). In a factor analytic study of first grade children, Berzonsky (1973) noted that the animism factor is specific to direct questioning about life attribution, and is relatively independent of operational thought, conceptions of physical causality in general, and Piagetian type problem solving.

Most, if not all, psychological studies of childhood animism omit background knowledge of the kind we are interested in here. Even when the background is supplied, Piaget's theory is not sufficient to explain the anomalous results such as reported in this chapter.

One might simply infer from our data that these Hawaiian children have a prevailing awareness of encompassing life in the form of plants and animals that is so strong that it eclipses the usual distinctions of living and dead. It also eclipses the kinds of distinctions that Piaget makes with his stages II and III (both based on movement) as in our sample, both for questions of what is living and for questions of what is dead; stages I and IV account for most of the variance, with decided emphasis on the latter. However, there are consistencies in the data. As has been pointed out, as we reach the higher age grades there is an approximation to data found from studies of children in the continental United States. Also, when the concept "dead" was clarified in experiment II, there was a clear monotonic decrease, with age, of stage IV items like plants, animals, and people, and a clear monotonic increase of dead things. Nevertheless, a very high percentage (70%) of stage IV items were listed as dead through age nine. At this point the percentage drops off drastically to 17% for the 10 to 12 year group. For this same age group a corresponding percentage increase is seen, from 28% to 56%, for things that are generally regarded as dead. These results suggest that for these Hawaiian children the distinction between living and dead does not become firm until sometime between 10 and 12 years of age.

One is left with the impression that the dichotomy of living versus dead may not be the relevant polarity for this group of children. It may be that another kind of verbal distinction would be relevant, but it has not yet been found. Another clear conclusion is that these children do include among things that are alive those things with which most adults in our own society would agree: plants, animals, and people. This seems to be true from the comparatively early age of 6 to 7, rather than the differentiation through the idea of movement.

A more definitive statement about animism among these rural Hawaiian children will have to await analysis of ongoing studies concerning causation, but we can speculate about the relevance of the living-dead dichotomy with respect to animism in this population. In the introduction, the traditional anthropological distinction between animism and animatism was noted, and it was observed that despite the nomenclature, psychological studies usually follow Marett's animatism rather than Tyler's animism. Inasmuch as animism is distinguished by the concept of a personal soul versus the concept of an impersonal force, one wonders whether there are quite different psychological dynamics involved. Identifying the concept of animism wholeheartedly with the diffuse notion of consciousness may not be adequate, at least in certain types of society. In this Hawaiian case, one can at least say that the children are more or less consistent with the adults. The adults show little or no animism, although there are some instances that could be so classified, as was noted earlier. The adults do have an overwhelming sense of the presence of living things—plants, trees, fish, animals, people—and a natural propensity toward conservation and ecology, which some think was manifest in the old *kapu* system. This obligation toward and respect for the natural world comes through in the children's responses. To confuse this awareness with philosophical notions attached to the concept of animism would be misleading.

ACKNOWLEDGMENTS

We wish to thank anthropology students Sandra Gaile, Jill Korbin, and Frank Newton for permission to use their field notes.

REFERENCES

Beckwith, M. 1970. Hawaiian Mythology. University of Hawaii Press, Honolulu.

Berzonsky, M. D. 1973. A factor-analytic investigation of child animism. J. Gen. Psychol. 122:287–295.

Billow, R. M. 1975. A cognitive developmental study of metaphor comprehensive. Dev. Psychol. 11:415–423.

Carr, E. 1972. Da Kine Talk. The University of Hawaii Press, Honolulu.

Dennis, W. 1943. Animism and related tendencies in Hopi children. J. Abnorm. Soc. Psychol. 38:21–36.

Gould, J., and Kolb, W. L. 1964. A Dictionary of the Social Sciences. Tavistock Publications Ltd., London.

Huang, I., and Lee, H. W. 1945. Experimental analysis of child animism. J. Gen. Psychol. 66:69–74.

Jahoda, G. 1958. Child animism: I. A critical survey of cross-cultural research: II. a study in West Africa. J. Soc. Psychol. 47:197–212, 213–222.

Kalakaua, D. 1972. In: R. M. Daggett (ed.), The Legends and Myths of Hawaii. Charles E. Tuttle Company, Rutland, Vermont.

Kastenbaum, R., and Aisenberg, R. 1972. The Psychology of Death. Springer, Inc., New York.

Klingberg, G. 1957. The distinction between living and not living among 7–10 year old children, with some remarks concerning the so-called animism controversy. J. Gen. Psychol. 90:227–238.

Klingensmith, S. W. 1953. Child animism: what the child means by "alive." Child Dev. 42:51–61.

Laurendeau, M., and Pinard, A. 1962. Causal Thinking in the Child: A Genetic and Experimental Approach. International Universities Press Inc., New York.

Looft, W. R. 1974. Animistic thought in children: understanding of "living" across its associated attributes. J. Gen. Psychol. 124:235–240.

Mead, M. 1932. An investigation of the thought of primitive children with special reference to animism. J. R. Anthropol. Inst. 62:173–190.
Nagy, M. 1959. The child's view of death. In: H. Feifel (ed.). The Meaning of Death. McGraw-Hill Book Company, New York.
Piaget, J. 1972. The Child's Conception of the World. Littlefield, Adams & Co., Totowa, N.J.
Pukui, M., and Elbert, S. H. 1971. Hawaiian Dictionary. University of Hawaii Press, Honolulu.
Pukui, M., Haertig, E. W., and Lee, C. 1972. Nana I Ke Kumu (look to the source). Queen Lilioukalani Children's Center, Honolulu.
Westervelt, W. D. 1963. Hawaiian Legends of Ghosts and Ghost-Gods. Charles E. Tuttle Company, Rutland, Vermont.

chapter 8

Observational and Experimental Methods in Studies of Object Concept Development in Infancy

Ina C. Uzgiris and Thomas C. Lucas

Research on infancy readily provides illustrations of strict experimental studies, descriptive observational studies, and studies exemplifying a blend of experimental and observational procedures. Discussions of research methods frequently tend to pose a polarity between experimental and observational approaches. However, these approaches may be better viewed as falling on a continuum, with complementary rather than opposing strengths, and it may be time to consider the most productive way to intermesh the two approaches in order to study human behavior in its full complexity.

Experimental and observational research is guided by assumptions that the investigator holds about the phenomenon under study, whether they are explicitly stated or not, although the hypothesis-testing aspect of experimental research may force a more explicit formulation of some of those assumptions. In both types of research there are some restrictions on what instances of the phenomenon are studied. The observer in the field selects the categories for observing behavior as well as the settings in which observations are to be made; the experimenter selects the settings to be established in the laboratory and the much smaller range of behavior to be recorded. The settings created in the laboratory are ultimately derived from prior observation (Fraisse, 1968). The experimental approach provides efficiency in yielding instances of the phenomenon under study and control over factors whose effects are of interest. These gains are offset in the observational approach by information regarding the range of factors that affect the phenomenon in question as well as the distribution of the phenomenon over a range of settings. In this chapter, we attempt to illustrate the complementarity of the information obtained with these approaches by focusing on studies of object concept development in infancy.

OBJECT CONCEPT DEVELOPMENT

The adult's conception of the physical world posits the presence of objects that persist through time as well as changes of position with respect to other objects, including ourselves. Such a conception requires presuppositions about nonperceived events grounded in knowledge of spatial, temporal, and casual relations. Thus, conception of objects is inherently tied to understanding of reality as a whole.

Piaget's (1954) theory of cognitive development holds that a series of distinct constructions precedes the adult conception of reality. The first such construction is elaborated at the sensorimotor level, during infancy, through a sequence of six stages. In Piaget's view, the infant's understanding of the physical world evolves not simply as a result of inherent growth processes, nor as a result of exposure to various aspects of the world, but essentially through activity in it. Consequently, Piaget has looked at infants' activities in different situations for evidence regarding his theory and used the pattern of such activities to infer the level of understanding of reality.

The construction of the object is considered by Piaget to be central to sensorimotor intelligence. He maintains that an objective understanding of spatial and causal relations is predicated upon the attribution of substantiality and permanence to objects. At the same time, the fully elaborated object concept entails the recognition that objects exist in relation to one another in a common space and that they are influenced by events independent of one's activity on them.

Many investigators seem to have grasped the centrality of the object concept to Piaget's theory of cognitive functioning in infancy. In recent years, probably more studies have been conducted on object concept development than on any other facet of sensorimotor intelligence. A number of studies have replicated the general sequence in object construction described by Piaget (Décarie, 1965; Casati and Lézine, 1968; Corman and Escalona, 1969; Uzgiris and Hunt, 1975), and many others have focused on the behaviors shown by infants at a particular stage in the sequence. The reported observations have been fairly consistent with Piaget's original descriptions, but Piaget's interpretation of the behavioral evidence has not gone unchallenged (e.g., Smillie, 1972; Bower, 1974; Moore, 1975). Since several extensive reviews of recent work on object concept development are available (Gratch, 1975; Harris, 1975), neither Piaget's theory nor the research it has generated regarding object construction in general will be presented here.

To delineate the six stages in object construction, Piaget used behavior shown by infants in response to the displacement and disappearance of objects. In this chapter, we deal with observations pertinent to the fourth stage. At this stage, the infant first begins to show active search for an object that has completely disappeared from view. Both the progress implied by this behavior and the limitations on its generality are important for Piaget's theory. The active search shown by the infant is interpreted to indicate that objects are now sufficiently differentiated from the actions in which they participate to be considered to exist independently at a specific location. However, Piaget reports that having found an object at a given location (A), the infant searches at this location even when the object is observed to disappear at a new location (B). This restriction on the infant's search activity is interpreted to indicate that the object is still conceived as tied to action at a particular location. The eventual elimination of the stage IV AB error is attributed to increasing differentiation and coordination of action schemes which also results in the elaboration of a coherent network of spatial relations among objects, so that the relation of one object to another in space does not depend on the perspective of the viewer. Only when such a network is constructed does the infant become able to take into account several displacements of a single object.

Piaget used observations of his own children to support his characterization of the stage IV level in object construction. These observations were carried out in quite informal circumstances; there was considerable variation in the objects used as screens, the placement of the screens with respect to the infant, the arrangement of the screens in space, and so forth. By letting many aspects of the test situations vary at random, Piaget probably was able to discern those aspects of the infant's behavior that were quite general and likely to be typical of that developmental level. In addition, he systematically explored some variants of the test situations, usually those necessary to refute other possible interpretations of the infant's behavior. But he did not systematically vary those factors which he held central for interpreting the infant's behavior. This task still remains.

To obtain consistency in procedure, both the more naturalistic Piagetian studies and the laboratory studies of object concept development have used only the most essential aspects of Piaget's test situations. They have dealt differently with all the seemingly extraneous variables associated with these situations. The longitudinal studies conducted in the homes of infants (Schofield and Uzgiris, 1969; Uzgiris, 1973; Lucas, 1975) retained much of the informality of Piaget's procedures: the infants were seated wherever convenient, often on the floor, the objects used as screens were arranged close to the infant, and the infants were allowed to search for the object as soon as it was covered from view. A number of factors that appeared unimportant from the Piagetian perspective were left uncontrolled: the particular toy that was being hidden, whether it did or did not form a hump under the screen, whether or not the two screens were identical or different from each other, and so forth. Only the infant's interest in the object being hidden was considered critical for evaluating his search behavior following its disappearance.

Most studies conducted in a laboratory setting were carried out by investigators who approached this phenomenon from a different theoretical orientation and, therefore, eliminated as many uncontrolled variables as possible from the testing situation. Gratch and his co-workers, for example, devised a box, later adopted by other investigators, for presenting the task of searching for an object hidden in one of two locations. The rectangular box (26 × 16 × 2 inches) contains two wells (7 × 7 × 1½ inches) spaced 12 inches apart into which a toy can be made to disappear. Two identical white wash cloths (12 × 12 inches) are used as screens to cover the wells. In order to prevent the infant from reaching prematurely, and to be able to impose a delay interval between hiding and search, the box is kept out of reach while the object is being hidden and is subsequently pushed forward to make it accessible to the infant. The use of such a box specifies not only a particular kind of location for hiding, but also a rigid alignment of the two locations being used.

The search for alternatives to Piaget's interpretation of the AB error exhibited by 8 to 10-month-old infants is tied to the laboratory method. The role of prior experience of finding an object at location A has been examined in several studies that employed the Gratch box as apparatus. Landers (1971) compared three groups of infants: those who found an object at A twice, those who found an object at A eight to ten times, and those who observed an object disappear and reappear at A six to eight times and then found it at A twice. When the object was hidden at B, a similar proportion of infants made the AB error in all three groups, but the infants in the second group persisted in making the error for a greater number of trials. Evans (1974) also compared groups of infants who either searched for the object at A two or five times or only observed the object disappear and reappear at A two or five times. He found little difference either in the proportion of infants making the AB error or in the persistence of the error across trials. Thus, it seems that the activity of searching for and finding the object at A does not, through some simple process of associative learning, account for the incidence of the AB error.

Other performance variables not intrinsically related to the notion of object have also been explored in relation to the AB error. In many of the studies (e.g., Gratch and Landers, 1971; Evans and Gratch, 1972; Harris, 1973), a short delay interval was used (typically 3 sec) between the hiding of the object and the search for it by the infant. Gratch, Appel, Evans, LeCompte, and Wright (1974) systematically investigated the effect of varying the length of the delay interval on the frequency of the AB error, using the Gratch box as apparatus. Groups of infants with a median age of 9 months were subjected to delays of 0, 1, 3, or 7 sec before getting to search for an object hidden at B. The majority of infants subjected to delay made the AB error; those in the 0-sec delay group essentially did not. The authors concluded that the error "involves forgetting in some sense," but did not reject outright Piaget's claim that the infant "forgets" precisely because he has difficulty in organizing the positions and displacements of the object in space. In a similar vein, Harris (1973) first suggested that proactive interference in short term memory might account for the AB error, but then concluded that positing limitations on the infant's ability to differentiate objects from their locations might better explain observed instances of search at A even when that location is visibly empty (Harris, 1974).

The use of the AB error to define a stage in the development of the object concept can be questioned on both empirical and theoretical grounds. Empirically, a number of studies have reported a low incidence of the AB error. In a longitudinal study of 14 infants, Schofield and Uzgiris (1969) found that only six of the infants made the error when tested in the same session in which they began to search for a completely covered object. Lucas (1975) found an even lower incidence of the error (3 out of 12) in another group of infants studied longitudinally. These infants persisted in making the error for no more than 2 weeks. In still another longitudinal study of 12 infants conducted by Uzgiris (1973), eight infants did not search directly at B upon first beginning to search for a completely hidden object. However, only five infants committed the AB error, and even for these infants, the error was short-lived. Finally, Bell (1968) reported that in a sample of 8½-month-old infants only 2 of 33 infants committed the AB error.

On the other hand, in a longitudinal study of 13 infants, Gratch and Landers (1971) found that 10 infants searched at location A when the object was first hidden at B. They also found that the great majority of infants committed the error in many sessions before searching only at B in two consecutive sessions. In addition, it must be remembered that a number of previously mentioned studies were successful in producing the AB error for study in the laboratory.

The interpretation of the AB error as stage-defining is challenged also by reports that the error is not confined to the period immediately following the achievement of active search for a hidden object. Instances of the error have been observed in older infants when they are presented with more complex displacements of objects (e.g., Moore, 1973). Thus, the AB error seems to have limited generality across individuals and across experimental situations, giving rise to questions concerning the empirical base for identifying stage IV in the development of the object concept on the basis of the AB error.

From a Piagetian position, the perspective taken here, performance on a single task should not be made synonymous with a level of development; only a pattern of performances on a variety of tasks allows an inference about the organizational characteristics of the infant's cognitive functioning at any given level of development.

In view of these empirical and theoretical considerations, the task in attempting to characterize the infant's notion of object during stage IV is twofold. First, to account for the inconsistent occurrence of the AB error in different contexts, various characteristics of the object-hiding situations that elicit the error need to be explored. In this connection, Piaget's claim of interdependence between the construction of object and of space, particularly immediately following the attribution of permanence to objects, suggests that the spatial arrangements of these object-hiding tasks be given special consideration. Such data might suggest a more satisfactory interpretation of the AB error.

Second, in order to obtain the converging evidence needed to support an inference about the infant's conception of the object at this level of development, his performance in a variety of hiding tasks must be examined Here again the presumed interdependence of object conception and spatial understanding may provide an important lead.

We wish to argue that the infant's search for objects in stage IV of object construction is a function of the spatial relations between objects (toy and screen) and of the displacements of these objects that are presented to the infant. Depending on the particular arrangement, search at A, search at B, search at yet another location, or no search may then be observed. Since the infant's understanding of displacements in space is still limited, this understanding is frequently insufficient to override perceptual pulls created by a particular hiding situation. With the development of a coherent spatial framework, more accurate specification of locations becomes possible, permitting the immediate retrieval of the object. The results of three studies in support of this contention are presented.

OBJECT HIDING IN NEAR AND FAR SPACE

In discussing the construction of space, Piaget distinguished "near space," the space within reach of a seated infant, from more distant space. This distinction is predicated on the assumption that infants in the middle of the first year of life interact more deliberately and persistently with objects within reach than with more distant ones. Piaget suggested that grasp of spatial relations is achieved first in near space. Because the studies on the AB error using the box devised by Gratch involved the disappearance of the object in what might be considered far space, a study was conducted (Boynton and Uzgiris, 1975) to investigate the role of that factor. It was expected that the frequency of AB errors would be greater when the object was hidden at B with the box out of reach. Furthermore, it was expected that infants would have greater difficulty in distinguishing spatial locations in any arrangement that was relatively less familiar from direct experience, such as a vertical stacking of two positions.

Subjects

Two groups of 16 infants between 8½ and 9½ months in age were tested in a laboratory at Clark University. The second group of infants participated in a replication of the first study.

Materials

A plywood box stained dark brown, having the same dimensions as those used by Gratch, was used to hide an object in one of two locations. A box was also made that had two locations arranged vertically, one on top of another. This vertical box measured 24¾ × 12½ × 12½ inches and contained a shelf 8 inches from the bottom surface, accessible through an open front. For the replication study it was slightly modified by the addition of a front panel. The boxes are illustrated in Figure 1. Two white wash cloths served as screens to cover the hiding locations. Small toys were used as objects for hiding.

Procedure

The infants were seated on a parent's lap at a table. A small toy was hidden in one well designated as location A until the infant found it successfully on two consecutive trials.

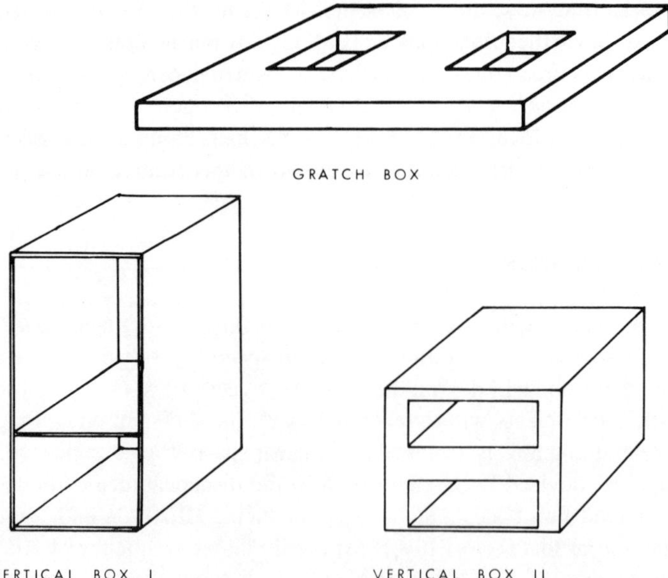

Figure 1. Boxes used in the horizontal and vertical arrangement of hiding locations.

The toy was then hidden at B. When the hidings took place with the Gratch box out of reach, the arrangement of the hiding locations was considered to be horizontal in far space (HF); when they took place with the Gratch box in front of the infant, the arrangement of the hiding locations was considered to be horizontal in near space (HN). In the HF condition, once the object was covered, the box was immediately pushed forward and the infant was allowed to search. This procedure approximates the 0-sec delay condition of Gratch et al. (1974). No delay was introduced in the other conditions. The vertical box was presented only in near space (VN) for the first group of infants studied.

The presentation of the HF and HN conditions was counterbalanced for the first group of 16 infants; the VN condition was always presented last. After each infant was tested once in all three conditions, the sequence was repeated. Because of difficulties with the vertical box, only 11 infants completed the requisite number of trials in the VN condition.

The 16 infants in the second group were randomly assigned to be tested with all hidings accomplished in either near space or far space. Each group of eight infants was presented with both a horizontal and a vertical arrangement of hiding locations, in a counterbalanced order. After two successful searches at location A, the object was hidden at B. This sequence of hidings was repeated three times in each condition. A 2-sec delay interval was used in all conditions in this replication.

Successful search at B was given a score of 3, whereas exclusive search at A was given a score of 1. Correction was permitted and was scored as an intermediate response.

Results

The first group of infants made practically no errors on the B trials in the HN condition; only one infant on one trial searched in both locations. In contrast, these same infants often searched at A when the object was hidden at B in the HF condition. The difference in performance between the two conditions was highly significant ($F = 25.79$, $df = 1, 15$, $p < 0.01$). The mean scores achieved in the two conditions are presented in Table 1.

The VN condition elicited few searches exclusively at A when the object was hidden at B, but a greater number of searches at both locations than in the HN condition. For the 11 infants who were tested in both HN and VN conditions, the difference in performance was significant ($F = 9.64$, $df = 1, 10$, $p < 0.05$).

Table 1. Mean scores for two "B" trials in three hiding conditions

Condition	*N*	Mean	s.d.	*p*
Horizontal near	16	2.97	0.12	<0.01
Horizontal far		2.00	0.75	
Vertical near	11	2.54	0.47	<0.05
Horizontal near (Subjects tested on VN)		2.95	0.15	

Table 2. Mean scores for three "B" trials in four hiding conditions

	Arrangement of location			
	Horizontal		Vertical	
Group	Mean	s.d.	Mean	s.d.
Near (N = 8)	2.92	0.24	2.46	0.50
Far (N = 8)	2.50	0.47	2.33	0.31

In the replication of this study with the second group of infants, similar results were obtained. Infants tested in near space searched more accurately overall. In the HN condition, only one of the eight infants searched at A before searching at B on two of the three trials when the object was hidden at B. Search was more variable in the VN condition. However, of the infants tested in far space, only three infants tested in the HF condition searched directly at B on all B trials. The mean scores for all four conditions are presented in Table 2.

A two-way analysis of variance was performed on these scores. It showed that the factor of near versus far space contributed significantly to performance in these tasks ($F = 5.08$, df = 1, 14, $p < 0.05$). In the HN condition the infants were significantly more accurate than in the HF condition ($t = 4.46$, df = 14, $p < 0.01$). In addition, performance in the HN condition was better than the VN condition ($t = 2.02$, df = 7, $p < 0.05$ one-tailed), as expected.

Discussion

The findings from the two replications of this study confirmed the expectation that infants would have greater difficulty in differentiating locations in space outside the immediate reach space. The finding that a vertical arrangement of the hiding locations also produced a greater number of errors implied that aspects of the procedure associated with hiding in far space, such as movement, delay, and intervening action by the experimenter are not likely to account completely for the results obtained. However, the effect of movement involved in pushing the box from far space into reach space following completion of hiding could not be discounted entirely. Moore (1975) has proposed that the ability to correctly locate an object that has been covered and then moved be considered the mark of a new stage in object concept development, one higher than the ability to find an object that remains in place after covering. Moore describes the tasks in terms of being presented "within reach" or "out of reach," but he does not consider the distance from the infant as a variable. Rather, he suggests that rules for recognizing the identity of objects transposed from place to place have to be acquired for successful search in the task involving movement of the covered object. We agree with the sequential ordering of the tasks, but suggest that movement of the hidden object per se is not the main factor responsible for the error in localization. Gratch et al. (1974) have argued also that movement in itself does not account for the AB errors observed in their studies, because they observed instances of the AB error when a delay interval was imposed by restraining the infants while keeping the box in place.

Of necessity, when hiding takes place in far space, some delay is involved between the disappearance of the object from sight and the opportunity to search for it. The delay is probably not the most significant variable, because the introduction of the 2-sec delay for all conditions in the replication study (equalizing the interval between hiding and search) did not substantially affect the accuracy of performance in the different conditions.

We concluded that particular arrangements of hiding locations posed difficulties for the infant's limited understanding of spatial relations and, thus, accounted for the greater frequency of AB errors found in studies using the Gratch box with hiding accomplished in far space.

THE USE OF A MARKER FOR THE PREVIOUS POSITION OF AN OBJECT

Piaget regards the AB error as an index of a much more general limitation on the stage IV infant's conception of reality. The infant's search errors are interpreted as evidence of a pervasive inability to construct a stable network of spatial relations among objects. It follows from this interpretation that the absence of such a network of relations ought to be reflected in the infant's performance on a variety of hiding tasks, in addition to the two-position situation emphasized in the research literature.

In a longitudinal study (Lucas and Uzgiris, 1975), infants between 6 and 9 months old were presented with a series of hiding tasks that used various spatial displacements of an object both to accomplish its disappearance and following its occlusion from view. The results of the two tasks involving a displacement of the object after it had been covered by a screen are reported here. In both tasks the displacement consisted simply in moving both object and the screen which covered it from their original location to a new location, roughly the same distance from the infant. This was accomplished using either two screens, one to transport the object and one to mark its previous location, or the transport screen alone. Considering the presumed inability of infants to organize the positions and displacements of objects in space, it was expected that infants who had just begun to search for hidden objects might localize the object at its place of disappearance and, thus, fail to take into account the displacement of the object while covered by the screen.

The use of a second screen to indicate the previous location of the object was designed to provide the infant with a visible landmark of the place in which the object had disappeared. The object was placed clearly *in front of* the marker screen before being covered by the transport screen. The introduction of the marker screen placed an additional requirement on the infant; he had to differentiate the spatial relations between the marker screen, the object, and the transport screen in order to accurately locate the object following its displacement. Since the infant is thought to lack precision in structuring complex spatial relations among objects during this period of development, it was expected that introducing the marker screen would delay the attainment of reliable search for the object in comparison with the single screen task.

Subjects

Twelve infants participated in the study. They were tested in their homes at weekly intervals, starting at 6 months of age and continuing until they reliably obtained the object in each of the hiding tasks, a period of 11.2 weeks on the average.

Materials

Four screens were used in this study. Two rectangular pieces of cloth served as horizontal screens. Two vertical screens were constructed of lightweight wood and were free standing. All four screens measured 10 × 8 inches.

Procedure

During testing the infant was seated on the parent's lap before a table. Testing sessions were comprised of four hiding tasks; the two involving the displacements of a covered object will be described. The spatial displacements involved in these tasks are illustrated in Figure 2 for the case of vertical screens.

Unmarked Task: Search for Object Covered and Laterally Displaced to New Location Using Single Screen A screen was positioned 15 inches to one side of the infant, and a toy was placed just out of reach in front of the infant. The screen was moved to cover the object, and both screen and object were then laterally displaced an additional 15 inches to their final location on the opposite side of the infant.

Marked Task: Search for Object Covered and Laterally Displaced to New Location Where Second Screen is Used to Mark Its Previous Location The marker screen was placed 12 inches to one side of the infant. The transport screen was positioned at the extreme edge of the table on the same side as the marker. A toy was placed directly in front of the marker screen, clearly separated from the marker by 2 to 3 inches. The transport screen was then moved to cover the object, and both the transport screen and the object were laterally displaced to their final location on the opposite side of the infant.

The order of presentation of these two tasks was counterbalanced across testing sessions. The criterion for reliably successful search was recovery of the object on three consecutive or four out of five trials. The infant's search in the task involving the marked location was judged to be successful only if the transport screen was removed directly, i.e., if the infant searched first at the marker screen and then at the transport screen, successful search was not scored.

Results

The findings reported here are based on the combined data for the vertical and for the horizontal screens, since the infant's performance in the two tasks was not differentially affected by the type of screen used to cover the object.

Infants who had just begun to search for hidden objects had little difficulty in obtaining an object covered and laterally displaced using a single screen. The mean age for the attainment of the unmarked task was 7 months 24 days. In contrast, reliable search

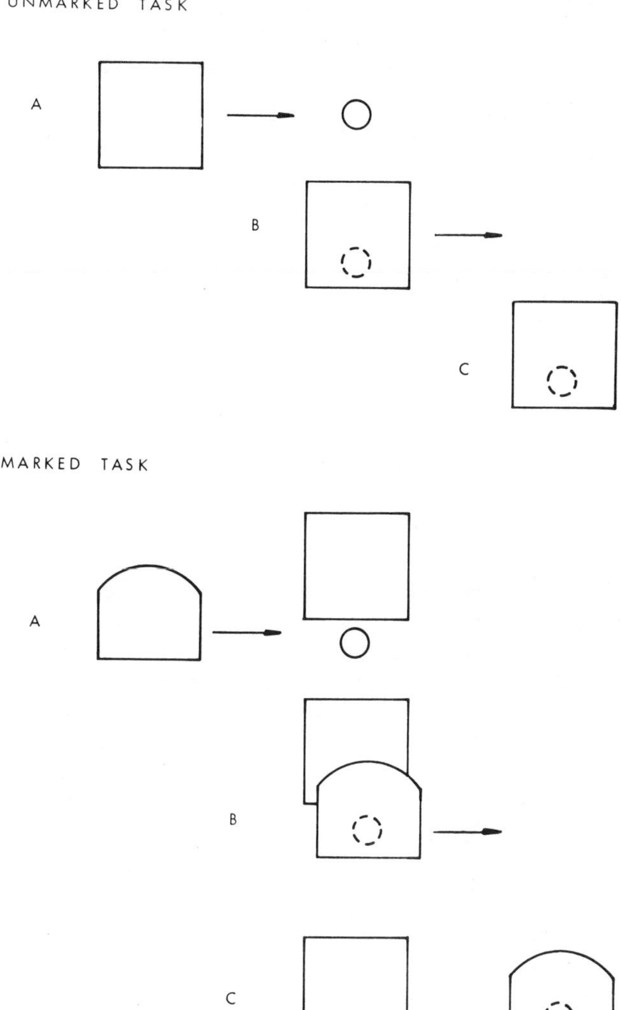

Figure 2. Spatial displacements involved in the unmarked and the marked tasks.

directly behind or under the transport screen was delayed considerably when the marker screen was introduced. The mean age for the attainment of the marked task was 8 months 19 days. The number of testing sessions separating the attainment of the marked from the unmarked task ranged from 3 to 8, with a mean of 5.1 sessions.

The infant's most frequent search response in the weeks preceding reliable search in the marked task was to look for the object behind or under the marker screen, the screen which had never occluded the object (see Table 3). In addition, when search at the marker proved unsuccessful, the infants were much more likely to abandon search than to infer

Table 3. Proportions of search behaviors prior to reliable search in the marked task

Weeks preceding reliable search	Removes neither screen	Removes marker screen only	Removes marker screen then removes transport screen and obtains object	Removes transport screen directly and obtains object
6	0.18	0.54	0.16	0.12
5	0.15	0.46	0.15	0.24
4	0.13	0.54	0.19	0.14
3	0.24	0.47	0.18	0.11
2	0.22	0.35	0.23	0.20
1	0.12	0.34	0.17	0.37
Reliable search	0.03	0.05	0.10	0.82

Table 4. Distribution of behaviors following marker screen removals preceding reliable search in the marked task

Weeks preceding reliable search	Proportion of marker screen removals that were followed by removal of the transport screen
6	0.22[a]
5	0.24[a]
4	0.26[a]
3	0.28[a]
2	0.40
1	0.33[a]
Reliable search	0.66

[a] $p < 0.05$, binomial test, two-tailed probability.

the location of the object behind or under the transport screen. The proportions contained in Table 4 represent the number of trials in which removal of the marker screen was followed by removal of the transport screen in comparison with the total number of trials in which the marker screen was removed. Because there are only two possible behaviors once the marker screen has been removed (i.e., the infant either abandons search or removes the transport screen), each of these proportions was subjected to a binomial test. The result of this analysis indicates that following removal of the marker screen, the probability of removing the transport screen was significantly smaller than chance in all testing sessions, excluding only the session 2 weeks before reliable search and the session in which reliable search was achieved.

Discussion

We propose that the error in the marked task is connected with lack of precision in spatial localization. Piaget and Inhelder (1967) have suggested that spatial relations among objects are conceived by the young infant in terms of their topological properties. Proximity, which corresponds to the "nearby-ness" of objects in the spatial field, is considered to be the most elementary of these topological properties and is said to dominate the young infant's conception of spatial relations. The period of development investigated in this study is regarded as a transitional one; space is still organized primarily in terms of topological relations, and under certain conditions, the relation of promixity may still predominate in the localization of objects in space.

We suggest that such conditions may have obtained in the marked task. The error of removing the marker screen may be interpreted as indicating that the infants structured the spatial arrangement of the object and the marker in terms of the topological relation of proximity; the separation of the object from the marker was not taken into account. Thus, the infants localized the object in a relatively undifferentiated manner, merely as being in the "general neighborhood" of the marker screen. Interpreting the error in this way accounts not only for its prevalence but also for the infants' failure to correct the error when it occurred. Since they had localized the object only in relation to the marker screen, the infants would not be expected to readily shift their search to the transport screen when search at the marker proved unsuccessful.

On this interpretation, then, the attainment of reliable search directly behind or under the transport screen provides evidence of a shift from more global to more precise differentiation of spatial relationships. Reliable search in the marked task does not necessarily index the attainment of a more advanced level in the development of the object concept. The difficulty of the task for the infant lies in the spatial relations inherent in the task, and the achievement of the task reflects the infant's capacity to discriminate between these relations with precision and accuracy. This suggests that if the spatial arrangement of the object and the marker screen were altered in such a way as to lead the infants to structure the relation between them in terms of their separation rather than their proximity, the error of removing the marker screen would not occur.

Follow-up Study

In a cross sectional replication study (Lucas and Uzgiris, 1977), the marked task was again presented to seven infants between the ages of 8 months 10 days and 8 months 22 days. In addition, a slightly modified version of this task was also presented: instead of being placed directly in front of the marker screen at the start of the task, the object was positioned forward and slightly to its side in the direction of the transport screen. As in the original marked task, a distance of 2 to 3 inches separated the object from the marker. However, repositioning the object in the modified version of the task ensured that from the infant's vantage point, the boundaries between the object and the marker screen were clearly distinguishable and the relation of separation between them was pronounced. It was expected that infants who committed the error of removing the marker screen in the marked task would search directly under the transport screen in the modified version of the marked task. For this study, to increase the discriminability of the marker screen from the transport screen, a horizontal screen was used to transport the object and a vertical screen was used to mark its previous location in both the original marked task and its modified version.

The results of the study were unambiguous. The error of removing the marker screen occurred significantly more often in the marked task than in the modified task; conversely, search directly under the transport screen occurred significantly more often in the modified task than in the marked task. The results in the marked task replicated the previous study. Averaged across infants, the mean proportion of marker screen removals was 0.70 compared with 0.63 in the previous study, when averaged for the 6 weeks prior to reliable search. In contrast, the mean proportion of marker screen removals in the modified task was 0.24. Conversely, the mean proportion of direct transport screen removals was 0.19 in the marked task and 0.66 in the modified task. As can be seen in Table 3, the proportion of direct transport screen removals did not exceed 0.40 in the previous study until reliable search was attained, whereas modifying the task to emphasize the separation between the object and the marker screen resulted in a considerably greater number of direct transport screen removals by the same infants who were making the error of searching at the marker screen in the unmodified task.

These findings clearly support our interpretation that lack of precision in spatial localization is responsible for the search error committed in the marked task. Increasing the apparent separation between the object and the marker by not overlapping them disrupted the proximal link between them and resulted in a substantial decrease in the occurrence of the error. These findings also indicate that the precision with which the infant differentiates spatial relationships increases gradually following the attainment of active search for hidden objects and his or her accuracy may vary considerably depending on the kinds of relationships involved.

FACTORS INFLUENCING IDENTIFICATION OF OBJECT LOCATIONS

The idea that infants at this level of development may have a strong tendency to code spatial relationships among objects in terms of topological properties suggested a rationale for the difficulty in localizing a hidden object when the Gratch box is used in far space. In a study undertaken to explore this factor (Flory and Uzgiris, 1975), it was reasoned that if an infant was relying on the proximity of the disappearing object to some distinct feature of the surround to note its location, the Gratch box as a whole was likely to serve as such a feature when the disappearances occurred at some distance from the infant. The distinctiveness of the two wells is reduced at a distance and the salience of the whole box as a figure in the surround increases. Consequently, it was expected that a change in the box to increase the separateness of the two hiding locations while in far space would reduce the incidence of the AB error.

In addition, the factor of movement from far to near space was further explored. One effect of the movement of the box might be to interest the infant in the spectacle of the moving object (box) and to disrupt the intention of recovering the hidden toy. It was reasoned that infants allowed to locomote toward the hidden object would be less subject to such disruption. Consequently, half of the infants in this study were permitted to crawl through space to recover the hidden object.

Subjects

Fifteen infants between 9 and 10 months of age who were able to crawl a distance of at least 3 feet with relative ease participated in the study. Their parents brought them to a testing room at Clark University for a single testing session.

Materials

A plywood box of the same dimensions as used by Gratch was employed in one of the testing conditions (GB). Two separate plywood boxes of the exact dimensions as the two wells in the Gratch box (7 × 7 × 2 inches, each) were constructed and employed in the other testing condition (SB). The two boxes were joined at the base by a thin metal bar to keep them exactly 12 inches apart. White washcloths covered the wells in both conditions. Small toys of interest to young infants were used for hiding.

Procedure

The study was conducted in a small room with a rug. During testing, the parent sat on the floor with the infant.

All infants were tested first in near space and then in far space. Far space was defined as 2½ feet from where the infant was seated. Seven of the infants were tested in near space using the Gratch box, and eight were tested using the separate boxes. All the infants were tested with both the Gratch box and the separate boxes in far space. First, each infant was tested in far space with the same box as used in near space, followed by a test with the other box. Testing consisted in hiding the object in well A until the infant was successful on two consecutive trials and then hiding the object at B. Only one trial was given at B.

When tested in far space, eight infants were permitted to crawl forward to find the object. For the other infants, the box was moved by the experimenter across the floor to be within reach. A 3-sec delay period was imposed during testing in near space, but a 5-sec delay period was imposed while moving the apparatus from far space toward the infants in order to approximate the time taken by those infants who were allowed to crawl to recover the hidden object.

Successful search at B was given a score of 5, search at A corrected to search at B was given a score of 3, and search exclusively at A was scored 1. Intermediate scores were given for variants of these search patterns.

Results

When the hidings were done in near space, the performance of infants tested with the GB or the SB was similar. Only one infant in each group did not search directly at B on the B trial. In addition, a similar number of trials had to be presented for each group in order to obtain two successful searches in succession at A. Only three of the 15 infants needed more than the minimum two trials.

For all infants, scores on B trials when the hiding took place in far space were somewhat lower than those in near space with the same type of box. Whether the infant was allowed to crawl or the box was moved toward the infant did not significantly affect performance. The mean scores obtained by the infants in near and far space with the two types of boxes are presented in Table 5.

Table 5. Mean "B" trial scores with the same type of box in near and far space

	Hiding in		
	Near space	Far space	
Separate boxes (*N* = 8)	4.5	Crawls (*N* = 4)	4.0
		Examiner moves (*N* = 4)	4.0
Gratch box (*N* = 7)	4.7	Crawls (*N* = 4)	2.7
		Examiner moves (*N* = 3)	2.6

Table 6. Mean "B" trial scores in far space with the two types of boxes

	Gratch box	Separate boxes
Infant crawls (N = 8)	2.4	4.5
Examiner moves (N = 7)	3.6	4.4

Table 7. Mean number of "A" trials given

	Hiding in					
Condition	N	Near space	N	Far space	N	Far space
Separate boxes	8	2.89	8	3.0	15	2.9
Gratch box	7	2.0	7	4.1	15	3.7

An analysis of B trial scores for the two testings in far space revealed a significant difference in performance in the SB compared with the GB condition for the same infants (F = 8.45, df = 1, 11, $p < 0.05$). Order of presentation of the conditions and the mode of gaining access to the box did not significantly affect the scores. The mean scores obtained for hidings in far space are presented in Table 6.

The number of trials given at A in order to accumulate two consecutive successful searches at A was also examined. The expectation that difficulties in distinguishing and localizing spatial positions would be reflected in the A trial data was confirmed. The infants were given a significantly greater number of trials when the hidings took place in far space (F = 10.52, df = 1, 13, $p < 0.01$) and there was a significant interaction between the type of box used for testing and the spatial location of the testing (F = 8.33, df = 1, 13, $p < 0.05$). The mean number of A trials for infants tested with the GB and the SB is presented in Table 7. Hiding in far space with the GB required a greater number of A trials to achieve two consecutive successes. Considering only the testings in far space, the infants needed an average of 3.7 trials to achieve two successful searches at A when the GB was used and 2.9 trials when the SB were used (t = 2.89, df = 14, $p < 0.05$). Neither the order of presentation nor the mode of gaining access to the boxes significantly affected the infants' performance.

Discussion

The main result of this study, showing that manipulation of the characteristics of hiding locations influences the accuracy of an infant's search behavior, adds support to our notion that AB error is a reflection of the infant's limited ability to understand spatial relations. To the extent that the infant tends to rely on topological properties in coding relations between objects in space, the accuracy of the infant's search can be influenced by making localization in terms of topological properties (such as proximity, separateness, etc.) sufficient or insufficient. The observation also suggests that the prevalence of the AB error observed in the first study when hiding took place in far space may be better accounted for by the fact that the use of the Gratch box in far space tended to reduce the separateness of the two wells rather than by the fact that the hiding took place in far space.

Several laboratory studies have reported a very low incidence of AB errors. For example, Harris (1973) found very few such errors in 10-month-old infants who had to search for a toy in one of two compartments with the two compartments only 4 inches apart; however, the two compartments were always within reach of the infant. Similarly, Butterworth (1975) found that only about half of the infants he tested in each of four conditions erred on the B trials despite manipulations that involved the movement of the containers between the A and B trials. The movement, though, was sideways, to the left or right, and did not involve movement between far space and reach space. The literature seems to be coming to the conclusion that the AB error is more accurately described as a tendency to search at both A and B when the object is hidden at B rather than as a strong tendency to search only at A. Certainly, the results of the three studies reported here support this conclusion. If this characterization is correct, it fits our contention that the infant has difficulty in accurately localizing the position of the hidden object rather than conceiving of the object as clearly located at A because of the infant's previous activity at A.

The finding that the manner in which the infant was allowed to reach the object hidden in far space did not affect accuracy of search was unexpected. However, it lends support to the interpretation that the difficulty of hidings in far space is due to factors other than the movement of the container per se. We have conducted some preliminary studies of search behavior in large space, in which the infant has to crawl to reach the hiding location of a desired object. The paths taken by infants to reach those locations may also serve as an indicator of their understanding of space in addition to their facility in finding hidden objects.

CONCLUDING REMARKS

Considered in relation to other studies in the literature, this work has several implications for understanding intellectual development in infancy. The first point to be made is methodological.

The pattern of results discussed in this paper demonstrates the importance of an active interchange between observational and experimental approaches for understanding developmental change. Experimental studies, by standardizing the testing situation and by greatly limiting the range of responses available to the infant, are in danger of overlooking aspects of that specific situation which may contribute significantly to the responses observed. The stability of the responses over a range of related testing situations is often unexamined. As a consequence, inferences regarding the infant's cognitive functioning based on such responses may be misguided. The use of the Gratch box to study the AB error in object construction may be a case in point. The particular arrangement of hiding locations in the box seems to contribute to the pattern of search and of gazing. Only the use of somewhat altered testing situations is leading investigators to consider interpretations of the performance of stage IV infants in terms of variables other than memory for the hiding location and prior activity at that location (e.g., Butterworth, 1975; Moore, 1975).

Observational studies, on the other hand, provide an opportunity to consider the infant's performance over a range of testing situations. The pattern of behavioral responses in these situations often provides suggestive leads with respect to the factors that affect performance. However, observational techniques generally do not permit isolation of the contribution of each of several co-occurring variables. Thus, our observational studies suggested that the factor of hiding in near versus far space may affect the accuracy of search at stage IV, but only the specific manipulation of the relations between the object, the screen, and the hiding locations permitted us to determine the means by which hiding at a distance from the infant influences accuracy of search. It is expected that further observations of the paths taken by infants in search for objects in large spaces will generate an even clearer understanding of the spatial world of infants within which the object must be constituted.

The point regarding the importance of integrating observational and experimental methods has been made many times before, but since this integration is so rarely implemented, it clearly warrants repetition.

The second point concerns the need to examine the links between object concept development and a much wider realm of the infant's experience in the world. The infant's ability to actively change his position through space either by crawling, by walking, or by other means may contribute significantly to the fabric of experience from which an objective understanding of reality is constructed. It may not be coincidental that the achievement of object search and the ability to crawl come in close temporal proximity. It seems reasonable that active movement in space would contribute to the infant's ability to differentiate spatial relations and to code them in more precise ways. It is suggested throughout this paper that a more differential comprehension of spatial relations is an important element for object construction in the period immediately following the achievement of object search. It has been noted that during this period infants engage in a great deal of spontaneous exploration of spatial relations between objects such as putting inside and taking out, building up and taking apart, and so forth (Uzgiris, 1973). At this same time, they also begin to actively locomote in large space. Walk's (1966) studies suggest that by the time infants begin to crawl, they clearly rely on visual depth cues to guide their locomotion.

Whether attribution of permanence to objects is systematically related to active locomotion has not been studied. However, it is instructive that in studies of blind infants, Fraiberg (1968) found no infant who learned to creep before beginning to reach for objects on sound cue, thus indicating that the blind infants already had some notion of an object when presented with an index of that object by the time they began to move actively through space. Furthermore, thalidomide-injured infants have been reported to achieve a concept of object without too great a delay (Décarie, 1969). These infants, although lacking limbs, generally do not lack experience in moving through space. The absence of limbs changes the form of their interaction with objects, but the infants do displace objects in space and also vary their own position with respect to stationary objects. Active locomotion through space may be a very important factor in achieving higher levels in object construction.

Interactions with other persons are also central to the infant's experience. Links between the development of attachment to familiar figures and object construction have been posited and examined in several empirical studies. Although no simple relationship between understanding of object permanence and attachment to familiar figures has been found, several studies support the assumption that ties between these two aspects of functioning exist (e.g., Bell, 1970; Décarie, 1974; Serafica and Uzgiris, 1971). Our studies of the relationship between spatial understanding and object conception and our speculations concerning the role of active locomotion in this relationship suggest still another tie. The infant's experience with familiar persons as they appear and disappear and change their position in space undoubtedly contributes to the construction of both space and object, especially in view of the salience of familiar persons and their importance as goal objects for the infant. In addition, we may cite the commonplace observation that active locomotion on the part of the infant is often instigated by the disappearance of significant persons.

Active locomotion through space and attachment to familiar persons are only two of many aspects of infant functioning which may be related to object construction. To gain a fuller understanding of the factors involved in the child's coming to know and understand reality, the child's experience in other domains of functioning must be examined. We suggest that the realm of infant experience relevant to achieving an understanding of reality is much broader than is commonly acknowledged.

ACKNOWLEDGMENTS

We thank Alec A. Pearsall, Psychology Research Shop, for the construction of the hiding boxes used in the studies reported. We are also grateful to L. Frey and G. Yablick for their comments on an earlier version of this paper.

REFERENCES

Bell, S. M. V. 1968. The relationship of infant-mother attachment to the development of the concept of object-permanence. Unpublished doctoral dissertation. The Johns Hopkins University.

Bell, S. M. 1970. The development of the concept of object as related to infant-mother attachment. Child Dev. 41:291–311.

Bower, T. G. R. 1974. Development in Infancy. W. H. Freeman & Company, San Francisco.

Boynton, J., and Uzgiris, I. C. 1975. Performance in the two-position hiding situation as a function of spatial organization. Unpublished manuscript, Clark University.

Butterworth, G. 1975. Object identity in infancy: the interaction of spatial location codes in determining search errors. Child Dev. 46:866–870.

Casati, I., and Lézine, I. 1968. Les étapes de l'intelligence sensori-motrice. Les Éditions du Centre de Psychologie Appliquée, Paris.

Corman, H., and Escalona, S. 1969. Stages of sensorimotor development: a replication study. Merrill-Palmer Q. 15:351–361.

Décarie, Th. G. 1965. Intelligence and Affectivity in Early Childhood. International Universities Press Inc., New York.

Décarie, Th. G. 1969. A study of the mental and emotional development of the thalidomide child. In: B. M. Foss (ed.), Determinants of Infant Behavior, Vol. 4. Methuen & Co. Ltd., London.

Décarie, Th. G. 1974. The Infant's Reaction to Strangers. International Universities Press Inc., New York.

Evans, W. F. 1974. The stage IV error in Piaget's theory of object concept development: an investigation of the role of activity. Dissertation Abstr. 34:5651.

Evans, W. F., and Gratch, G. 1972. The stage IV error in Piaget's theory of object concept development: difficulties in object conceptualization or spatial localization? Child Dev. 43:682–688.

Flory, K., and Uzgiris, I. C. 1975. The role of topological relationships in the infant's understanding of the two-position hiding task. Unpublished manuscript, Clark University.

Fraiberg, S. 1968. Parallel and divergent patterns in blind and sighted infants. Psychoanal. Study Child 33:264–300.

Fraisse, P. 1968. The experimental method. In: P. Fraisse and J. Piaget (eds.), Experimental Psychology: Its Scope and Method, Vol. 1. Basic Books Inc., New York.

Gratch, G. 1975. Recent studies based on Piaget's view of object concept development. In: L. B. Cohen and P. Salapatek (eds.), Infant Perception: From Sensation to Cognition, Vol. 2. Academic Press, New York.

Gratch, G., and Landers, W. F. 1971. Stage IV of Piaget's theory of infant's object concepts: a longitudinal study. Child Dev. 42:359–372.

Gratch, G., Appel, K. J., Evans, W. F., LeCompte, G. K., and Wright, N. A. 1974. Piaget's stage IV object concept error: evidence of forgetting or object conception? Child Dev. 45:71–77.

Harris, P. 1973. Perseverative errors in search by young infants. Child Dev. 44:28–33.

Harris, P. L. 1974. Perseverative search at a visibly empty place by young infants. J. Exp. Child Psychol. 18:535–542.

Harris, P. L. 1975. Development of search and object permanence during infancy. Psychol. Bull. 82:332–344.

Landers, W. F. 1971. Effects of differential experience on infant's performance in a Piagetian stage IV object-concept task. Dev. Psychol. 5:48–54.

Lucas, T. C. 1975. Spatial factors in the development of the object concept. Unpublished masters thesis, Clark University.

Lucas, T. C., and Uzgiris, I. C. 1975. Space and object concept in infancy. Paper presented at the meetings of the American Psychological Association, Chicago, Illinois.

Lucas, T. C., and Uzgiris, I. C. 1977. Spatial factors in the development of the object concept. Dev. Psychol. 13:492–500.

Moore, M. K. 1973. The genesis of object permanence. Paper presented at the meetings of the Society for Research in Child Development, Philadelphia.

Moore, M. K. 1975. Object permanence and object identity: a stage developmental model. Paper presented at the meetings of the Society for Research in Child Development, Denver.

Piaget, J. 1954. The Construction of Reality in the Child. Basic Books Inc., New York.

Piaget, J., and Inhelder, B. 1967. The Child's Conception of Space. W. W. Norton & Company Inc., New York.

Schofield, L., and Uzgiris, I. C. 1969. Examining behavior and the development of the concept of object. Paper presented at the meetings of the Society for Research in Child Development, Santa Monica, California.

Serafica, F. C., and Uzgiris, I. C. 1971. Infant-mother relationship and object concept. Paper presented at the meetings of the American Psychological Association, Washington, D.C.

Smillie, D. 1972. Piaget's constructionist theory. Hum. Dev. 15:171–186.

Uzgiris, I. C. 1973. Patterns of cognitive development in infancy. Merrill-Palmer Q. 19:181–204.

Uzgiris, I. C., and Hunt, J. McV. 1975. Assessment in Infancy. University of Illinois Press, Urbana.

Walk, R. D. 1966. The development of depth perception in animals and human infants. Monogr. Soc. Res. Child Dev. 31, No. 5 (Serial No. 107): 82–108.

OBSERVATIONAL METHODS IN THE STUDY OF LANGUAGE DEVELOPMENT:

Comparison with Ethological Methods in the Study of Animal Communication

Introduction

Patricia Black-Cleworth

The possible relationships between animal vocalizations and human language have been discussed extensively in the past; see Lenneberg (1967) and Thorpe (1972) for review. A comparison of the methodologies used to study both phenomena should reveal what similarities have evolved and which methods one discipline might profitably borrow from the other. In the field of developmental linguistics, vocalizations are relatively simple in structure, at least with regard to adult language; thus, they should enable some degree of comparison with certain aspects of ethological theory and methodology, especially where those aspects are concerned with animal communication and social behavior. Dale (chapter 9) has thoroughly described the methods used in developmental linguistics; therefore, this discussion concentrates on a brief description of relevant ethological methods and a comparison between the two. A more detailed review of animal communication including some discussion of methodology can be found in Cullen (1972).

Most animals have relatively discrete vocalizations, facial expression and postures, and chemical products or pheromones that serve in social communication. The young often have additional patterns not produced by adults. The ethologist interested in social communication in a given species wants to define more or less precisely what these patterns consist of, what their communicative significance is, and how they function in assuring existence and reproduction. There is a clear distinction between the sending and receiving of animal signals (Smith, 1965). The sending animal produces a signal, defined as the "message," which reflects some aspect of the state of its central nervous system, or its mood, such as a feeling of aggression or fear. That the animal produces such a signal, however, does not necessarily, or even usually, mean that it is consciously trying to communicate its feelings. The recipient processes this signal along with all other environmental information, and then may or may not produce a response that reflects the "meaning" of that signal at that time to that animal. If a signal does not produce an overt response, that does not necessarily mean there was no meaning, but such meanings are difficult if not impossible to ascertain.

Before communicative significance can be assessed, it is necessary to compile an ethogram, that is, a description of the various behavior patterns produced by a given species. It has proven difficult to define exactly what constitutes a pattern; usually it includes whatever seems to be a repeatable unitary event. For example, scratching can vary in both the muscles that are used and the intensity of the movement, but it is recognizable in all cases. In the case of vocalizations it is often easier to define the beginning and end of the event, whereas the precise physical structure of a sound can only be determined using a sound spectrograph.

Analyzing the communicative value of behavior patterns initially involves a series of observations of their production and reception under conditions as natural as possible, with the aim of making correlations between these patterns and more obvious types of behavior such as feeding, copulation, or attack. The ways in which ethologists analyze the motivation or causation of the animals' displays (i.e., the message) have been defined by Tinbergen (1959). They include 1) comparison of the individual movements of similar components of the display with components of acts such as actual attack or escape, in order to identify similarities that could indicate underlying motivation; 2) temporal analysis; and 3) situation analysis.

Temporal analysis assumes that an animal's environment, and hence motivation, usually changes more slowly than its behavior patterns, so that behavior patterns occurring close together in time are likely to have the same underlying motivation. This motivation can then be inferred from the more obvious behaviors. Thus, if an animal facing another individual produces a display and then attacks the other animal, the display was very likely a threat. This principle underlies the statistical technique of sequential analysis. Situation analysis compares situations in which displays of unknown function are produced with situations in which more obvious types of behavior such as attack and escape are produced. Further discussion of these methods and a comparison of the results obtained by applying each of them to the displays of the great tit can be found in Blurton-Jones (1968).

The investigation of the meanings of behavior patterns generally proceeds along similar lines. For example, in the same situation given above, if one animal produces a display and the other responds either by attacking or fleeing, it would mean that the second animal interpreted the display as a threat. By collecting many observations of this type and subjecting them to statistical analysis, one can often obtain a reasonably reliable interpretation of the meanings of signals (Altmann, 1965; Hazlett and Bossert, 1965).

Whenever possible, the results obtained from observation should be tested with controlled experiments. As Blurton-Jones (1968) has pointed out, observational methods *suggest plausible hypotheses,* but experiments are necessary to prove or disprove these hypotheses. The classic ethological experimental technique has been the use of models or their acoustical counterparts, playbacks. Physical models of a male or female bird, for example, can be placed in the territory of a male and his resulting behaviors can be interpreted as threat and courtship displays, respectively. Tape recordings of various vocalizations can be played back to individual animals in natural or appropriate laboratory environments and their reactions used to test the meanings of the recorded vocal signals.

Analysis of the development of communication in infant and juvenile animals has centered around a few basic areas of interest. One of these has been the patterns that serve for communication between parent and offspring. Often the young produce distinctive patterns, such as cries for food, to which the adults respond with specific actions. Similarly, the young respond specifically to certain parental signals, such as alarm cries. These types of interaction have been studied by the same methods described above; and (as exemplified by many of the conference papers) this approach is now being used successfully to study human mother-infant interactions.

Another type of study involves the age at which adult communication signals and responses are established in the young. These studies also address the question of whether the young initially use and respond to signals in the same way as adults or whether they require some developmental period. These questions can be studied by observations over time, or by setting up situations that will elicit the appropriate behavior in adults and examining the behavior of young animals of different ages.

A third area of interest that has developed from the study of young animals has been their use of metacommunicative signals, which involve communication about communication. The best studied examples are signals used as an invitation to play or emitted during play: they signal that all of the behavior that occurs during the interaction is not to be taken seriously, but playfully (Bekoff, 1972).

Unlike human language, many animal signals appear in the adult form the first time they are used by young animals. In many cases this seems to be related to the relative simplicity of the signals. Such signals may also be entirely under genetic rather than cultural control. An exception is the development of song in certain species of birds such as chaffinches and white-crowned sparrows. Birds of these species do not develop the normal species-specific song if they are raised in isolation, but instead produce a more simple song. The song is even more abnormal if the birds are deafened at an early age. In contrast, birds such as chickens develop all of their typical calls even if they are deafened within a few days of hatching. If a chaffinch is kept in isolation after the age of 4 months it will develop a normal song even though it does not begin to sing a complete song until the age of 10 months. This finding has been interpreted as evidence for the existence of a "critical period" for song learning. Moreover, chaffinches deafened after a season of singing will maintain their song, whereas birds deafened just as they are developing their full song will regress to a more primitive level. Thus, auditory feedback is also critical in song development. In addition, the neural control of bird song in these species is lateralized, as is the case with human language control. If the bird's left hypoglossal nerve is cut, from 70% to more than 90% of the song elements, depending on the species and the complexity of the song, disappear (see Nottebohm, 1970 and Nottebohm in Lenneberg, 1974 for a review). A combination of observational and experimental methodologies has been necessary to establish this information.

An analysis of the methodologies currently used in animal communication and developmental linguistics reveals a certain degree of convergence, particularly noticeable in recent linguistic studies. Ethological techniques have developed gradually and intuitively for 50 to 60 years, and a theoretical framework began to emerge only 20 years ago. Similar observational methods seem to have developed independently in linguistics over the last 15 years.

Linguistics has always made a strong logical distinction between syntactics, semantics, and pragmatics, which have been translated into the terms form, content, and use for the benefit of the layman. It was apparent at the conference that these terms are still not easy for the layman to grasp. Hood has defined them more simply as 1) form: the way something is said, 2) content: meaning, and 3) use: the purpose for which the sentence or phrase serves. These distinctions are less easily made in animal communication studies. Form or structure amounts to a physical description of the parts of the act. In the case of vocalizations, it consists of a sound spectrogram or a description, with similarities and differences, of a series of sound spectrographs including frequencies, intensities, and temporal structures. In linguistics the structure exemplifies grammatical relations that are logical to the human mind and which then admit a great deal of additional analysis. In animal communication this description serves chiefly as a precise identification. In descriptions of bird song it is also used to classify consistent differences between species and populations; terms such as syllables, elements, and phrases are used to describe a species-specific song or local dialect. However, one cannot say that one structure is better or more correct than another as one can in linguistic analysis, where the correct grammatical form can be defined and collected examples compared to it. Instead, the variations in song are collected, analyzed, and interpreted in terms of different levels of function as indexed by differences in behavioral outcomes.

In the past, ethologists often ignored the distinction between content and use, but it is now well appreciated. A clear differentiation has been made by Smith (1968) in his discussions on message, meaning, and context. He defines the semantic level as the message and the pragmatic level as the meanings. He also points out that a given signal or message can have several different meanings depending on the context in which it is used and the identity of the recipient animal.

Ethology has a fourth level of functional analysis that has been its chief guiding light over the years: the evolutionary function of a signal; how it enables a species to survive, prosper, and reproduce. The species-specific bird songs of the chaffinches and white-crowned sparrows discussed above are excellent examples of both how ethological thinking operates in this regard and how ethological evolutionary concepts have sometimes been applied to language. Some of the ecological functions of bird songs are to advertise that a single male bird is in possession of a territory, is in reproductive condition, and is seeking a mate. These birds are singing a song that is distinctive to their species and even to their population. It is hypothesized that female birds are especially attracted by the song that they grew up hearing, i.e., the species-specific or population-specific song. Baptista (1976) notes that when white-crowned sparrow females sing, they sing the population-specific song. If females select mates that sing a song with which they were raised, this acts as a reproductive isolating mechanism, i.e., members of the same population or species breed with each other, resulting in populations of sparrows that are well adapted to the local conditions in their habitat. Ecological evidence supporting this hypothesis comes from finches in the Azores, Madeira, and the Canary Islands. There is usually only one or, at the most, two species of finches living on any one of these islands, in contrast to the variety of closely related species living on the mainland. Correspondingly, the island song is much simpler, resembling the song of chaffinches raised in isolation. This is interpreted to mean that with the disappearance of the need for a mechanism to enable accurate distinction between many species in order to ensure reproductive isolation, the learned complexity of the song has disappeared (Marler and Hamilton, 1966).

Nottebohm (1970) has gone so far as to suggest that human language-learning abilities could have the same effect. Human beings learn language very easily at certain early ages, after which it becomes more difficult. During this sensitive or "critical period" children tend to be living with their parents in a given cultural group. Later, when they come to select their mates, it is more difficult for them to learn a different language and hence they will probably select a mate that speaks the same language. This assures that human beings will tend to remain in the same group with which they were raised. Lenneberg (1967) also discusses the evolutionary implications of the same critical period phenomenon, which he calls resonance. His conclusion, however, is that this type of system enables a complex precise signaling system to exist without the need for precise genetic coding. It would require a great deal of genetic material to specify the details of bird song, not to mention human language, and a complex genetic system would be exceedingly prone to errors, and hence to loss of individuals with genetic mistakes. He thus envisions the critical period learning system as evolutionarily efficient in promoting complex signaling systems with a minimum of genetic information.

Certain conceptual parallels between ethological distinctions and linguistic concerns can be identified. One is distinguishing between production and comprehension in linguistics, which is generally analogous to distinguishing between the message and meaning in ethology. The distinction is certainly important in both fields. For example, as related by Sackett at the conference, the facial expressions produced by monkeys raised in isolation are quite different from those produced by normal monkeys. To determine whether this was caused by a deficit in production or in reception, the isolates were taught to respond with simple reactions to video taped facial expressions of normal monkeys in order to avoid shock. The results demonstrated that these monkeys had a deficit in their ability to interpret monkey facial expressions, in addition to their obvious problems in producing them. Dale has pointed out that naturalistic observations have been used to characterize the development of language production in recent years, but that it has proven more difficult to adapt naturalistic observations to study comprehension.

Another interesting development in linguistics is the use of context and situational analysis in manners similar to the way they have been applied in ethology. This is exemplified by Hood et al. (chapter 10), who present transcripts of children's language accompanied by descriptions of the nonlinguistic situation, and use the latter to interpret the meaning. It is also evident in recent studies of pragmatics, described by Dale, in which the situation is used to understand the intent and motivation of the child. This type of analysis should be useful in studying comprehension as well.

Some similarities between linguistics and ethology can also be seen in the comparative approach. Of course, the comparisons originate from very different sources. In linguistics, languages learned in different cultures are compared; in ethology, phylogenetic differences in signal production and reception between related species are studied. One of the primary purposes of both approaches is to construct taxonomies: in the one case, of language relationships; in the other, of species relationships. In addition to classifying differences, the comparative approach is useful in revealing similar or universal characteristics that occur across species or larger groupings. Ethologists, for example, have found that vocalizations accompanying similar motivational situations have similar physical characteristics in many birds and mammals. Threat vocalizations usually are low pitched, harsh continuous sounds whereas attraction vocalizations of many parents to young are soft, low pitched, brief, and repetitive. Alarm calls, on the other hand, tend to be high pitched and harsh (Collias, 1960). These characteristics persist in our own vocalizations.

The comparative approach to linguistics should also be useful for validating what appear to be universals in children's learning of English. Dale mentions that children develop 14 grammatical elements in a nearly invariant sequence. If these or similar sequences were found to apply to other languages as well, it would suggest that certain patterns of language acquisition might be a general rule in the human species rather than just peculiar to English.

The comparison of verbal language with various forms of nonverbal communication is also an intriguing area. It is somewhat analogous to comparison of the features of signals of different modalities in ethology, such as gestures, vocalizations, chemical products, and even such unusual modalities as electrical signal production and reception (Black-Cleworth, 1970). These nonverbal forms in humans include a wide variety of normal and compensatory reactions, usually in the visual mode, such as the expressions and nonverbal signals accompanying speech and the gestures used by children who are at preliminary stages of language development, and by adults who do not speak the same language. The development and use of a complete gestural sign language in deaf people results from their sensory loss, which affects both comprehension and production of speech. Sign language, however, is similar to spoken language in the way it is acquired by children and used grammatically by adults, and in having lateralized neural control (Klima and Bellugi, in Lenneberg, 1974). Other more restricted examples of compensation have been mentioned. Dale tells of a man with extreme cerebral palsy who could not speak and was eventually able to demonstrate his knowledge of language only with a foot-operated typewriter; Landesman-Dwyer describes the unique nonverbal signals of a mentally retarded woman who kicked her foot whenever a familiar adult appeared.

These cases are interesting and enlightening for the study of language in that they indicate a number of pragmatic approaches to language teaching that can be or have been undertaken. The interrelationships between language and nonverbal communication show that language is only a part, although usually the major part, of the desire to express oneself, to communicate feelings and information, and to obtain desired ends. Thus, the study of language out of the context in which it is produced will lose the impact of these powerful motivations and be unable to assess them. Naturalistic observation techniques and experimental testing yield discrepant ages at which production of particular linguistic elements are achieved; these discrepancies almost certainly result from the different motivations present in the different situations; i.e., children in a natural situation are more motivated to communicate, as demonstrated by Bloom (1974).

The ways in which persons compensate for defective comprehension or production of language demonstrate the plastic capabilities of the nervous system, given the appropriate motivation. They also show that some of the postulated prerequisites for language development are either not essential or can take different forms, e.g., babbling would seem to be of little use to a deaf person learning sign language, although early use of the hands might act as a substitute (Eibl-Eibesfeldt, 1970). Moreover, babbling does not occur in persons who comprehend but cannot produce normal language, and thus cannot be considered as essential for language comprehension (Lenneberg, 1967).

The ease with which visual signals or symbols can substitute for verbal language, both in human communication and in chimpanzees, has led to a number of pragmatic attempts to use such systems in teaching language to those with impairments in language learning abilities. Very often these systems have tried to switch the learners to verbal language at a later stage. Sign language has often been taught to the deaf. More recently, as Charlesworth has pointed out, attempts have centered on teaching only verbal language to deaf children in schools, with the common result that they learn sign language on their own and use it extensively in their private lives. Sign language has also been taught to autistic children and has been transferred to verbal behavior (related by Dale in the discussion). A certain degree of proficiency in American sign language can also be achieved by chimpanzees (Gardner and Gardner, in Ploog and Melnechuk, 1971; and Thorpe, 1972).

One of the most successful systems for teaching language principles to the severely retarded has been the system described by Carrier, which was designed using the visual system developed by Premack for teaching chimpanzees. This system has been remarkably effective and has resulted in about a 70% spontaneous transfer to verbal language.

Up to now we have been considering what can be taken from normal human development or from other related fields and applied to the problems of the mentally retarded. However, it is not always necessary or desirable to study normal development first and then look at differences in the development of the mentally retarded. Instead, Begab has suggested that study of the retarded first might lead to a better understanding of normal development. This principle has been confirmed in other areas, particularly in physiology. For example, the anatomical organization of the human sensory and motor cortex was proposed by Jackson (1875) after he observed the anatomical spread of focal epilepsy. A similar approach was used by Eibl-Eibesfeldt (1970) in studying the facial expression of children born blind and both deaf and blind. He found that these children show almost all of the characteristics of normal children in smiling, crying, and other expressions and has used this natural deprivation experiment as an argument for the innateness of human facial expressions. The natural development of language in the mentally retarded might provide another example; the features known to date are amply discussed by Dale in chapter 9.

REFERENCES

Altmann, S. A. 1965. Sociobiology of rhesus monkeys: II. stochastics of social communication. J. Theor. Biol. 8:490–522.

Baptista, L. F. 1976. Song dialects and demes in sedentary populations of the white-crowned sparrow (*Zonotrichia leucophrys mutalli*). Univ. Calif. Publ. Zool. 105:1–52.

Bekoff, M. 1972. The development of social interaction, play, and metacommunication in mammals: an ethological perspective. Q. Rev. Biol. 47:412–434.

Black-Cleworth, P. 1970. The role of electrical discharges in the non-reproductive social behaviour of *Gymnotus carapo* (Gymnotidae, Pisces). Anim. Behav. Monogr. 3:1–77.

Bloom, L. 1974. Talking, understanding, and thinking. In: R. L. Schiefelbusch and L. L. Lloyd (eds.), Language Perspectives—Acquisition, Retardation, and Intervention. University Park Press, Baltimore.

Blurton-Jones, N. G. 1968. Observations and experiments on causation of threat displays of the great tit (*Parus major*). Anim. Behav. Monogr. 1:75–158.

Collias, N. E. 1960. An ecological and functional classification of animal sounds. In: W. E. Lanyon and W. N. Tavolga (eds.), Animal Sounds and Communication. Publ. No. 7, pp. 368–391. AIBS, Washington, D.C.

Cullen, J. M. 1972. Some principles of animal communication. In: R. A. Hinde (ed.), Non-verbal Communication, pp. 101–122. Cambridge University Press, New York.

Eibl-Eibesfeldt, I. 1970. Ethology: The Biology of Behavior, Holt, Rinehart & Winston, New York.

Hazlett, B. A. and Bassert, W. H. 1965. A statistical analysis of the aggressive communications systems of some hermit crabs. Anim. Behav. 13:357–373.

Jackson, J. H. 1875. Cases of partial convulsion from organic brain disease, bearing on the experiments of Hitzig and Ferrier. Med. Times Hosp. Gaz. 1:581–585.

Lenneberg, E. H. 1967. Biological Foundations of Language. John Wiley & Sons, Inc., New York.

Lenneberg, E. H. 1974. Language and brain: developmental aspects. Neurosci. Res. Prog. Bull. 12:513–656.

Marler, P., and Hamilton, W. J., III. 1966. Mechanisms of Animal Behaviour. John Wiley & Sons, Inc., New York.

Nottebohm, F. 1970. Ontogeny of bird song. Science 167:950–956.

Ploog, D., and Melnechuk, T. 1971. Are Apes Capable of Language? Neurosci. Res. Prog. Bull. 9:600–700.

Smith, W. J. 1965. Message-meaning analyses. In: T. A. Sebeok (ed.), Animal Communication. pp. 44–60. Indiana University Press, Bloomington.

Thorpe, W. H. 1972. The comparison of vocal communication in animals and man. In: R. A. Hinde (ed.), Non-verbal Communication. pp. 27–47. Cambridge University Press, New York.

Tinbergen, N. 1959. Comparative studies of the behaviour of gulls (Laridae): a progress report. Behaviour 15:1–70.

chapter 9

What Does Observing Language Mean?

Philip S. Dale

A developmental psycholinguist might come to a conference on observational methods with a feeling of righteousness. In few other areas of developmental psychology are observational methods so firmly established as the central methodology. The major advances in our understanding of language development in the past 15 years have to an enormous extent come from the observational studies of Brown and his co-workers on Adam, Eve, and Sarah; of Bloom and her associates on Kathryn, Gia, and Eric (and later children); of Bowerman on the Finnish-speaking children Seppo and Rina; and others.

To be sure, the limitations of the observational approach are well recognized: sampling problems, problems of sorting utterances that reflect general patterns from utterances that are idiosyncratic or slips of the tongue, the missing knowledge of what a word or construction actually means to a child, and many others (see Dale, 1976). And there is general agreement on the need for controlled and standardized procedures to supplement the findings of naturalistic research. Nevertheless, there is something approaching a consensus that the child shows best what he knows when allowed in a familiar and unconstrained situation to express himself on a topic of his own choosing in the manner he favors. Just two illustrations of this point will be provided here. The first is from Brown's landmark work, *A First Language,* in the context of a discussion of the emergence of inflections.

> Experimental studies generally ''date'' the acquisition of inflections at much later chronological ages than does our naturalistic study. This seems to be not a fundamental disagreement on the facts but a seeming disagreement arising from such factors as the following:
>
> 1. Differences in the criterion of acquisition including percentages of children as opposed to percentages of contexts for one child.
> 2. The use of invented or synthetic stems as opposed to real stems.
> 3. The creation, in the interests of experimental design, of quite unusual problems in sentence processing which probably throw off habitual routines.

Preparation of this chapter was supported in part by Contract HD-3-2793 from the National Institute of Child Health and Human Development entitled ''An Investigation of Certain Relationships between Hearing Impairment and Language Disability.''

> To these which have been rather clearly established, I would add the general problem of the experimental method which requires us to direct and hold the child's attention as one need not in the naturalistic study of spontaneous speech. It is, I have found, a very general fact extending far beyond the study of the grammatical morphemes that assessments of particular kinds of linguistic competence based on experimental findings "date" the competencies in question later than do assessments based on naturalistic data. The performance on which the estimates are based are always different especially with regard to the need to direct and hold attention. I think the naturalistic data can yield a truer estimate in the sense of an estimate that is less dependent on performance skills not routinely developed in the child. But the experimental data, needless to say, can often be complete, where the naturalistic data are seriously fragmentary. The two methods, together give us the best chance of discovering the truth (Brown, 1973, p. 293).

A study by Prutting, Gallagher, and Mulac (1975) provides very clear empirical evidence for Brown's generalization. They compared the results obtained with the expressive portion of the Northwestern Syntax Screening Test (Lee, 1969), which requires children to look at pictures and "name" them, with the results of an analysis of spontaneous speech for a group of 4 and 5-year-old language-delayed children. Thirty percent of the structures that were failed on the test were produced in spontaneous speech. Like Brown, Prutting et al. (1975) argue that the test requires psychological operations beyond mastery of specific grammatical construction.

This view of the relationship between natural performance and performance in the laboratory is the exact opposite of a widely held view in cognitive development, the "production deficiency" hypothesis (see Butterfield, chapter 6, for a review). Under constrained laboratory conditions, children can perform many complex tasks with skilled strategies which they do not do when unconstrained. The production deficiency hypothesis (Flavell, 1970) is an attempt to account for this discrepancy in favor of the laboratory. However, in many areas of language performance, the discrepancy favors the natural setting.

It is the point of this chapter that feelings of superiority on the part of the developmental psychologist, like most such feelings, are unjustified; that there are some serious questions about the nature and use of observational research in child language development; and that these questions call for innovative research of a type that cannot easily be labeled "methodological" or "substantive." Before turning to these questions, the present state of research is considered.

WHAT DOES OBSERVING LANGUAGE MEAN (NOW)?

There are no fully standardized procedures that a novice investigator could use for observational research on language development. Bloom (1970, chapter 2 and appendix A) and Bowerman (1973, chapter 2) provide more complete information than most published works. The present remarks are based on my own general impressions of the field. In general, the psycholinguist becomes a participant-observer in the child's daily life, interacting with the child in the home setting during a variety of familiar activities. Most often the observer brings a few new toys and books each visit to elicit speech from the child. A justification for observing the child's language in interaction with the investigator is that it holds the input to the child relatively more constant than if each child were observed in interaction with family members. A tape recorder is used to record utterances of the child and those interacting with him, but notes by the observer are often necessary to decode the child's unintelligible utterances. Transcription of the tapes is always difficult as it must steer between two problems. On the one hand, the untrained ear is likely to hear sentence elements that are required in adult English but not produced by young children (such as articles and inflections), and a skeptical attitude is necessary. On the other hand, young children have deviant phonological systems which may obscure elements that are present. Reliability of transcription is seldom assessed, and in fact it is not clear how best to do so.

Clinicians often wish to collect language samples under more constant conditions, both to enhance efficient assessment and to allow comparison with norms. Lee (1974) presents a good description of eliciting samples under slightly less natural conditions for clinical assessments. Clinicians also face the problem of necessary sample size, as many children must be seen, and many language-disabled children are not as talkative as normal children. There is essentially no research on the role of sample size in determining conclusions about a child's language. Clinicians generally use samples of 50 or 100 utterances, whereas the most thorough research studies typically collect 300 to 700 utterances at each developmental point. It seems clear that larger samples are needed to characterize the language of more advanced children, but no quantitative conclusions can be made at this time.

Once the transcript is obtained, the real work can begin. The child's discourse must be segmented into distinct utterances, both for a calculation of mean length of utterance (the most widely used overall index of development; see Brown, 1973), and for grammatical analysis. Even this preliminary step is difficult (Crystal, 1974). Given a list of utterances, the investigator can attempt to determine the underlying patterns. Just how to express these patterns remains a fundamental problem (see Brown, 1973, for a review), but it most often amounts to some kind of list of patterns or schemas. Bloom (1970) and Bowerman (1973) initiated the practice of reporting lists of utterances that do not fit the general patterns induced from the sample.

Bloom (1970) introduced a major change in our concept of "observing language." Earlier, most research focused on a distributional analysis of the child's utterances, for example, determining whether adjectives regularly preceded or followed nouns. Bloom pointed out that a great deal of structure may be obscured by such a narrow approach. The utterance "baby blanket" contains two nouns, but the nature of the relationship between the two is not yet specified. The utterance can be a possessive ("baby's blanket"), an agent-object construction ("baby is pulling the blanket"), or a locative ("baby is under the blanket"). An adequate description of the child's language must include the range of relationships the child is expressing, and often only the context clarifies a particular utterance. Thus, Bloom (1970) showed how rather complete records of the context could decode utterances in this way, and revealed the use of a small stock of basic relationship types in early child language. One implication of her research was to change our definition of "observing language" from one requiring only audiotaped utterances to one requiring contextual information as well.

Nevertheless, just how much context to record and how to record it is far from standardized, or even explicitly formulated by various researchers. In Bloom's ongoing research project, very complete records are taken of the child's actions and events. Other researchers, such as Brown and Bowerman, appear to record far less. Though it is probably true that "the more information the better," no research has been addressed to comparisons of various schemes for coding contextual information for the express purpose of facilitating language analysis.

Through naturalistic research of this type we have learned that early child language is patterned and creative, and that it is remarkably uniform among children. During the period that Brown calls stage 1, as mean length of utterance (MLU) rises from 1.0 to 2.0, inflections and grammatical morphemes (such as articles) are missing from speech. Instead, content words are joined according to a fairly small stock of patterns such as recurrence ("more milk"), possessive ("mommy chair"), agent-action ("Eve read"), objective-locative ("sweater chair"), and about a dozen others (Brown, 1973). Gradually children come to combine two or more of the basic relationships as in "sit daddy chair" ("sit in daddy's chair") which joins a possessive and a locative relationship. Genuinely new elements enter the language system as MLU approaches 2.0 in the form of certain inflections and grammatical morphemes. Brown (1973) and de Villiers and de Villiers (1973) have shown that 14 of these elements enter in a nearly invariant sequence: -ing, on, in, the plural -s, and so on. The addition of these elements renders the child's utterances far less ambiguous. As MLU approaches 3.0, the child begins to learn distinctive patterns for the basic sentence types of the language. For example, simple questions that were first expressed simply with a rising intonation ("mommy see doggie?") now are produced with proper auxiliary-subject inversion ("do you see the doggie?"). For more details, see primary sources such as Brown (1973), Bloom, Hood, and Lightbown (1974), and Bowerman (1973), or reviews such as Bloom (1975) and Dale (1976).

In recent years, the common observation that words do not mean the same thing to a child as to an adult has been translated into a flourishing research effort. Diary studies and other intensive observational records have been used (Nelson, 1973; Clark, 1971) to demonstrate the important role played by factors of action and change and by static perceptual features in determining which words are learned first and what the early meanings will be. Determining the exact meaning of a word for a child is extremely difficult, and requires extensive observation of the child's use of the word (and also the non-use; the widespread belief that overgeneralization is the most frequent phenomenon in early child semantics undoubtedly is due largely to the fact that overgeneralization errors are errors of commission—calling a horse a dog—and thus are more conspicuous than overrestriction errors—failing to call a chihuahua a dog—which are errors of omission. Bowerman (1976) and others have shown that overrestrictions and mixed cases are also highly frequent.)

Beyond descriptive information about child language and its development, naturalistic research has provided a wealth of information illustrating the role of various environmental and other explanatory factors. We have learned that direct instruction is rare and generally unsuccessful; that many putative reinforcers are in fact not relevant because they are not properly contingent on the form of the child's utterance (Brown and Hanlon, 1970); that imitation does not appear to play a central role in syntactic development, since many children do not spontaneously imitate much parental speech; that the actual input to the child is a special kind of language (the term "motherese" is increasingly used) which may play an important role in aiding language development (de Villiers and de Villiers, 1976). The question of inferences about explanation based on observation is discussed later.

SOME UNCONFRONTED QUESTIONS

The discussion above presents a positive picture of the use of observational methods in the study of language development, but some serious questions have been avoided or treated carelessly. The requirements and implications of observational research have not been thoroughly considered. Four questions are discussed in this chapter.

What Constitutes Productivity?

Knowing language is knowing patterns, or rules. As a branch of cognitive psychology, our goal is not to describe and measure the frequency of individual responses, but to characterize the underlying schemas that generate them. To put this another way, if one considers the schemas as responses, then the question is whether the response (say pronouns, or relative clauses, or plurals) is present at all. There is a growing interest in conditions and frequencies of use of various constructions (Bloom, Miller, and Hood, 1975) but the simple question of existence in the child's language repertoire is primary.

The relationship between general pattern and particular instance is described in meticulous detail by the linguist of adult language. His description, however, does not carry over directly to children. The problem is that children cheat. That is, one of the ubiquitous phenomena of child language is the production of various forms by simpler means than those used by adults. Phrases are often unanalyzed wholes, that is, single lexical items. Adam, studied by Brown's group, occasionally produced the expression "just checking." In adult English "checking" is a combination of two morphemes. The principle evidence for this analysis is that -ing may be added to a broad class of verbs. However, Adam never used -ing except in the compound checking, and it would be entirely unwarranted to credit Adam with mastery of the -ing morpheme. Adam undoubtedly picked up the entire phrase "just checking" from a parent as a single unit. But how often must a child use a morpheme or construction, and in how many different contexts, before we are justified in crediting him with mastery?

Between the single lexical item generation of a phrase, and generation by adult rules, many intermediate stages can occur. There are convincing arguments that sentences resembling adult complex forms may result from far simpler rules (Clark, Hutcheson, and van Buren, 1974; Ingram, 1975). The sentence "Let's go see Baby Ivan have a bath" (Clark et al., 1974) is relatively complex in adult English, with at least three distinct sentences in deep structure. However, this sentence was produced by a boy less than 3 years old, as part of a longer utterance: "Baby Ivan have a bath, let's go see Baby Ivan have a bath." A more complete examination of the child's language reveals that the sentence is the juxtaposition of "let's go see," which is used as a single word which introduces sentences, as with the simple sentence "Baby Ivan have a bath." Similarly, "I want I eat apple" stems from the addition of "I want" to a simple sentence.

Ingram (1975) has proposed that we require truly productive use of a rule (in particular transformational rules which generate complex sentences, but the argument applies more broadly), not just the production of a few instances of the structure before we credit the child with knowledge of the rule. He points out that this will have the effect of shifting the effective data of mastery considerably upwards in some cases. The problem, of course, is deciding what constitutes productive use.

Most commonly, some numerical criterion is established for mastery of a construction. In the work of Bloom and her associates, five is most commonly used. Brown, Cazden, and Bellugi (1969) and Bowerman (1975) have called attention to a ''trap'' in the use of such a criterion. The various constructions of English are used with unequal although consistent frequency by adults. In many cases the constructions within the child's competence are used with a similar frequency profile. The trap is that ''when children emit constructions with unequal frequencies, the use of an *arbitrary frequency* criterion to establish that a form is productive for a child could cause the more frequently produced constructions to *appear* to become productive earlier than the less frequently produced constructions, even though this might not be the case'' (Bowerman, 1975). In particular this raises questions about observed regular sequences of development in children. ''The student of child speech might then conclude that the hypothesis of simultaneous development was false when it could indeed be true'' (Brown et al., 1969). Brown et al. propose that child frequencies be compared with adult frequencies to set less arbitrary frequency criteria. Yet even this is not as simple as it sounds, because it is often not clear just what to count in adult speech for constructions comparable to child speech. Bloom, Hood, and Lightbown, (1974) in their reply to Bowerman's critique, devised a chi-square analysis which revealed that constructions were used with frequencies in the lumped samples *before* the apparent criterion was met, which were significantly different from the lumped frequencies of all samples *after* the criterion was met. This test reveals that *some* change in frequencies is occurring over the span of the samples, but does not specifically identify the point of criterion mastery as reflecting the greatest change.

Traditionally one appeals to probability and statistics to settle questions like these, which concern evidence for general conclusions. But it is a mark of our lack of understanding of the underlying principles relating children's knowledge of language to their actual productions that we do not know how to use statistics in this domain.

How Can We Study Comprehension?

Observational research on child language is virtually always the observation of children's productions. Comprehension is probably more significant a subject of research than is production. Some children comprehend language without being able to speak at all (Lenneberg, 1962), although no children learn to produce meaningful speech without being able to understand other people. The child's learning must ultimately be based on his or her partial or complete comprehension of the speech of others. Of particular interest is the question of whether children comprehend specific aspects of language before they are able to produce them. Yet comprehension is typically studied by a very different means, standardized testing in the laboratory.

The rationale for such an approach stems from the multiple cues available in the natural setting. When a child hears a sentence, he has several sources of information as to the meaning: a) knowledge of words and syntactic structure; b) the linguistic context, that is, preceding utterances; c) the nonlinguistic context, the objects and events in the situation; and d) general knowledge of the world. In the laboratory we can eliminate all but the first cue, for example, by having the child point to pictures or act out sentences with dolls. In the natural setting, comprehension of the plural morpheme in "bring the books over here" is not crucial if there are, in fact, two books lying before the child. In the test setting, the child can be asked to point to the picture of "dogs," where one picture portrays one dog and the second picture two dogs. In this way we can arrive at a "pure," "uncontaminated" comprehension assessment. But we may have thrown out the baby with the bath. When all "extraneous" cues are eliminated, the comprehension task is no longer comparable to production. In the production task, the plural morpheme is elicited by the actual presence of a plurality of objects, which is hardly an "extraneous cue."

The importance of context for production is illustrated by an observation of Bloom (1974). She presented several sentences for Peter to imitate. In response to "I'm trying to get this cow in here," Peter produced "cow in here," converting a complex sentence to a simple one. Other sentences were correspondingly simplified. Yet all the sentences presented for imitation had in fact been produced on the preceding day. The example sentence was produced as Peter tried to get a toy cow's feet to fit into a barrel. The contrast between production of the full sentence one day and simplification the next is clearly due to the missing context on the second day. Children generally talk about the here and now; contextual support, together with the child's own behavior and intentions, plays an important role in the formulation of sentences. These contextual factors do not "contaminate" our assessment of production, they are essential to it. Similarly, the child's ability to use contextual factors constitutes a major component of his comprehension skills. There is no one "pure" comprehension skill, but many; each relative to a particular constellation of syntactic, semantic, and contextual factors. Comparisons of various comprehension abilities would probably be far more enlightening than the continued, and thus far highly inconclusive, attempts to compare *the* comprehension with *the* production (Dale, 1976).

Thus, observational studies of comprehension in the natural context are not hopeless, but essential. Yet there really is no appropriate methodology at the present time. The closest approach is to do experiments in the home, as done by Shipley, Smith, and Gleitman (1969), who studied the spontaneous responses of young children to commands produced by their mothers according to a script prepared by the investigators. They found that children past the one-word stage responded appropriately more often when the command was well formed ("throw me the ball") than when it was simplified to resemble early child language ("throw ball"), suggesting that comprehension is in advance of production. Although this finding is intriguing, it is basically an experimental finding, with concessions to the nature of 2-year-olds as experimental subjects.

One possible approach to the study of natural comprehension would be to use adult performance to assess the information available to the child. When a child hears a sentence, he has, as has been seen, a complex package of information available to him. Much of this information would be preserved on a video tape of the scene up to and including the speaker's gestures, but not the actual sounds uttered. Adult viewers could be asked to guess the meaning intended by the speaker. Some utterances would be more easily identifiable than others, and they are also likely to be ones which are responded to appropriately by the child. I also venture the prediction that, although performance may not be very high on the task as outlined, simply providing one or two key content words from the sentence will raise performances enormously. The most interesting cases are those in which adult viewers, without knowledge of the sentence, cannot provide the meaning, but to which the children do respond appropriately.

One major problem for implementing such a line of research is the same as that raised earlier in the context of using situational information to decode child utterances: It is not known how much of the situation is relevant, and we do not have any standardized procedures for specifying what is relevant.

Whether this is a fruitful approach can only be determined empirically. What is clear is that no observational science of child language can be considered complete unless it includes the study of comprehension skills.

How Are Language and Language Use Related to the Total Structure?

Anyone who has observed child language has learned that children talk differently, both quantitatively and qualitatively, in different situations. Although this is easily demonstrated, it is typically done only in group comparisons to illustrate the role of some situational factor. For example, 4 and 5-year-olds talk more about a toy than about a still photograph of the toy. Kindergarten children ask more questions about stories and pictures that are novel or surprising than about familiar, unsurprising ones. They produce more advanced and increased speech in housekeeping play and group discussion than in play with blocks, dance, and woodworking (all examples from Cazden, 1970). In contrast, the longitudinal studies of individual children which make up the mainstream of developmental psycholinguistics use a very narrow range of situations, as discussed above.

The situational variable that has been most intensively investigated is the nature, and particularly the age, of the listener. From an early age, children are responsive to the particular identity of the listener. Four-year-olds produce simpler speech to 2-year-olds than to adults, both in free speech and in descriptions of a new toy (Shatz and Gelman, 1973). Four-year-olds without younger siblings make this adjustment as well as those with younger siblings, demonstrating that the simplification is not based directly on parental modeling. Speech to adults is not distinguished from speech to peers of that age on the quantitative and structural variables used by Shatz and Gelman. However, children are clearly responsive to this distinction in other respects. For example, 3 and 4-year-olds are more likely to give true imperatives ("give me the doll") and negative directions ("don't do that!") to other children; whereas adults are more likely to be given the polite and respectful declaratives ("I wonder if we have any ice cream?") and embedded imperatives ("Would you like to play house with me?") (Ervin-Tripp, 1974).

Sachs and Devin (1976) added two role-playing conditions to their study of the effects of the listener on the speech of preschool children. Their subjects generally simplified their language when speaking to a baby doll, or when pretending to be a baby. The implications of such results are captured in their conclusions:

> Finally, these results suggest that the child's utterances should not be viewed simply as a sample of the output of his grammar; the utterances that occur in a particular situation are

partly a result of the communication characteristics in that situation. Descriptions of the young child's linguistic ability must be rich enough to capture the developing awareness of appropriateness of speech for various communication situations. The problems involved in such descriptions will be similar to the problems encountered when working with adults' speech . . . (Sachs and Devin, 1976, p. 97).

Despite the aptness of these comments, it remains true that the only situational variable that has thus far been taken seriously is age of the listener. Furthermore, the situation as a whole is generally taken to be a global and static, rather than dynamically changing, variable. We assume that the child is "in" a situation for some period of time, during which we can record him, then moves on to another situation, and so on. Yet situations are not as discrete and external as scenes in a play. The situation changes, and often it changes as a function of the child's own behavior. Change is far more salient than continuity to a child. A child at the one-word state is most likely to speak at transition points either in his activity or in the events he is observing. For example, in the film *Early Words* (Bruner, May, and Greenfield, 1973), Matthew sees an airplane, points to it, and when it disappears, says "byebye." The technology for viewing the situation as a dynamically changing whole *is* being developed, as other papers in this volume attest. The problem for developmental psycholinguistics is to integrate these two currently distinct lines of observation.

Probably more important even than the physical setting, the nature of the listener, and other nonlinguistic situational factors in determining the language used by the child, is the nature of the linguistic interchange in which the child's speech is embedded. Children's imitations are not identical with their spontaneous speech (Bloom et al., 1974) and spontaneous utterances that begin a topic are different from those that continue a topic already mentioned (Bloom et al., 1975). It is characteristic of the human use of language that every language act is affected by an extraordinarily wide range of events and processes; young children are not exception.

In many ways, the most encouraging development in recent years has been the emergence of the study of pragmatic development (Dore, 1974; Bates, 1974). (See de Villiers and de Villiers, 1976, for an insightful review.) The term "pragmatics" has been defined as "the study of the use of language in context, by real speakers and hearers in real situations" (Bates, 1974, p. 277). In fact, the research thus far has been narrower than the definition might imply. Much has centered on the very earliest stages of development, in an attempt to demonstrate a continuity between prelinguistic communication systems and early language. And for the most part, it has focused on what the child is trying to do with language: to request, greet, protest, and so on. Thus far the situation is primarily used to clarify the intent of the child, but at least there is an attempt to observe language use in the context more specifically than before. It should be pointed out, though, that in many studies of "pragmatics," classification systems are imposed on young children's behavior which are of unknown reliability and completely undetermined functional reality.

Is Language Use an Interaction or a Collective Monolog?

Even "situational" research as described above typically views one speaker at a time: how he is affected by the situation, and what he wishes to get from the situation by speaking. Piaget's vivid phrase "collective monolog" describes the picture perfectly. Yet language use is not *always* truly a collective monolog. How can we begin to look at the interaction as a whole, rather than as two speaker-listener pairs?

Several investigators have proposed that young children are more capable of genuine conversational interaction than would be expected from the widespread characterization of them as "egocentric." Mueller (1972) introduced pairs of preschoolers to each other and observed their play. In general, the children played and communicated successfully. Over 80% of their remarks received replies or at least attracted the listener's attention. This finding does not, of course, tell us much about the exchange of information going on. Keenan (1974) recorded the early morning dialogs of her twin boys, age 2 years 9 months, and concluded that "young children are able to sustain a coherent dialogue over a number of turns" (p. 163). However, this coherence was most often manifested by each speaker responding to a sequence of sounds in the other's last utterance, or by reproducing a constituent, possibly modified, from the other's utterance in his own comment. Thus the coherence of the dialog is restricted in two ways: first by the relationship being restricted to links between successive utterances; and second, by the links taking the form of simple reproduction (possibly with modification) of a portion of one utterance in the next. What is lacked in judging children's conversational ability is a framework for structurally analyzing dialog.

Riegel (1976) has recently presented a developmental theory of dialog. In this theory, thus far untested empirically, the fundamental dimension of development is the growing extent of links between utterances. Gradually each utterance comes to be related to previous utterances of each partner in the conversation. A hypothetical dialog at each of Riegel's levels 3, 5, and 7 will give the flavor of his account (all examples and structural analyses from Riegel's Table 1):

Level 3		Level 5		Level 7	
C:	Coat	M:	Where is your coat?	C:	Cookie
M:	Put your coat on.	C:	Upstairs	M:	No, you can't have a cookie before lunch
C:	Where going?	M:	Go and get it	C:	Hungry
M:	We are going to the store	C:	Get it	M:	We will be eating soon
		M:	Watch your steps	C:	Lunch soon
C M C M		M C M C M		C M C M C	

Riegel's model has promise as a start for a much needed metric of discourse structure, although for the present it remains vague on the nature and identification of links between utterances (the lines in the diagrams).

Interestingly, more research has been done on the structure of communication interactions of preverbal infants with their mothers than on interactions in the language-learning period. For example, Kaye (1975) has used powerful statistical techniques to map the growing interrelation of infants' sucking over the first 2 weeks of life, and pausing during feeding and maternal responses (such as jiggling). Freedle and Lewis (1976) have studied prelinguistic vocalization interactions through a transition probability analysis, and have shown that mother-infant pairs develop distinctive styles of interactions; that there are sex differences and situational differences; and that there is some predictability from aspects of prelinguistic "conversations" to aspects of child language at age 2. Vietze et al. (chapter 5) have used a similar procedure to trace the growing reciprocal nature of mother-infant interaction, and have found developmentally delayed infants to engage in patterns of interaction similar to younger normal infants. Research of this type could provide a useful model for research on true linguistic interaction. However, it is doubtful that the study of child language is ready for the powerful statistical models which have been developed for interaction in other domains, because we have yet to determine the appropriate behavioral categories for analysis. It is no coincidence that studies of interaction have begun with prelinguistic infants, for the relevant behavior-vocalization is easy to identify, but is not easily susceptible to further subdivision.

This section is an attempt to show that although observation is a basic tool of developmental psycholinguistics, we are far from having an observational science of child language. We do not know how to go from particular utterances to general patterns; we are ignoring one category of language behavior almost entirely; we are just beginning to explore the relationship of language to the situation as a whole; and we have virtually no way to characterize the distinctive qualities of one of the most human of all activities: dialog.

THE QUESTION OF "HOW?"

Is observational evidence only useful for describing children's knowledge as a function of development, or can it provide explanations? To say that it might provide *only* descriptions would be misleading. Attempts to construct theories are highly constrained by the nature of the descriptions available; the converse is also true. Witness the change in prevailing theories of language learning as characterizations of child language shifted in the early 1960's from an impoverished and error-prone version of adult language to a highly structured grammatical system; and in the early 1970's to a system of syntactic semantic schemas for the expression of meaning. Nevertheless, the question remains as to how, or how *best,* to use observational methods to arrive at explanations of language development.

In language development, as in almost all psychology, there are two broad approaches to constructing explanations: the individual differences approach and the universals approach. In the former, some factor, most likely environmental, is hypothesized to be crucial for language development, and a correlation is obtained between the incidence of this factor and the rate of language development. In the universals approach, some factor is hypothesized to be crucial that is always (or nearly always) present, and hence accounts for the near universal acquisition of language. Obviously the individual differences approach is favored by those who are impressed by the diversity of language development and the universal approach by those who are impressed by its uniformity.

Expansions provide a good example of the former approach. Many parents, especially middle class ones, imitate their children's productions, providing a more complete form for the child's presumed meaning, e.g., responding to "sat wall" with "he sat on the wall" (Brown and Bellugi, 1964). These interchanges would appear to be ideal teaching situations. There is a very modest amount of evidence that children whose parents expand more frequently proceed at a faster rate. To avoid the ambiguity of such a correlational finding, experiments have been conducted on the effect of expansions. Two studies (Cazden, 1965; Feldman, 1971) failed to obtain evidence for a positive effect. On the other hand, Nelson, Carskaddon, and Bonvillian (1973) did find an advantage for children being given what they called "recast sentence" training, in which incomplete sentences were expanded, and completed sentences were recast in a new form, e.g., "the bunny chased fireflies" was responded to with "the bunny did chase fireflies, didn't he?" Nelson et al. (1973) argue that this condition provides a greater variety of linguistic forms to the child than do expansions, which are tied closely to the form of the child's utterance. Thus the present research on expansions is inconclusive. Furthermore, as Cazden (1972) points out, it is difficult to judge the relevance of these experiments for an understanding of parental responses. Parental responses often combine the categories so carefully distinguished in experiments. A parent might respond to the child's "dog bark" with "yes, the dog's barking at kitty." On the other hand, it may be just the fact of this variability that makes parental responses helpful in language acquisition.

The nature of the linguistic input to children exemplifies the universals approach. It has been argued that the remarkable similarities among children learning language result from the equally uniform nature of their linguistic environment, which provides an essential aid to learning. Part of Macnamara's (1972) very thoughtful analysis of language learning is the claim that at the beginning it is essential that the meanings of utterances addressed to the child be obvious. For the child to begin to break the code, the events and objects in the environment being talked about must be clear and match directly what is said. Only later will the child be able to learn by inference from what has been said before, just as adults can interpret novel utterances about remote events. Macnamara assumes all parents do this. Clearly this is a question that deserves further research.

Another example is the hypothesis that cognitive development, in particular the development of object permanence, is an essential foundation for language development (Bloom 1973). The rough coincidence between object permanence and the beginning of language *is* striking, although so far no correlation has been found between the achievement of object permanence and various language measures (Corrigan, 1976).

"Universalist" explanations are far more difficult to evaluate than "differences" explanations. Virtually all the machinery of modern statistics has been developed for the latter. The major tool available for the former is scaling procedures for identifying the existence of invariant sequences of development, such as those developed by Guttman (Green, 1956; Edwards, 1957) and Coombs and Smith (1973). Nevertheless, the fact that *A* occurs invariably before *B* is at best circumstantial evidence that *A* is necessary for *B*, and certainly does not imply that *A* is sufficient for *B*. Another solution to the problem of evaluating universalist explanations is to resort to a differences strategy focusing on aspects of language, rather than on individual children. That is, a hypothesized factor may be present in the environment or developmental history of all children, but be more directly tied to some element of language than others, so that we can test predictions about sequences of development. Thus Brown evaluated the role of simple presentation rate in facilitating the acquisition of 14 grammatical morphemes of English by correlating the sequence of acquisition of these morphemes with their frequency in parental speech; he found only a weak correlation (0.26).

The formal nature of maternal speech to children has been studied extensively (de Villiers and de Villiers, 1976), and it is clear that this "motherese" (Newport, 1976) is simpler and more regular than speech direct to adults. It is also clear, however, that maternal speech is considerably more complex than the language of children to whom it is addressed. Maternal speech gradually becomes more complex as the child's language develops. But Newport (1976) has argued that while maternal speech is grossly adjusted to the child listener, it is in no sense "fine tuned" in the sense of having particular aspects of language tuned to a particular child's mastery of that aspect. "In short, although speech to children is . . . somewhat simpler in syntactic structure than is speech to adults, it is imperfect indeed in its tuning to the differing syntactic sophistication of children" (Newport, 1976, p. 44). I have argued elsewhere (Dale, 1976, pp. 142–146) that the child controls the linguistic input through differential attention; that speech which exceeds the child's comprehension (not just production level) will not be attended to, and hence extinguished in the adult. Thus fine tuning of the sort discussed by Newport is not to be expected. There is a very small amount of experimental evidence that children do attend more to maternal speech than to adult-directed speech. However, note that the crucial variable is whether speech is comprehended *in context*. We are back to the problem raised earlier: how to study natural comprehension of language.

Imitation illustrates another way in which observational evidence can inform theorizing. Many children simply do not produce any significant number of spontaneous imitations (Bloom et al., 1974), so that imitation cannot be a necessary process of learning. Furthermore, when children do imitate they typically simplify the sentence imitated to conform with their own grammars (Bloom et al., 1974; Kemp and Dale, 1973). Thus, new features can hardly enter a child's language when it is just these new features which are omitted in imitations. Patterns that have only begun to enter the language system are most likely to be imitated, but imitation is clearly not responsible for the initial acquisition.

In conclusion, observational studies can provide a characterization of the information available to the learner, and special conditions of language use that may be important for learning. They can also rule out possible mechanisms of learning, such as imitation. In many cases experiments may seem necessary for conclusive evaluation, but in these experiments one must preserve the essential aspects of the phenomena observed naturally, as in looking at contextual support for language use, or at the complexity of parental responses.

Furthermore, laboratory experiments seldom resolve issues by themselves. As other chapters in this volume point out, and as emphasized repeatedly in conference discussions, laboratory effects do not always generalize to normal development. What *can* be done is not always what actually happens. Only an integration of observational and experimental evidence, perhaps along the lines suggested by Butterfield (chapter 6), can give an adequate process account of language development.

THE LANGUAGE OF THE MENTALLY RETARDED

This section is concerned more with methodological questions than with a survey of research on language development in retarded individuals. Reviews are available in

Schiefelbusch (1972), Schiefelbusch and Lloyd (1974), and Lenneberg and Lenneberg (1975).

On the whole, the prevailing tendency has been to apply standardized tests of comprehension, and to a lesser extent, equally standardized and controlled tests of production, rather than studying language use naturally. The reasons for this imbalance are clear. Ingenious tests have been developed for the study of language development in normal children, such as Carol Chomsky's work on the "easy to see" construction (Chomsky, 1969). It is hard to resist the temptation to try them out with other groups of children. Furthermore, standardized tests fit into a cross sectional design; (stratified either by chronological or mental age), guaranteeing quicker publication. Although it seems inadvisable for researchers in the field of mental retardation to undertake longitudinal research (it takes long enough with normal children, and will take still longer with the developmentally delayed), the only kind of evidence with substantial implications for explanation is the longitudinal type, which permits an examination of the changing interplay of child and environmental variables.

The most frequently asked question about language development in the retarded is whether it is simply retarded; that is, a delayed version of normal development, or whether it follows a qualitatively different path. To expect a single answer to this question is simplistic. The situation varies from child to child; on the whole the relatively moderate and "clean" retardation conditions, such as Down's syndrome, are associated more with delay than difference, whereas more severe handicaps are more likely to result in grossly different patterns of development. More to the point, the answer may vary from one aspect of language to another. The goal ought to be to characterize the domains of delay and difference. For this purpose, information about sequence is far more important than information about rate. Many recent findings about normal language development concern (nearly) invariant sequences of milestones, and these sequences are particularly suggestive for research with other populations. For example, Brown's (1973) observation of a nearly universal sequence of mastery of 14 grammatical morphemes provides a well defined field for theorizing about the role of various factors such as frequency in parental speech (negative), syntactic complexity (some role), and semantic complexity (some role).

In the Child Language Acquisition Study at the University of Washington the sequence of development of these morphemes in Down's syndrome and hearing-impaired children is being examined. Our hope is to disentangle the role of perceptual, syntactic, and semantic-cognitive factors. We are explicitly assuming that each element of language has prerequisites of all types, but that the balance among them differs from morpheme to morpheme. Thus morphemes that are syntactically simple but semantically complex, such as the articles, should be delayed even more than other morphemes in Down's syndrome children. To the extent that the articles, being syllabic, are easier to perceive than morphemes like the plural, despite their semantic complexity, they should be mastered earlier *in the sequence* by hearing-impaired children, although still delayed absolutely.

Coggins (1976) has recently studied the earliest multiword utterances (Brown's stage I) in Down's syndrome children, and has concluded that the beginnings of structured language are essentially identical in Down's syndrome and normal children. Lackner (1968) studied five children at a more advanced point in development: writing transformational grammars. He concluded that the same kinds of phrase structure and transformational rules described retarded and normal children. He did find, however, that language development tended to fall behind general mental age (MA) assessment after about MA = 4 years. Lackner's analysis, however, was of a purely formal nature, and did not take into account contextual information in the way first proposed by Bloom. In addition, both Coggin's and Lackner's studies were cross sectional in design. Although limited inferences about sequence can be drawn from cross sectional evidence by scaling analyses *if the sample size is large enough,* longitudinal evidence is, again, essential for a deeper understanding. The difficulties of integrating situational information into an account of language development have been discussed above, but they are even more challenging for retarded individuals who are often no longer at home but in a very different environment, i.e., institutions.

Perhaps the most challenging question of all is the relationship between processes of normal development and therapeutic methods for exceptional children. For example, that imitation does not play a major role in the syntactic development of normal children does not imply that it may not be of great value for the therapist or trainer. Children are language-impaired precisely when the normal processes fail. The papers on language remediation included in Schiefelbusch and Lloyd (1974) illustrate very well the debate over whether training should follow natural sequences of development. Miller and Yoder argue for following normal sequences; Guess, Sailor, and Baer for finding an optimal sequence which may not be "normal"; and Bricker and Bricker for an intermediate position.

Ultimately this question is an empirical one, not to be settled by a priori arguments. But as a working hypothesis, I propose that *conditions that are sufficient for language learning for normal children are likely to be necessary for language-disabled children.* Three examples include, first, the primacy of meaning in communicating with children. Children are attempting to communicate meaning, and they expect the response to be addressed to that meaning. In a classic observational study, Brown, Cazden, and Bellugi (1969) compared the correctness of those child utterances that were followed by signs of approval from parents with those child utterances that were followed by signs of disapproval. In general, the grounds on which an utterance was approved or disapproved were not linguistic at all, but were based on the correspondence between utterance and reality.

> It seems, then, to be truth value rather than (well-formed syntax) that chiefly governs explicit verbal reinforcement by parents—which renders mildly paradoxical the fact that the usual product of such a training schedule is an adult whose speech is highly grammatical but not notably truthful. (Brown, Cazden, and Bellugi, 1969, p. 71).

Brown and Hanlon (1970) performed a similar analysis for relevant replies, as opposed to approval/disapproval; their conclusion was that parents fit some meaning to even the most fragmentary utterances and respond as best they can. In both cases, form is virtually ignored. In fact, Nelson (1973) observed in a longitudinal study of the early development of 18 children that mothers who engaged in selective reinforcement for good and bad pronunciation and word choice had children who developed more slowly than those whose mothers were more accepting. Therefore attention to meaning is part of a sufficient set of conditions, and attention to form is not. Attention to form may well have to be added to training programs for language-impaired children, but meaning must not be removed. Yet many training programs include extensive imitation drills, entirely removed from context.

A second example is the importance of a variety of objects and events to talk about. Most of the words of our language refer to a complex range of phenomena; witness the difficulty of composing a dictionary. It is tempting to simplify the problem for the child. Yet children *are* able to focus their attention on particular words and structures, and to gradually refine their concepts. Simplification may actually be misleading. Cook (1976) has provided a good illustration in her study of the development of the meaning of "big" and "long." She points out that assessing the meaning of "big" by asking the child to select between A and B:

A □ B □

while assessing the meaning of "long" by asking the child to select between C and D:

C ▯ D ▯

confounds perceptual features and semantic features. *A* is longer than *B*, as well as bigger; and *C* is bigger than *D*, as well as longer. It is necessary to assess the meaning of both "big" and "long" with stimuli that include both the pairs above, as well as A and C:

A □ C ▯

Her longitudinal study of normal children revealed that at first both "big" and "long" refer to area; gradually they both come to refer to extension (length); and only much later are the two words properly distinguished. A small group of Down's syndrome children were also tested cross sectionally, and appeared to be proceeding through the same sequence of development. The implications for training should be obvious: typically "big" is taught with stimuli like pair A-B; and "long" with stimuli like pair C-D. These stimuli by themselves will not be of any use in the crucial differentiation between "big" and "long."

A third member of the set of sufficient conditions is the ability of the child to control the sequence of acquisition to some extent. This is a pervasive feature of language development. The first nouns acquired by children are not the most frequent in parental speech, but are selected on the basis of size and the child's ability to act on them (Nelson, 1973). The sequence of acquisition of the 14 grammatical morphemes is only weakly correlated with frequency in parental speech (Brown, 1973). It reflects organizing strategies of the child. The nature of maternal speech itself appears to be determined by the child's response (Dale, 1976). Again, it may be necessary to add highly structured teaching sequences for language-disabled children, but some domain of child selection is probably also necessary. If a theoretical justification for this is needed, one need look no further than Piaget's emphasis on the natural tendency of children to focus on problems that are just a bit beyond their level of comptence. Rondal (1976) has recently studied maternal speech addressed to young Down's syndrome children and has found it to be generally indistinguishable from maternal speech to mental age-matched normals, though of course very different from speech to chronological age-matched normals. Rondal's finding demonstrates the ability of Down's syndrome children to exert an effect on their linguistic environment.

To conclude, the promise of observational studies of language development for mental retardation, as is the promise of such methods generally, is to provide information that is less fractionated and has greater ecological validity. However, delivery on that promise will require that developmental psycholinguistics look at its methods more critically.

REFERENCES

Bates, E. 1974. Acquisition of pragmatic competence. J. Child Lang. 1:277–281.

Bloom, L. 1970. Language Development: Form and Function in Emerging Grammars. M.I.T. Press, Cambridge.

Bloom, L. 1973. One Word at a Time. Morton & Co., The Hague.

Bloom, L. 1974. Talking, understanding, and thinking. In: R. L. Schiefelbusch and L. L. Lloyd (eds.), Language Perspectives—Acquisition, Retardation, and Intervention. University Park Press, Baltimore.

Bloom, L. 1975. Language development. In: F. D. Horowitz (ed.), Review of Child Development Research 4:245–303. University of Chicago Press, Chicago.

Bloom, L., Hood, L., and Lightbown, P. 1974. Imitation in language development: if, when and why. Cog. Psychol. 6:380–420.

Bloom, L., Miller, P., and Hood, L. 1975. Variation and reduction as aspects of competence in language development. In: A Pick (ed.), Minnesota Symposium on Child Psychology, pp. 3–55, Vol. 9. University of Minnesota Press, Minneapolis.

Bowerman, M. 1973. Early Syntactic Development: A Cross-linguistic Study with Special Reference to Finnish. Cambridge University Press, Cambridge.

Bowerman, M. 1975. Commentary on: L. Bloom, L. Hood, and P. Lightbown. Structure and variation in child language. Monogr. Soc. Res. Child Dev. No. 160, 40:80–90.

Bowerman, M. 1976. Word meaning and sentence structure: uniformity, variation, and shifts over time in patterns of acquisition. In: F. D. Minifie and L. L. Lloyd (eds.), Early Behavioral Assessment of the Communicative and Cognitive Abilities of the Developmentally Disabled.

Bricker, W. A., and Bricker, D. D. 1974. An early language training strategy. In: R. L. Schiefelbusch and L. L. Lloyd (eds.), Language Perspectives—Acquisition, Retardation, and Intervention, pp. 431–468. University Park Press, Baltimore.

Brown, R. 1973. A First Language: The Early Stages. Harvard University Press, Cambridge.

Brown, R., and Bellugi, U. 1964. Three processes in the child's acquisition of syntax. Harvard Educ. Rev. 34:133–151.

Brown, R., Cazden, C., and Bellugi, U. 1969. The child's grammar from I to III. In: J. P. Hill (ed.), Minnesota Symposium on Child Psychology, pp. 28–73, Vol. 2. University of Minnesota Press, Minneapolis.

Brown, R., and Hanlon, C. 1970. Derivational complexity and order of acquisition. In: J. R. Hayes (ed.), Cognition and the Development of Language, pp. 11–53. John Wiley & Sons Inc., New York.

Bruner, J. S., May, A., and Greenfield, P. 1973. Early Words: Action and the Study of Language. (Film). John Wiley & Sons Inc., New York.

Cazden, C. 1965. Environmental assistance to the child's acquisition of grammar. Unpublished doctoral dissertation, Graduate School of Education, Harvard University, Cambridge.

Cazden, C. 1970. The neglected situation in child language research and education. In: F. Williams (ed.), Language and Poverty, pp. 81–101. Markham, Chicago.

Cazden, C. 1972. Child Language and Education. Holt, Rinehart & Winston, New York.

Chomsky, C. S. 1969. The Acquisition of Syntax in Children from 5 to 10. M.I.T. Press, Cambridge.

Clark, E. V. 1971. On the acquisition of the meaning of "before" and "after." J. Verb. Learn. Verb. Behav. 10:266–275.

Clark, R., Hutcheson, S., and van Buren, P. 1974. Performing without competence. J. Child Lang. 1:1–10.

Coggins, T. 1976. The classification of rational meanings expressed in the early two-word utterances of Down's syndrome children. Unpublished doctoral dissertation, University of Wisconsin, Madison.

Cook, N. 1976. The acquisition of dimensional adjectives as a function of the underlying perceptual event. Presented at the Stanford Child Language Research Forum, April, Stanford University, Stanford.

Coombs, C. H., and Smith, J. E. K. 1973. On the detection of structure in attitudes and developmental processes. Psychol. Rev. 80:337–351.

Corrigan, R. 1976. The relationship between object permanence and language development: how much and how strong? Presented at the Stanford Child Language Research Forum, April, Stanford University, Stanford.

Crystal, D. 1974. Review of R. Brown, a first language: the early stages. J. Child Lang. 1:289–334.

Dale, P. S. 1976. Language Development: Structure and Function. 2nd Ed. Holt, Rinehart & Winston, New York.

de Villiers, J. G., and de Villiers, P. A. 1973. A cross-sectional study of the acquisition of grammatical morphemes in child speech. J. Psycholinguistic Res. 2:267–278.

de Villiers, J. G., and de Villiers, P. A. 1976. Semantics and syntax in the first two years: the output of form and function and the form and function of the input. In: F. D. Minifie and L. L. Lloyd (eds.), Early Behavioral Assessment of the Communicative and Cognitive Abilities of the Developmentally Disabled.

Dore, J. 1974. A pragmatic description of early language development. J. Psycholinguistic Res. 4:423–430.

Edwards, A. L. 1957. Techniques of Attitude and Scale Construction. Appleton-Century-Crofts Inc., New York.

Ervin-Tripp, S. 1974. The comprehension and production of requests by children. Papers and Reports on Child Language Development, Committee on Linguistics, No. 8, pp. 188–196. Stanford University, Stanford.

Feldman, C. 1971. The effects of various types of adults responses in the syntactic acquisition of two- to three-year-olds. Unpublished paper, Department of Psychology, University of Chicago, Chicago.

Flavell, J. H. 1970. Developmental studies of medicated memory. Adv. Child Dev. Behav. 5:182–211.

Freedle, R., and Lewis, M. 1976. Prelinguistic conversation. In: M. Lewis and L. Rosenblum (eds.), Communication and Affect. John Wiley & Sons Inc., New York.

Green, B. F. 1956. A method of scalogram analysis using summary statistics. Psychometrika 21:79–88.

Guess, D., Sailor, W., and Baer, D. M. 1974. To teach language to retarded children. In: R. C. Schiefelbusch and L. L. Lloyd (eds.), Language Perspectives—Acquisition, Retardation and Intervention, pp. 529–563. University Park Press, Baltimore.

Ingram, D. 1975. If and when transformation are acquired by children. In: D. P. Dato (ed.), Georgetown University Round Table on Languages and Linguistics, pp. 99–127. Georgetown University Press, Washington, D.C.

Kaye, K. 1975. Toward the origin of dialogue. Presented at the Loch Lomond Symposium, September, University of Strathclyde, Scotland.

Keenan, E. O. 1974. Conversational competence in children. J. Child Lang. 1:163–183.

Kemp, J. C., and Dale, P. S. 1973. Spontaneous imitation and free speech: a grammatical comparison. Paper presented to the Society for Research in Child Development, March, Philadelphia.

Lackner, J. R. 1968. A developmental study of language behavior in retarded children. Neuropsychologia 6:301–320.

Lee, L. 1969. Northwestern Syntax Screening Test. Northwestern University Press, Evanston.

Lee, L. 1974. Developmental Sentence Analysis. Northwestern University Press, Evanston.

Lenneberg, E. H. 1962. Understanding Language without the ability to speak. J. Abn. Soc. Psychol. 65:419–425.

Lenneberg, E. H., and Lenneberg, E. 1975. Foundations of Language Development: A Multidisciplinary Approach. Academic Press, New York.

Macnamara, J. 1972. Cognitive basis of language learning in infants. Psychol. Rev. 79:1-13.

Miller, J. F., and Yoder, D. E. 1974. An ontogentic language teaching strategy for retarded children. In: R. L. Schiefelbusch and L. L. Lloyd (eds.), Language Perspectives—Acquisition Retardation, and Intervention, pp. 505-528. University Park Press, Baltimore.

Mueller, E. 1972. The maintenance of verbal exchanges between young children. Child Dev. 43:930-938.

Nelson, K. 1973. Structure and strategy in learning to talk. Monogr. Soc. Res. Child Dev. 38, No. 149.

Nelson, K., Carskaddon, G., and Bonvillian, J. D. 1973. Syntax acquisition: impact of experimental variation in adult verbal interaction with the child. Child Dev. 44:497-504.

Newport, E. L. 1976. Motherese: the speech of mothers to young children. In: N. J. Castellan, D. G. Pisoni, and G. R. Potts (eds.), Cognitive Theory, Vol. II. Lawrence Erlbaum Associates, Publishers, Hillsdale.

Prutting, D. A., Gallagher, T. M., and Mulac, A. 1975. The expression portion of the NSST compared to a spontaneous language sample. J. Speech Hear. Disord. 40:40-48.

Riegel, K. F. 1976. The temporal structure of dialogues. Unpublished paper, University of British Columbia, Vancouver.

Rondal, J. A. 1976. Maternal speech to normal and Down's syndrome children matched for mean length of utterance. Unpublished doctoral dissertation, University of Minnesota, Minneapolis.

Sachs, J., and Devin, J. 1976. Young children's use of age-appropriate speech styles in social interaction and role-playing. J. Child Lang. 3:81-98.

Schiefelbusch, R. L. 1972. Language of the Mentally Retarded. University Park Press, Baltimore.

Schiefelbusch, R. L., and L. L. Lloyd (eds.). 1974. Language Perspectives—Acquisition, Retardation and Intervention. University Park Press, Baltimore.

Shatz, M., and Gelman, R. 1973. The development of communication skills: modifications in the speech of young children as a function of listener. Monogr. Soc. Res. Child Dev. 38, No. 152.

Shipley, E. G., Smith, C. S., and Gleitman, L. R. 1969. A study in the acquisition of language: free responses to commands. Language 45:322-342.

chapter 10

Observational, Descriptive Methodology in Studying Child Language: Preliminary Results on the Development of Complex Sentences

Lois Hood,[1] *Margaret Lahey,*[2] *Karin Lifter, and Lois Bloom*

The purpose of this chapter is twofold: 1) to describe the preliminary results of a study of how 2 to 3-year-old children learn to express related thoughts in complex sentences; and 2) to illustrate the use of observational methodology in language development research by describing the paradigm as fully as possible and by discussing its advantages and limitations. Thus, both methodological issues and the results and interpretations related to a specific aspect of language development are presented.

The research of the past 10 years has clearly demonstrated that when children begin, at about 1½ to 2 years of age, to put two words together to form a primitive sentence, they are doing more than simply conjoining words. The relation between the words that are combined are varied and complex (e.g., Bloom, 1970; Schlesinger, 1971; Brown, 1973). That is, "Mommy book," when said by a 2-year-old, rarely expresses merely a conjunctive relation between Mommy and book. It more often expresses a more complex relation, such as between "Mommy" as agent and "book" as the object affected by some action, or between "Mommy" as possessor and "book" as the object possessed. It is reasonable

---

This research was supported in part by National Science Foundation Grant Soc 74-24126 and NIH grant HD03828 to Lois Bloom, and a Release Time For Research Grant from Montclair State College to Margaret Lahey.

[1]The authors are all affiliated with Teachers College, Columbia University. Lois Hood is also at the Rockefeller University.

[2]Also affiliated with Montclair State College and Hunter College, CUNY.

to ask whether the same situation exists when older children, from 2 to 3 years of age, begin to combine simple sentences in longer, complex sentences. That is, do children's earliest sentence combinations express a variety of different meanings, as do their first word combinations?

The results presented here are only a small part of a larger study of how children learn to express more than one thought in a sentence, at first by juxtaposing sentences, and later through rules of grammar for conjoining and embedding two or more clauses in longer, complex sentences. The study was begun before the children had started to combine clauses, or to use conjunctions and relative pronouns. The portion of the study presented here begins at a later point in development, with the use of syntactic connectives in the language development of four 2-year-old children, both in terms of form (i.e., the particular conjunctions and relative pronouns used) and in terms of content (i.e., the particular semantic relationships between the clauses that these forms connect).

BACKGROUND

Our study was concerned with both linguistic form and content (or meaning) in the development of complex sentences. Regarding language content, there are at least two major questions: 1) what kinds of events do children talk about in their complex sentences, both before and after they start to use connectives, and 2) what are the time relations between the two (or more) reference events about which the children talk? The first question is addressed in this chapter. The second will be discussed in a forthcoming paper (Bloom, Hood, Lifter, and Lahey, in preparation).

The two main aspects of the development of the form of complex sentences have to do with particular lexical items such as conjunctions, and various syntactic constructions such as coordination, subordination, and embedding. The present study traces the acquisition of conjunctions and relative pronouns as syntactic connectives.

The interrelation of form and content was examined in terms of the development of categories of semantic relations between clauses or sentences, and the acquisition of connectives vis-à-vis the semantic relations they code. Eventually, the influence of various factors of language use on the development of complex sentences will also be explored. At the least, it is important to determine if any of the form/content interactions observed are facilitated or constrained by aspects of discourse. This and other influences of language use on content and form are currently under investigation.

Other Studies of Complex Sentences

Most other studies have focused on the form of children's complex sentences. The first type of complex construction that Limber (1973) observed in the speech of children from 1½ to 3 years of age was object complements, followed by relative clauses, and then coordinate and subordinate sentences with conjunctions.

Chambaz, Leroy, and Messeant (1975) dealt with both kinds of connectives and the types of construction, presenting longitudinal data from four French-speaking children from approximately 3 to 6 years of age. They focused on two types of connective:

''introducteurs de complexité,'' such as *qui, que, quand, parce que, si,* etc., and ''petits mots,'' such as *et, alors, apres, mais*. The first type appears to be used for subordination; the ''petits mots'' are purposely given an imprecise term, because they are used sometimes to link clauses and sometimes just as fillers. As part of a study of the development of logical and linguistic connectives, Beilin (1975) reported the occurrence of *and, or, but,* and *not* in the speech of 2 to 3-year-old children, with no indication of how they were used. The speech samples that were examined were extremely short, an average of 24 min for the eight 2-year-olds and 13.5 min for the eight 3-year-olds.

''And'' is the first conjunction that English-speaking children have used in the studies of Bohn (1914), Clark (1970), Limber (1973), Jacobsen (1974), and Beilin (1975); it is also the first conjunction used by children learning other languages, for example, Swedish (Johansson and Sjölin, 1975), Italian (Clancy, 1974) and German (Werner and Kaplan, 1963). Information concerning conjunctions other than ''and'' is much more limited, and for the most part is based on data from children over 3 (e.g., Menyuk, 1969; Clark, 1970).

The interaction of form and content in the development of complex sentences by children older than 3 years has been described in two studies that deal with how children encode the temporal relation between events, in English by Clark (1970; 1973) and in French by Ferreiro and Sinclair (1971). Only one study to date has been concerned with the kinds of meaning relations that children express when they begin to combine clauses between 2 and 3 years of age. Clancy, Jacobsen, and Silva (1976) examined the acquisition of conjunction in four languages: English, German, Italian, and Turkish. Their analysis was based on both longitudinal and cross sectional data from a variety of sources, including children in the Berkeley Cross Linguistic Language Development Project, Roger Brown's subject, Adam, and diary studies. They noted the age at which the first utterance expressing a specific conjunction occurred, whether there was an explicit connective in the utterance, and changes in formal expression, such as use of an explicit connective, different order of clauses, etc. They did not note the onset of particular connective forms, nor the sequence of their emergence in any systematic way. In addition, they did not include frequency data, and there is no way of knowing which conjunction types were the most frequent, or even which conjunction types were productive for each child.

In summary, most of the studies of complex sentences in children's spontaneous speech are limited in that they deal with either form or content, and not the interrelation of the two. Language consists of three components: content, form, and use. Although the three are interrelated, research has most often focused on one to the exclusion of the other two. This has been true, until very recently, in studies of early language development. Studies in the early 1960's concentrated primarily on language forms. The emphasis then shifted to language content or semantics, and the trend in the early 1970's has been to study language use or pragmatics. Only in the past year or so has there been an attempt to integrate the three components of language in studies of acquisition (e.g., Bloom, Miller, and Hood, 1974; Bloom, Rocissano, and Hood, 1976). Whereas language development at any particular stage obviously represents the integration of these three components, it is helpful to retain the distinction between content, form, and use in describing children's behavior in order to infer what they know of language—in this instance, complex sentences in the course of development—as well as to put previous research into a meaningful framework.

An additional limitation of previous studies of complex sentences is that by and large they were based on relatively little data, in most cases no more than an hour per sample, collected in only seminaturalistic situations (e.g., preceding an experimental task). The next section describes the observational paradigm for collecting and analyzing large amounts of longitudinal child language data.

PROCEDURES

Subjects and Data Collection

The four subjects—Eric, Gia, Kathryn, and Peter—were first born children of white, upper middle income, college-educated parents living in New York City. They were chosen with these social and birth limitations in an effort to reduce variability in their linguistic behavior that could result from either sibling interference or cultural differences. The children were visited in their homes at periodic intervals, and their speech was audio-recorded along with descriptions of relevant nonlinguistic context and behavior, using the procedures described by Bloom (1970, pp. 234–239). The same group of toys was used with all of the children (described by Bloom, 1970, pp. 239, 240), with toys dropped and added as each child's interests changed with development. Eric, Gia, and Kathryn were seen for approximately 8 hr every 6 weeks. Peter was added later and he was seen at shorter intervals (every 3 weeks) for shorter periods (4 to 5 hr), which proved to be more advantageous; it provided about as much observation time, with less time lapse between sessions. Eric, Gia, and Kathryn were visited by Lois Bloom; Peter was visited by Lois Hood and Patsy Lightbown. The interactions were primarily between investigator and child, to reduce the possible variable effects of different persons talking to the children.

The children were part of a longitudinal study of language development, and were observed from approximately 19 to 36 months of age. The data base for this study of syntactic connectives consists of the observations when the children were 25 to 36 months old. Other aspects of their language development have been reported elsewhere (Bloom, 1970; Bloom, Hood, and Lightbown, 1974; Bloom, Lightbown, and Hood, 1975; Bloom, et al., 1975; Bloom, et al., 1976; Hood, 1977). Table 1 presents a summary description of the speech samples used in the present study in terms of duration of observations, age, mean length of utterance (MLU), and number of child utterances.[3]

[3]The total number of utterances in each sample was estimated using the single stage cluster sampling technique (Cochran, 1963). Each page of transcription was considered a cluster. Twenty five clusters—or fifty if the full transcription was greater than 250 pages—were randomly sampled from the transcription and the sum of the child utterances was recorded for each cluster. All utterances, including single word and unintelligible utterances, were included in this sum. The total was then estimated using the following equation:

$$\text{Total: } \frac{N}{n} \left(\sum_{i=1}^{n} X_i\right)$$

where N = total number of pages in the transcription, n = number of pages sampled, X_i = sum of the utterances on the sampled page.

Table 1. Summary description of speech samples

Child and time		Hours	Age (months, weeks)	MLU	Total number of utterances[a]
Eric:	V	8	25,1	2.63	3,587
	VI	8	26,3	2.84	3,697
	VIII	8	29,3	3.45	2,457
	X	8	33,0	4.21	2,172
	XII	8	36,0	3.49	3,800
Gia:	V	7.5	25,2	2.30	3,099
	VII	9	28,1	3.07	4,663
	VIII	9	29,3	3.64	4,144
	XI	9	34,2	3.71	4,390
Kathryn:	III	9	24,2	2.83	4,635
	IV	7.8	26,1	3.30	4,041
	VI	9	29,1	3.35	3,291
	VIII	9	32,1	3.70	2,808
	X	9	35,1	4.23	5,250
Peter:	VIII	4.5	25,3	2.0	2,279
	X	4.5	27,0	2.63	2,501
	XII	4.5	28,2	2.90	2,352
	XIV	4.5	30,0	2.53	2,085
	XVI	4.5	31,2	3.58	2,453
	XVIII	4.5	33,3	3.30	2,456
	XIX	4.5	35,0	3.05	2,501
	XX	3	38,0	3.57	2,397

[a]The total was estimated using the single stage cluster sampling method where each page of transcript was considered as a cluster.

Before describing the procedures specific to the present study, it might be helpful to present a general summary of the methodology at successive stages within the paradigm.

Transcription

The actual data consist of annotated transcriptions of each of the longitudinal observations of the children that were tape recorded at periodic intervals. Each transcription includes all of the child speech, all of the speech to the child, and a description of the accompanying behavior and situations that form the nonlinguistic context. All of the transcriptions were done immediately after the recordings were made. The linguistic record was transcribed in traditional orthography, with phonetic notation used in cases where speech could not be understood. A standardized notation convention was used for recording the interaction between linguistic behavior and nonlinguistic information about the context of each utterance (Bloom, Lightbown, and Hood, 1974).

The following procedures were used to establish confidence in the transcriptions. All of the data from Peter were transcribed by one investigator (either P. Lightbown or L. Hood) and subsequently checked by the other until agreement between them was established in the transcript. In the few cases where agreement could not be reached, the utterance was considered unintelligible. All of the data from the three other children were transcribed by L. Bloom. Samples of 100 utterances from the data of each of those three were retranscribed by L. Hood and then compared with L. Bloom's original transcription of the same utterances. The proportion of agreement between the two transcriptions (each utterance scored as same or different) was 0.97, 0.95, and 0.98 for the three children.

Coding

Coding procedures begin with an initial hypothesis about the regular features that might be expected to exist in the data. For example, one hypothesis was that "and" would be the first connective used by the children; another was that coordination would precede subordination. In the course of coding each of the behaviors, the initial hypothesis may be extended (to include other relevant features of the event), revised, or even abandoned. Each revision in the hypothesis makes it necessary to revise the coding with all of the data again. Coding typically begins with a sample of 200 child utterances from each of the children at the same MLU level. If the children are not consistent with one another, then a second 200-utterance sample in each observation from each of the children is coded; most often, as in this study, the coding is then applied to all of the data in a particular sample. When regularity among the children is observed, or when the variation among the children appears to be patterned, then subsequent observations are coded, with hypotheses about regularity again revised, as necessary, to account for developmental change.

Each utterance is examined and the semantic-syntactic relations among words are identified by observing the relationship between the utterance and aspects of the child's behavior and the situational context in which the utterance occurred. Obviously, one cannot be confident that an adult's interpretation of an utterance does indeed equal the child's intent. At the least, it is necessary to establish that 1) any utterance can be identified by other observers as a separate behavior (from the other linguistic behaviors that occur), and 2) given the same information about the utterance and nonlinguistic context and behavior, different observers can assign the same interpretation to it. Interpretation of each speech event is made by at least two of three investigators independently. For this study, the proportion of agreement between independent codings for major categories ranged from 0.80 to 0.90.

Descriptive Taxonomies

By examining each speech event (which included the utterance, and behaviors by the child and others relative to the utterance), and considering its relation to other speech events in terms of similarities and differences, it is possible to identify categories of utterances that are presumably functional for the child. A criterion of productivity has been established to support the assumption that the categories derived from the children's behavior do indeed represent their underlying linguistic knowledge: a category is considered productive (i.e., derived according to an underlying rule system) if a particular child within a sample displays five or more utterance types (different utterances) in that category.

The frequency of a category within a given time span is relevant to determining productivity in any paradigm for the study of child language that assumes a developmental model. That is, at an early point in time the child does not know or use some rule, and at some later time he does. Setting the number of required utterances at precisely five was an arbitrary decision. Although one can never be sure of the exact moment of onset, given the time span of each observation and the number of speech events observed, the criterion of five different utterances was presumed to represent evidence of linguistic knowledge. We have less confidence that four or fewer utterances clearly shows the absence of such knowledge.

The taxonomy of productive categories includes absolute frequencies, but by far the most relevant interactions are proportional. In every instance, the large regularities are those that consume proportionately large amounts of the data and are considered important according to how they appear 1) developmentally, in successive samples from the same child, and 2) in intersubject comparisons, in samples from the different children with MLU held constant.

Data Base

For this study the longitudinal data were sampled in the following way. Beginning with the last observation of each child (at approximately the third birthday) and working backward, every other sample was coded and analyzed, to the point at which connectives were not yet productive. In one exception the difference between Peter's samples XVIII and XX was so great that we also had to include sample XIX. In all, the data base consisted of five samples from Eric, four from Gia, five from Kathryn, and eight from Peter (see Table 1). Utterances used in the analysis were those that contained conjunctions, relative pronouns and wh- adverbials. Each utterance was copied from the transcription, along with preceding and subsequent utterances by both child and adult as well as relevant nonlinguistic context, onto Indecks coding cards for repeated and revised sorting.

RESULTS

Presented here are two major results having to do with 1) the development of *form* in terms of the acquisition and development of connectives that were conjunctions, relative pronouns, and wh- adverbials, and 2) the development of *content* in terms of semantic relations between connected clauses.[4]

The Acquisition and Development of Connectives

The children's use of connectives increased dramatically over time, in absolute frequency, in the number of different connectives used, and in the proportion of connectives used in different categories of interclausal semantic relations. The results are presented in terms of the sequence of development of 1) overall use of connectives, 2) interclausal use of connectives, and 3) interclausal use of particular connectives.

All Connectives Table 2 presents the number of connectives used, whether or not the connective form was used to connect two clauses, in absolute frequency and as a

[4]See Bloom, et al. (in preparation) for the development of form in relation to content and use in terms of the intersection of different connectives with different semantic relations in different contexts.

Table 2. Number of connectives used

Child	Time	Total connectives: Frequency	Total connectives: Proportion of all utterances[a]	Interclausal connectives: Frequency	Interclausal connectives: Proportion of total connectives
Eric:	V	24	0.007	2	0.08
	VI	185	0.005	81	0.44
	VIII	297	0.12	159	0.54
	X	227	0.10	122	0.54
	XII	400	0.11	219	0.55
Gia:	V	21	0.006	2	0.10
	VII	177	0.04	76	0.43
	VIII	229	0.06	125	0.55
	XI	346	0.08	214	0.62
Kathryn:	III	9	0.002	1	0.11
	IV	70	0.02	32	0.46
	VI	194	0.06	133	0.69
	VII	371	0.13	192	0.52
	X	565	0.11	396	0.70
Peter:	VIII	5	0.002	2	0.40
	X	53	0.02	16	0.30
	XII	35	0.015	11	0.31
	XIV	91	0.04	50	0.55
	XVI	93	0.04	51	0.55
	XVIII	147	0.06	61	0.41
	XIX	354	0.14	174	0.49
	XX	235	0.10	163	0.69

[a]These are approximate proportions since a small number of utterances contained two connectives.

proportion of the total number of utterances in each sample. The number of times connective forms were used increased for each child: no child used connectives more than 25 times in the first sample, and all children used connectives at least 200 times by the last sample. Kathryn and Gia showed a steady increase over time, whereas Eric and Peter showed some variability in the overall pattern. The proportion of total utterances containing connectives also increased over time, but reached a plateau at about 0.10 of all the utterances in a given sample. The proportion in the first sample for each child was less than 0.01. This proportion gradually increased over time for Gia, Kathryn, and Peter, leveling off at approximately 0.10 in the last two samples for Kathryn and Peter. For Eric, however, the proportion was less than 0.01 at the first two samples, increasing to at least 0.10 in the remaining samples.

Interclausal Connectives The use of connectives to join two clauses increased both in absolute frequency, and as a proportion of all connectives that were used (see Table 2). There was slight variability for all the children except Gia; however, by the last sample all children used connectives interclausally at least 0.50 of the time.

Particular Interclausal Connectives The different connectives used by each child at each time are presented in Table 3. Some of these are combinations of connectives, for example, "and," "then," and "and then" were considered as different connectives.

There was a dramatic increase in the number of different connectives used, from only one or two in the first samples to as many as 27 different connectives for Kathryn X. Many of the connectives, however, were used only one or two times in a sample, and thus were not considered productive. The number of different connectives used productively also increased, from one to a maximum of eleven (see top half of Table 3). This increase was not gradual; a comparison of the last two samples for each child shows doubling in the number of different productive connectives for Eric and Gia, and greater than a 0.50 increase for Kathryn and Peter.

The connectives used productively are listed in Table 3 according to the number of samples in which they were productive. Thus, the first connective, "and," was used productively in the most number of samples (17 of 22), whereas the 17th, "like," was used productively in only one of the 22 samples. By the last session all the children productively used the following connectives: "and," "because," "what," "when," "but," and "that." "If" and "so" were productive for three of the children by the last sample, but not for Gia. The pattern of productivity was variable for some of the connectives, i.e., some connectives, although used productively at one time, were not productive at a later time, as in "and then" for Kathryn and Peter.

In addition to being the most frequently used connective, "and" was also the first to appear in the children's speech, the first to be used as an interclausal connective, and the first to be productive. Whereas the absolute frequency of "and" used interclausally was variable, it was always more frequent than any other connective, although its use decreased proportionately to other connectives. "And" was often used in combination with other connectives. For example, the connective "then" was not used productively until the combined form "and then" became productive. Combinations of other connectives with "and" were not productive in any of the samples.

It should be noted that many of these same connective words have other uses in the language, and for certain of these words other uses precede their connective function. For example, "that" occurred in the children's speech to encode existence (as in "that's a ball") well before it was used as a relative pronoun. Similarly, "what" and "where" occurred in the children's first questions; their function in noun-phrase complements was a much later development. It remains to be determined whether other forms are used in other ways before they function as connectives.

Development of Semantic Relations between Clauses

An initial pass through the data suggested that there were at least three categories of semantic relations expressed in utterances with connectives: concomitance, causality, and specification. It soon became clear, however, that a much finer categorization was necessary to capture the developmental complexity and diversity of utterances in these categories as well as other utterances. Successive and repeated passes through the data yielded a total of eleven categories of semantic relations. Several of these categories, in turn, had subcategories. The result was a taxonomy of the different semantic relations between connected clauses in the children's sentences and longitudinal development of these semantic relations.

Table 3. Connectives used in interclausal semantic categories

	Connectives used productively									
Connective	Eric V	Eric VI	Eric VIII	Eric X	Eric XII	Gia V	Gia VII	Gia VIII	Gia XI	Kathryn IV
and	0.50 (1)[a]	0.88 (72)	0.70 (119)	0.53 (63)	0.31 (69)	1.0 (2)[a]	0.82 (76)	0.46 (61)	0.30 (65)	0.93 (37)
because		0.09 (7)	0.05 (9)	0.11 (13)	0.26 (58)		0.02 (2)[a]	0.01 (1)[a]	0.20 (42)	
what	0.50 (1)[a]		0.02 (3)[a]		0.09 (20)			0.02 (3)[a]	0.11 (23)	
and then				0.04 (5)	0.03 (6)		0.02 (2)[a]	0.15 (20)	(1)[a]	0.05 (2)[a]
when			0.03 (5)		0.04 (8)		0.04 (4)[a]	0.17 (23)	0.10 (22)	
so		0.03 (2)[a]	0.04 (7)	0.10 (12)	0.06 (14)					
but			0.02 (4)[a]	0.03 (4)[a]	0.03 (7)				0.03 (7)	
if			0.02 (4)[a]	0.08 (9)	0.05 (12)					
that				(1)[a]	0.02 (5)		0.01 (1)[a]	0.02 (3)[a]	0.03 (6)	
where			0.02 (3)[a]	(1)[a]	0.03 (6)			0.02 (2)[a]	0.02 (5)	
how										
then							0.02 (2)[a]	0.06 (8)		0.03 (1)[a]
til								0.01 (1)[a]	0.02 (5)	
for			0.03 (5)		0.01 (2)[a]		0.03 (3)[a]		0.06 (12)	
if-then										
when-then								0.04 (5)	0.02 (4)[a]	
like									0.02 (5)	
Number of connectives used productively	0	2	5	5	10	0	1	5	10	1

Connective	Kathryn VI	Kathryn VIII	Kathryn X	Peter VIII	Peter X	Peter XII	Peter XIV	Peter XVI	Peter XVIII	Peter XIX	Peter XX
and	0.59 (71)	0.28 (58)	0.26 (107)	1.0 (2)[a]	1.0 (16)	0.36 (4)[a]	0.78 (38)	0.66 (33)	0.54 (33)	0.55 (94)	0.18 (34)
because		0.18 (39)	0.28 (112)					0.06 (3)	0.25 (15)	0.15 (25)	0.14 (27)
what	0.05 (6)	0.02 (5)	0.02 (7)			0.45 (5)	0.08 (4)[a]	0.16 (8)	0.05 (3)[a]	0.07 (12)	0.13 (25)
and then	0.09 (11)	0.11 (23)	0.02 (8)							0.10 (17)	0.02 (4)[a]
when	(1)[a]	0.03 (7)	0.03 (12)					0.02 (1)[a]	0.05 (3)[a]	0.03 (5)	0.04 (7)
so	0.07 (9)	0.09 (20)	0.02 (9)							0.01 (1)[a]	0.09 (16)
but	0.05 (6)	0.08 (18)	0.17 (68)						0.02 (1)[a]	0.02 (3)[a]	0.03 (5)
if		0.02 (4)[a]	0.05 (19)							0.01 (1)[a]	0.12 (23)
that	0.02 (3)[a]	0.02 (4)[a]	0.02 (7)							0.01 (1)[a]	0.03 (5)
where		0.04 (9)	(2)[a]								
how	0.04 (5)	(2)[a]	0.03 (11)								
then	0.07 (9)	(2)[a]	0.04 (17)								
til											
for											
if-then											
when-then			0.01 (6)								
like											
Number of connectives used productively	7	8	11	0	1	1	1	2	2	5	8

[a]Connectives not used productively at that time.

Connectives not used productively

Connective	Eric V	Eric VI	Eric VIII	Eric X	Eric XII	Gia V	Gia VII	Gia VIII	Gia XI	Kathryn IV
after									(1)	
and if				(1)						
and so									(1)	
and then if				(1)						
and when										
because when									(1)	
before									0.01 (2)	
except				0.02 (2)						
first then								0.01 (1)		
for										
for when					(1)					
from										
how					(2)				0.02 (4)	
if							0.01 (1)	0.02 (3)	0.01 (2)	
like				(1)	(1)					
or			(1)							
so							0.02 (2)	0.02 (2)	0.01 (3)	
so that										
then				(1)	0.01 (3)					
then-and										
then if										
to			0.02 (3)		(2)				(1)	
unless				(1)						
until (til)			(1)	(1)	(2)					
whenever					(1)					
when-then										
where										
while				(1)						
without				(1)						
who			0.02 (3)	(1)					0.01 (2)	
why				(1)						
Total number of different connectives used	2	3	13	19	18	1	9	13	21	3

Connective	Kathryn VI	Kathryn VIII	Kathryn X	Peter VIII	Peter X	Peter XII	Peter XIV	Peter XVI	Peter XVIII	Peter XIX	Peter XX
after		0.02 (4)	(2)								
and if											
and so											
and then if											
and when			(1)								
because when											
before			(2)								
except											
first then											
for		(1)	(2)					0.02 (1)		0.01 (1)	
for when											
from			(1)								
how											
if							0.02 (1)		0.02 (1)	0.01 (2)	0.02 (4)
like		(1)	(1)								
or			(2)							0.01 (2)	0.01 (1)
so											0.01 (2)
so that			(1)								0.01 (1)
then							0.02 (1)	0.02 (1)		0.01 (1)	
then-and			(2)								
then if			(1)								
to		0.01 (4)	(1)				0.06 (3)				0.01 (1)
unless											
until (til)									0.02 (1)	0.01 (1)	
whenever											
when-then			(2)								
where						0.18 (2)	0.04 (2)	0.04 (2)	0.05 (3)	0.02 (3)	0.01 (2)
while		(1)	(1)						0.02 (1)		
without											
who			(3)							0.01 (2)	0.02 (3)
why								0.02 (1)		0.01 (1)	0.02 (3)
Total number of different connectives used	9	17	27	1	1	3	6	8	9	17	17

Table 4. Categorization of semantic relations

Interevent relations		Intraevent relations
Concomitance (no new meaning)	Superordinance (new meaning)	(no new meaning)
1. Same verb in two clauses 2. Different verb in two clauses	1. Causality 2. Antithesis 3. Time specification	1. Epistemic 2. Object-specification 3. Notice-complement 4. Other-complement

The final step was categorization of the semantic relations in this taxonomy on the basis of focus in events and whether a new meaning resulted when the two events were coded in complex sentences, as presented in Table 4. There were both interevent relations in which there was a focus on two events, and intraevent relations in which there was a focus on one event (with "event" defined simply as a happening or state of being).

There were two kinds of interevent relations. In *concomitance,* the combination of the two clauses did not result in any new meaning, or one plus one equalled two, for example, "You sit here and I sit there," or "That's a car and that's a plane." In *superordinance,* the combination of the two clauses did result in a new meaning such as causality, as in the sentence "Bend the man so he can sit," or antithesis, as in the sentence "I was trying to get my crayons but I fell." In such sentences one plus one equalled more than two, in that the combination of the two meanings of the clauses, for example, "bend the man," and "he can sit" resulted in a larger meaning, in this case, causality. *Intraevent* relations were those in which there was focus on one event, no new meaning resulted from the combination of clauses, and one plus one equalled one, for example "This can go in corner where sofa is" (focus on *corner*) and "I know what else is in it" (focus on *else*).

The proportion of utterances in these categories of semantic relations (once productivity was attained) is presented in Table 5 and Figure 1, according to the sequence of development for each child. The same sequence of development was observed for all four children: within the interevent relations, concomitance preceded superordinance; and both interevent relations preceded intraevent relations. That is, children used connectives when talking about two-focus events before they used connectives when talking about a one-focus event; when talking about two-focus events they first joined two clauses, which did not create new meaning.

For all children, the proportion of concomitance decreased from over 0.60 at the first sample in which there was productivity to less than 0.30 by the last samples. Superordinance increased developmentally, and by the last sample it had superceded concomitance. Intraevent relations also increased developmentally, but never accounted for more than 0.22 of the utterances of Eric, Gia, and Kathryn.

The proportion of intraevent relations for Peter was high in the first and last samples (0.64 at Peter XII; 0.36 at Peter XX) and was variable throughout. This difference can be accounted for by one of the subcategories, epistemic (see definition below). Utterances in this subcategory were largely confined to variations of one type, for example, "know

Table 5. Major categories of semantic relations

		Concomitance		Superordinance		Intraevent relations		
Child	Time	*p*	*f*[b]	*p*	*f*	*p*	*f*	Total[a]
Eric	V							2
	VI	0.69	56	0.16	13	0.07	6	81
	VIII	0.63	100	0.27	43	0.09	15	159
	X	0.39	47	0.39	47	0.17	21	122
	XII	0.27	59	0.45	98	0.21	46	219
Gia	V							2
	VII	0.62	47	0.18	14	0.08	6	76
	VIII	0.52	65	0.33	41	0.10	13	125
	XI	0.26	55	0.48	102	0.22	48	214
Kathryn	III							1
	IV	0.88	28					32
	VI	0.64	85	0.17	22	0.04	5	133
	VIII	0.33	63	0.50	96	0.11	21	192
	X	0.27	108	0.57	227	0.12	46	396
Peter	VIII							2
	X	0.62	10					16
	XII					0.64	7	11
	XIV	0.62	31			0.12	6	50
	XVI	0.47	24	0.10	5	0.22	11	51
	XVIII	0.43	26	0.30	18			61
	XIX	0.56	98	0.29	50	0.09	16	174
	XX	0.21	35	0.36	58	0.36	58	163

[a]The total includes utterances from nonproductive categories as well as productive categories.
[b]The frequencies, and corresponding proportions of the total, are of the productive categories, only.

what this is.'' Only in the last two samples were Peter's epistemic utterances more varied, although the other children's were varied from the beginning (see examples page 256).

The subcategories of inter and intraevent relations along with representative examples from the children at different times are defined below.[5]

Interevent Relations: Concomitance Utterances in this category referred to events and/or states that were bound together in space or time. Each clause was meaningful by itself and independent of the other, and the two clauses together did not create a meaning that was different from the meaning of each of the clauses separately. Within this category, utterances could be differentiated on the basis of whether the same or different verbs occurred in the two clauses. There was one type of concomitance in which the same verb was used in both clauses, and three types of concomitance in which there were different verbs in the two clauses.

Same Verb These utterances consisted of clauses that had the same verb, or if no

[5]Utterances on the right were spoken by the child. Material in parentheses on the left describes the situational context, and utterances from the adults are presented on the left without parentheses. The connective used as an illustration is underlined, to highlight it and differentiate it from other connectives in the same utterance not under immediate discussion.

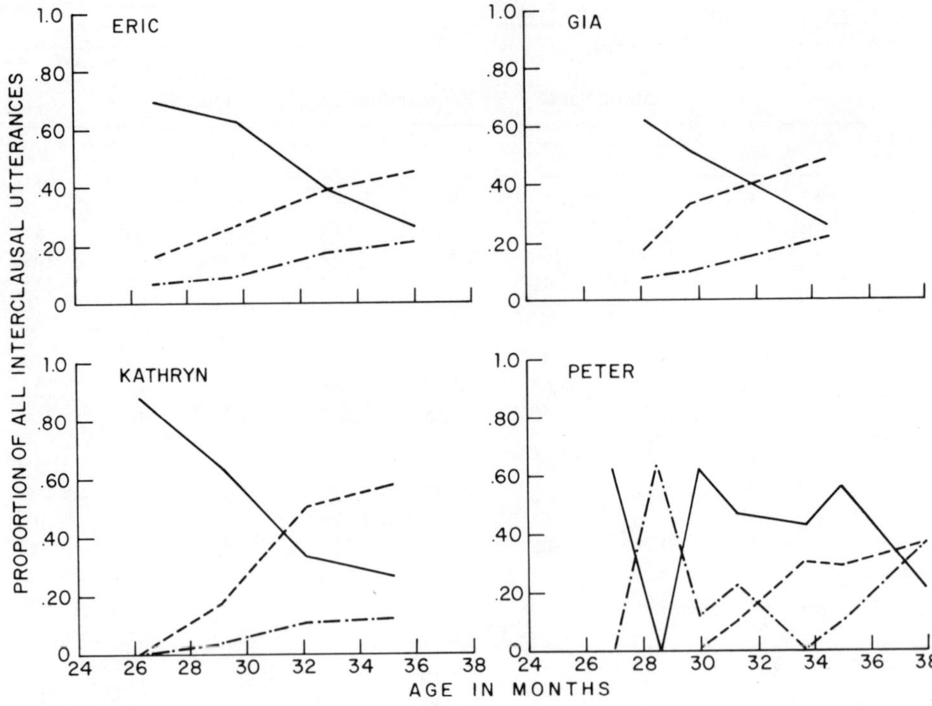

Figure 1. Major categories of semantic relations. Interevent relations: concomitance (——); interevent relations: superordinance (– – –); intraevent relations (·—·).

verb was explicit, had the same verb implied. At least one major sentence constituent (subject-verb-complement) in each clause had the same referent.

Peter XIV (pointing to and touching furniture in doll house)	That's full *and* that's full too
Kathryn VIII	I'm sitting here *and* you can sit there and rest
Gia XI (referring to two different animals)	I put this on the train *and* this lamb on the train

Different Verb: Interclausal These utterances consisted of clauses with different verbs, but at least one of the other major sentence constituents had the same referent.

Eric VIII (pointing to lamb)	That one is eating *and* now he's lying down
Peter XVI	I'm gonna put this away/ *then* I'm gonna ride my bike
Kathryn X (referring to imaginary party guests)	and they'll come too *and* bring the cake.

Different Verb: Extraclausal In these utterances, all the referents for the major sentence constituents were different for each clause.

Eric VIII (looking at picture in book)	They're taking a vacuum cleaner to wipe *and* puppy dog's running
Kathryn X	now you drive *and* I be waiting over here
Peter XX Adult: Yeah Lynn's gonna stay with me	*and* I'm gonna go get my toys out here and play with them

Different Verb: Precausal In these utterances reference was made to sequential actions by the same actor; in most cases, the first (and first mentioned) action was expressed with a locative action verb (which entailed *place* as a complement), followed by a simple action or state verb. These utterances were considered to be precausal, because the relation between the clauses was *potentially* one of action and result.

Gia VII	I gonna get my blanket *and* sleep on my blanket
Peter XVI	Daddy's gonna come in here *and* put out the fire
Gia XI Adult: On the stool?	I wanna put a blanket on here/ yes/ *and* the lambs can rest

Interevent Relations: Superordinance There were three major subcategories of superordinance. While these utterances all focused on two events, they could be differentiated on the basis of the type of new meaning that was created when the clauses were joined.

Causality Utterances in this subcategory expressed a dependence between two events and/or states. Most often, the relation was intentional or motivational, with one clause referring to an intended or ongoing action or state, and the other clause giving a reason for or result of it.

Gia VII	it's on too tight/ *so* I fix my shoe
Peter XVI Adult: Why?	don't touch this camera *cause* it's broken
Eric X	I'm blowing on this *cause* it's hot
Eric VIII Adult: Why isn't it open?	it's not open/ *cause* it's locked
Gia VII	I gonna step in the puddle with sandals/ *and* get it all wet
Peter XX	she put a bandaid on her shoe/ *and* it maked it feel better

Time Specification Utterances in this subcategory expressed a dependency relation between two events and/or states, in which the dependency was one of temporality, referring to one event or state occurring prior to or simultaneous with the other.

Gia VIII	*when* I go out I wanna blow bubbles here
Kathryn VIII	I'm gonna put it in my room so I can see it *when* I'm sleeping
Peter XX	you better look for it/ *when* you get back home
Kathryn X	now *while* I hide it you stay here
Eric XII	and I can't eat it *til* Mommy comes home

Antithesis Utterances in this subcategory expressed a dependence between two events and/or states by means of contrast between them. Most often, the relation between the clauses was one of opposition, in which one clause negated or opposed the other, or of exception, in which one clause qualified or limited the other.

Kathryn VI	I gon' do this/ *but* this don't fits
Eric X	it sound like a tunnel *buts'* a bridge
Kathryn X	I was trying to get my crayons *but* I fell
Eric X	that train broke down/ *and* dis train did not broke down
Peter XX	he's trying to find some food *but* the wind blew it and he got outa his mouth!

Intraevent Relations There were four subcategories of utterances referring to intraevent relations. No new meaning was created in intraevent relations; rather, the two clauses merged to focus upon one referent.

Object Specification In this subcategory the two clauses combined described an object or person mentioned in the first clause. Most often, the person or object was a predicate complement constituent, either object or place. The most common types of object specification described the object or person by function, place, or activity.

Eric VIII Adult: What's that?	a toilet *where* you poopoo
Kathryn VIII	this can go in a corner *where* sofa is
Gia XI Adult: Who's that?	the man *who* fixes the door
Kathryn X	it looks like a fishing thing *and* you fish with it
Kathryn X (holding stick)	it's just a thing *that* I hold

Epistemic Utterances in this subcategory coded certainty or uncertainty about a particular state of affairs. The two clauses together focused on the object of certainty or uncertainty.

Gia XI	now I know *how* to take this off
Eric XIII	I know *what* else is in it
Gia VIII	I going see *if* there's more tape
Kathryn X	I don't know *what* this color is
Peter XVI	know *where* the playhouse is

Notice Complement Utterances in this subcategory served to call attention to a state or event. The joining of the clauses, the first of which contained a notice verb, resulted in focus on the object of attention, which was most often the complement of the second clause.

Eric XII	now look *what's* in here
Kathryn X	watch *what* I'm doing
Gia XI	look *what* my Mommy got me

Other Complement There were instances of complements other than notice complements, which did not fit the pattern of other semantic relations.

Kathryn VIII	that's *what* you can do
Eric XII	tell Iris *that* I wet my bed
Eric X	make sure *that* nothing happens to that train

Other Categories All the above subcategories of semantic relations included utterances in which a connective form was used to join two clauses. In addition, intraclausal, concatenative, and undetermined uses of connectives were tabulated and included in the total number of connectives (Table 2).

Intraclausal Connectives The most frequent intraclausal use of a connective was to link the constituents of a predicate complement. For example,

Peter XX	have big ones *and* little ones
Eric XII	I was playing with the sprinkler *and* the fountain

Concatenative There were also frequent occurrences of "and" used to join two verbs, such as "go" and "get." These were not counted as interclausal, because they seemed to function as two-part verbs. For example,

Kathryn IV	I'll go *and* get a plate for it
Peter XIV	come *and* watch TV
Peter XX	I better open up *and* see

Uncategorized The remaining instances in which connectives were used could not confidently be placed within any of the above semantic categories. The most frequent seemed to function as introducers; the connective occurred at the beginning of a child utterance and appeared to have no consistent relation to the previous utterance. For example,

Peter XIX	I want cookies on a plate/ *and* don't leave that Lucy baby

Other utterances that were not categorized included those in which part of the utterance was incomplete, or the connective occurred as a single word utterance. Also uncategorized were anomalous or otherwise uninterpretable utterances and routines, such as segments of songs, nursery rhymes, and stories.

Development of Specific Subcategories of Semantic Relations The frequency and proportion of the productive subcategories of semantic relations for each child at each time are presented in Table 6. There were both similarities and differences among the children in the sequence of emergence of subcategories. First, no child had any productive subcategories in the first sample. Second, when productivity was attained, concomitance with the same verb was the most frequent (and for Peter it was the first productive subcategory). However, the children varied in their rate of acquiring productivity; Eric and Gia

Table 6. Productive subcategories of interclausal semantic relations

Subcategory	Eric IV	Eric VIII	Eric X	Eric XII	Gia VII	Gia VIII	Gia XI	Kathryn IV	Kathryn VI
Causality	0.16[a] (13)[b]	0.18 (28)	0.32 (39)	0.35 (76)	0.18 (14)	0.10 (13)	0.25 (53)		0.12 (16)
Epistemic		0.03 (5)	0.09 (11)	0.15 (33)		0.06 (7)	0.06 (12)		
Concomitance: different verb interclausal	0.23 (19)	0.22 (35)	0.09 (11)	0.10 (22)	0.19 (15)	0.26 (33)	0.13 (27)	0.19 (6)	0.28 (37)
Concomitance: same verb	0.31 (25)	0.26 (42)	0.15 (18)	0.15 (32)	0.23 (18)	0.16 (20)	0.11 (23)	0.69 (22)	0.27 (36)
Object specification	0.07 (6)	0.06 (10)	0.08 (10)	0.06 (13)	0.08 (6)	0.05 (6)	0.07 (14)		
Antithesis		0.06 (9)	0.07 (8)	0.06 (13)			0.04 (8)		0.05 (6)
Time specification		0.04 (6)		0.04 (9)		0.22 (28)	0.19 (41)		
Concomitance: precausality	0.15 (12)	0.08 (12)	0.06 (7)	0.02 (5)	0.22 (17)	0.10 (12)	0.02 (5)		0.09 (12)
Concomitance: different verb extraclausal		0.07 (11)	0.09 (11)						
Notice complement							0.05 (11)		
Other complement							0.05 (11)		0.04 (5)
Total number of interclausal relations[c]	81	159	122	219	76	125	214	32	133
Number of productive subcategories	5	9	8	8	5	7	10	2	6

	Kathryn VIII	Kathryn X	Peter X	Peter XII	Peter XIV	Peter XVI	Peter XVIII	Peter XIX	Peter XX
Causality	0.36 (69)	0.35 (137)				0.10 (5)	0.30 (18)	0.18 (32)	0.31 (50)
Epistemic		0.02 (8)		0.64 (7)	0.12 (6)	0.22 (11)		0.09 (16)	0.31 (50)
Concomitance: different verb interclausal	0.14 (26)	0.13 (51)			0.14 (7)	0.25 (13)	0.08 (5)	0.21 (37)	0.11 (18)
Concomitance: same verb	0.06 (12)	0.06 (25)	0.63 (10)		0.48 (24)	0.22 (11)	0.34 (21)	0.27 (47)	0.06 (10)
Object specification	0.06 (12)	0.06 (22)							0.05 (8)
Antithesis	0.08 (15)	0.18 (71)						0.07 (12)	0.05 (8)
Time specification	0.06 (12)	0.05 (19)						0.03 (6)	
Concomitance: precausality	0.13 (25)	0.04 (14)						0.04 (7)	0.04 (7)
Concomitance: different verb extraclausal		0.05 (18)						0.04 (7)	
Notice complement		0.04 (16)							
Other complement	0.05 (9)								
Total number of interclausal relations[c]	192	396	16	11	50	51	61	174	163
Number of productive subcategories	8	10	1	1	3	4	3	8	7

[a]The proportion represents the proportion of the total number of utterances in the subcategory.
[b]The number in parentheses represents the frequency of utterances in the subcategory.
[c]The total includes utterances from nonproductive categories.

expressed several meaning relations at once, going from no productive subcategories in the first sample to five in the next. Kathryn and Peter progressed more slowly, going from none in the first sample to one (Peter) or two (Kathryn) in the next.

By the last sample, the children showed striking similarity in the relative frequency of subcategories (see Table 6). The rank order of the five most frequent subcategories in the last sample was the same for all four children, with the two exceptions that are noted:

1. Causality
2. Epistemic (for Eric and Peter; time specification for Gia; antithesis for Kathryn)
3. Concomitance: different verb-interclausal
4. Concomitance: same verb (reverse 3 and 4 for Eric)
5. Object specification

In terms of the major categorization, then, the most frequent concomitance subcategory was different verb-interclausal; the most frequent superordinance subcategory was causality; and the most frequent intraevent subcategory was epistemic.

DISCUSSION

The results of this study are discussed in terms of 1) previous findings in the literature on the development of complex sentences and 2) the more general issue of a common process within different aspects of language development.

Comparison of Results with Other Studies of Connectives

The sequence of development of connective forms is in general agreement with results reported elsewhere. "And" was the first and most frequent connective used by the children, as has been observed repeatedly (e.g., Clark, 1970; Limber, 1973; Jacobsen, 1974; Beilin, 1975). The sequence in which the connectives appeared in the children's speech between the second and third years of age—"and," "because," "what," "when," "but," "that," "if," "so"—is essentially similar to the relative frequencies of connectives observed by Clark (1970) with 3½-year-old children: most frequent were "and," "and so," and "and then"; next were "when" and "because"; last was "if." Chambaz et al. (1975) found that the most frequent "introducteur de complexité" for French speaking children (3 to 6 years old) was *parce que* (because) followed by *quand* (when). Menyuk (1969) reported that "because" was used with greater frequency than "so" and "if" by first grade children. Thus, the sequence of development reported here in children from 2 to 3 years of age reflects the frequency with which connectives are reportedly used by older children.

The results of the analysis of the meaning relations coded by the connectives are not as easily compared with previous literature. Most other studies have been limited to a particular type or types of complex sentence relation. For example, Clark (1970; 1973) and Ferreiro and Sinclair (1971) were concerned with how children code temporal relations only. They observed that the use of "and" or "then" characterized the first stage in describing temporal events (in children from about 3½ to 10 years old); the most advanced stage was the use of "when" or "before." In the present study, "when," as a means of coding time specification, was already productive for all the children before the age of 3; "before" was never productive.

More generally, Clancy et al. (1976), in a study of the acquisition of conjunction in English, German, Italian, and Turkish, reported a general trend. In all four languages, juxtaposition without, and later with, a surface connective expressed four basic kinds of relationships: coordination, sequence, antithesis, and causality. Coordination was the first to emerge in all languages; the order of the remaining relationships was variable. Whereas Clancy et al. referred to semantic relations expressed both with and without connectives, and the present study was concerned only with relations expressed *with* connectives, the kinds of relations observed and their sequence were similar. That is, concomitance (coordination) occurred before superordinance (causality and antithesis). "Sequence" is not directly applicable to any of the relations observed in the present study; it seems to encompass both concomitance and time specification.

Developmental Continuity

In previous studies of the development of the same four children, there were changes in form and in the content of their language (Bloom, 1970; Bloom et al., 1974; Bloom et al., 1975; Bloom et al., 1975; Bloom et al., 1976). Two major developmental interactions between form and content have been observed: 1) when forms become progressively more complex but content does not change; and 2) where new forms result in the expression of new semantic relations.

Children's first word combinations can encode the same kinds of conceptual notions that were represented by their earlier single word utterances; for example, the combination of "more" and "cookie" does not encode a new relation. Thus, the appearance of certain multiword utterances can be seen as a change in the form of child language, with little or no change in content. Similarly, in the development of negation, children learn new, more complex forms to express the same negation concepts (nonexistence, rejection, and denial) that they expressed earlier with single word and two-word utterances. When children first add syntactic complexity to their early two-word utterances, they do so by combining the semantic relations that were coded in earlier two-word utterances, so that form changes but again content essentially does not. For example, the relations of recurrence, attribution, and possession are frequently embedded in an action relation, e.g., "Mommy eat more raisins," "play big truck," "Daddy drink my juice." Such combinations of semantic relations focus on single events, where one relation is embedded in or subordinated to another.

This same developmental relationship between form and content was found in the results of the present study. When MLU passed 2.0 and the children began to use syntactic connectives, the first connective simply joined two independent clauses that had previously occurred separately and no new meaning was introduced (concomitance). For example, the meaning of "I sit here and you sit there" is no more and no less than the meaning of each clause separately. Here again, although form changes, content does not. The difference between this later complexity, in which two independent clauses are joined and the earlier complexity, in which one semantic relation is embedded in another, is that the child is now focusing on two events in a single sentence.

A later development was again a change in form, with no new meaning. Intraevent interclausal relations were a syntactically more complex change in form, in which one clause was embedded in another, and no new content emerged. The occurrence of intra-event interclausal relations observed in the present study can be viewed as a syntactically more complex illustration of the same process that occurred when children combined such early semantic relations as recurrence, possession, and attribution in predicates (for example, "eat more raisin"). Semantic relations are again combined by adding complexity in the predicate, but here it is through the embedding of another clause. Thus, "put in corner where sofa is" means the same thing as "put there near sofa" or "put over there/sofa over there." The focus is still on one event, and no new meaning is derived from the combination of the clauses. Further, just as "put there" expresses a locative relation, "put in corner where sofa is" does also.

The second developmental interaction between form and content, when new forms result in the expression of new content, is observed in such early word combinations as "Mommy eat." Here the resulting semantic relation of agent-action is not encoded by either word alone but by the two combined. The same development was found in the present study with the appearance of superordinate interclausal relations. New content (e.g., causality, antithesis, time specification) resulted from the combination of clauses with new connective forms (e.g., because, but, when). In the combination of clauses represented in the utterance "bend the man so he can sit," the resulting relation of causality is not encoded by either clause alone, but by the combination of the two.

The interactions between form and content observed in the present study can be summarized as follows. First, new connective forms were used to focus on two events without encoding any new meaning or involving syntactic embedding. Next, new connective forms were used to focus on two events that resulted in a new meaning, but which did not also involve syntactic embedding. Last, new connective forms were used to focus on one event without encoding any new meaning, but involving syntactic embedding. Thus, as with earlier development of form and content, syntactic embedding, which is the more complex form of linguistic conjoining, develops last, after the children have learned to express meaning or content with simpler forms.

In conclusion, there was a sequence in the development of both interclausal syntactic connectives used by the children in this study and in the semantic relations coded by these connectives. This sequence is in accord with findings reported about older children's use of connectives in particular, and with the earlier developmental interactions of form and content in general.

ACKNOWLEDGMENTS

We wish to thank Kathleen Fiess and Barbara Schecter for their help in data processing, and Owen Whitby for his help in statistical matters.

REFERENCES

Beilin, H. 1975. Studies in the Cognitive Basis of Language Development. Academic Press, New York.

Bloom, L. 1970. Language Development: Form and Function in Emerging Grammars. M.I.T. Press, Cambridge.

Bloom, L., Hood, L., and Lightbown, P. 1974. Imitation in language development: if, when, and why. Cog. Psychol. 6:380–420.

Bloom, L., Hood, L., Lifter, K., and Lahey, M. The integration of form, content, and use for the acquisition of syntactic connectives. In preparation.

Bloom, L., Lightbown, P., and Hood, L. 1974. Conventions for transcription of child language recordings. Unpublished manuscript, Teachers College, Columbia University.

Bloom, L., Lightbown, P., and Hood, L. 1975. Structure and variation in child language. Monogr. Soc. Res. Child Dev. No. 160.

Bloom, L., Miller, P., and Hood, L. 1975. Variation and reduction as aspects of competence in language development. In: A. Pick (ed.), Minnesota Symposium on Child Psychology, Vol. 9. The University of Minnesota Press, Minneapolis.

Bloom, L., Rocissano, L., and Hood, L. 1976. Adult-child discourse: developmental interaction between information processing and linguistic knowledge. Cog. Psychol. 8:521–552.

Bohn, W. 1914. First steps in verbal expression. Pedagogical Seminary, 21:578–595.

Brown, R. 1973. A First Language, the Early Stages. Harvard University Press, Cambridge.

Chambaz, M., Leroy, C., and Messeant, G. 1975. Les "petits mots" de coordination: etude diachronique de leur apparition chez quatre enfants entre 3 et 4 ans. Langue Française, Apparition de la Syntaxe Chez l'enfant, 27:38–54.

Clancy, P. 1974. The acquisition of conjunction in Italian. Unpublished manuscript, University of California, Berkeley.

Clancy, P., Jacobsen, T., and Silva, M. 1976. The acquisition of conjunction: a cross-linguistic study. Paper presented at the Stanford Child Language Research Forum.

Clark, E. V. 1970. How young children describe events in time. In: G. B. Flores d'Arcais and W. J. M. Levelt (eds.), Advances in Psycholinguistics. American Elsevier, New York.

Clark, E. V. 1973. How children describe time and order. In: C. A. Ferguson and D. I. Slobin (eds.), Studies of Child Language Development. Holt, Rinehart & Winston, New York.

Cochran, W. G. 1963. Sampling Techniques, 2nd Ed. John Wiley & Sons Inc., New York.

Ferreiro, E., and Sinclair, H. 1971. Temporal relationships in language. Int. J. Psychol. 6:39–47.

Hood, L. 1977. A longitudinal study of the development of the expression of causal relations in complex sentences. Unpublished doctoral dissertation, Columbia University, New York.

Jacobsen, T. 1974. On the order of emergence of conjunctions and notions of conjunctions in English-speaking children. Unpublished manuscript, University of California, Berkeley.

Johansson, B. S., and Sjölin, B. 1975. Preschool children's understanding of the coordinations "and" and "or." J. Exp. Child Psychol. 19:233–240.

Limber, J. 1973. The genesis of complex sentences. In: T. Moore (ed.), Cognitive Development and the Acquisition of Language. Academic Press, New York.

Menyuk, P. 1969. Sentences Children Use. M.I.T. Press, Cambridge.

Miller, W. 1973. The acquisition of grammatical rules by children. Paper presented at the meeting of the Linguistic Society of America, 1964. Reprinted in C. A. Ferguson and D. I. Slobin (eds.), Studies of Child Language Development. Holt, Rinehart, & Winston, New York.

Schlesinger, I. 1971. Production of utterances and language acquisition. In: D. Slobin (ed.), The Ontogenesis of Grammar. Academic Press, New York.

Werner, H., and Kaplan, B. 1963. Symbol Formation. John Wiley & Sons Inc., New York.

chapter 11

Design and Application of a Data System for Development of a Set of Language Programs

Joseph K. Carrier, Jr.

Language training has a history of relying heavily upon subjective impressions of teachers, clinicians, and parents as major determiners of a child's abilities to learn and of the success of instructional efforts. This is partially a function of naiveté or disregard by professionals of data management practices as they can be applied to language training, but there are other reasons as well. The traditional mystique surrounding language—the view that it is a covert process—has in a sense denied its appropriateness as objectively determined data. The unlimited complexity of language has further confounded the issue, as has the fact that language learners (in therapy or classroom instruction) most often acquire numerous skills beyond the scope of those directly taught. And finally, professionals' efforts to use a data base to evaluate linguistic abilities and skill acquisition are severely limited by a dearth of carefully designed training programs, and by the fact that standardized language tests are seldom directly appropriate to the training that children have undergone. None of this, however, precludes the feasibility of direct use of carefully collected training data for the purposes of defining child abilities and language acquisition.

Carefully collected child training data have a variety of functions critical to any systematic language training. First, if the training sequences or steps follow a systematic model, data provide answers to questions about child failure; "Why didn't Billy learn to use verbs?," "Why is Mary taking so long to learn to label with nouns?" etc. Second, data provide the basis for concluding that a child has indeed learned a class of skills, or is still in the process of acquisition. Data, in addition to these most critical functions, assist us in determining weaknesses in training procedures, weaknesses in child modalities (input and output), and the effectiveness of specific parameters of various training paradigms. Training data might very well be the vehicle whereby language training can be removed from the realm of an art, placed under the constraints of science, and then systematically improved to the point where success and failure are carefully defined and can each serve as indicators of subsequent training, rather than as subjective bases for teacher exultation or exasperation.

The purpose of this chapter is to describe the use of data in one attempt to develop programs for teaching communication skills to severely and profoundly retarded individuals. Data formed the basis for nearly all critical program development decisions and, now that a program is completed, the data form the foundation upon which others can administer the same procedures and make decisions about their own training and their own children. These direct applications of data to the issues involved in developing a language program are presented in such a manner that others may be able to use this information as an aid in planning data systems appropriate to their own training or program development efforts.

The first issue in planning data collection and management is to determine the functions the data are expected to perform. For the program presented in this chapter, the task was to develop a set of programs for teaching communication skills (language) to severely and profoundly retarded individuals. The proposed training strategy was to use geometric shapes as symbols (a circle would represent "woman," a square would represent "boy," etc.), to teach children to use these symbols meaningfully, and to sequence these symbols to construct communicative phrases and sentences. The theoretical bases and procedural tactics were taken in part from work done by Premack (1970, 1971) in which a similar system was used to teach language to a chimpanzee. Our task was to adapt such a system to the severely retarded.

NATURE OF SKILLS TO BE TAUGHT

The necessary data functions in such an undertaking required a careful analysis of the specific classes of skills to be taught. (It should be pointed out that data systems, without careful consideration of how and what is to be taught, are no better than programs without data systems. The two must go hand in hand or the resultant information is without substance.) Premack's functional analysis of language (1970) and Skinner's (1957) *Verbal Behavior* suggested the key components to such an analysis. It was hypothesized (Carrier, 1973; 1974a) on the basis of Premack, Skinner, and a cross section of linguistics literature, that a child must learn certain classes of skills in order to master language:

1. Discrimination among environmental events, i.e., telling the difference between categorized entities in the environment such as "man," "woman," "baby," etc.
2. Discrimination among the symbols to be used to represent those events, i.e., telling the difference between various spoken words, manual signs, or geometric shapes.
3. Use of symbols to represent events, i.e., saying "boy" when shown a boy or selecting the square shape representing boy when shown a boy, etc.
4. Production of sequential responses, e.g., article-noun-verb, etc.
5. Discrimination among different sequences, e.g., "The boy can run" versus "Can the boy run?"
6. Discrimination among occasions calling for different sequences, e.g., events to be labeled such as "The boy is sitting" versus events calling for interrogatives such as "Is the boy sitting?"

7. Matching sequences appropriately to the occasions calling for different sequences.
8. Generalizing concepts appropriately, i.e., labeling all boys with the symbol for "boy," all girls with the symbol for "girl," etc.
9. Use of symbol functions as cues for the locus of the symbol in a sequence, i.e., nouns serve as subjects, objects, etc. and can occupy only certain spaces in each sequence or sentence. Verbs have other functions and occupy other spaces, as do prepositions, etc.

The child must be able to use all of these skills in combination. Each can to some extent be sorted from the others and treated separately in an appropriate experimental design, but the child must ultimately be able to combine all classes of skills in their complexity to produce actual communicative, symbolic responses.

PREPARING TRAINING PROGRAMS ON PAPER

With this list of skills in hand, the next major undertaking was to design proposed teaching strategies (training program on paper). This was done following some preliminary pilot work (Schmidt et al., 1971; Carrier, 1973; 1974a) and yielded a set of carefully sequenced trainer instructions that, after being tailored to data management needs, would be ready to be tested with children. It should be strongly emphasized that at this point the "program" was not a program except as it appeared on paper. Pilot data, indications from the literature, and professional experience suggested that the "paper program" was reasonably likely to evolve into a viable teaching tool, but there were as yet no substantive data reflecting the actual application of these training procedures. The collection and management of data had to be carefully undertaken if this compilation of ideas on paper was to become an actual training "program."

DETERMINING DATA SYSTEM'S NEEDS

Once the paper program was in hand, the development of appropriate data collection and management systems required consideration of three basic research issues:

Effectiveness of training procedures was the first and foremost consideration. Could children learn the skills to be taught, using these procedures? When could we conclude that a child had learned a class of skills? When could we conclude that a child was not learning the skills using these procedures? In essence, the issue of effectiveness asks whether or not a set of training procedures does indeed teach a child the target skills.

Efficiency is a second issue that must be faced by all professionals teaching children, and must be dealt with in the development of viable training programs. How long does it take to teach a child a particular skill? How many responses are required before training is completed? What is the error rate? The answers to these questions determine the ultimate dollar cost of training and, in reality, the feasibility of a program. An effective but inefficient program is not a viable program and therefore program development efforts must consider efficiency.

Replicability is a final issue that is also basic to program development. In the case of this set of programs, the initial data were collected in a carefully controlled research laboratory by a few well trained, heavily supervised trainers. What happens when clinicians in clinical settings or parents in homes use the same programs? This issue must also be clarified with data if a ''paper program'' is to become a viable teaching tool.

DETERMINING DATA SOURCES

The considerations listed above—effectiveness, efficiency, and replicability—were basic to the design of a data collection/management system. It was determined after careful study of these issues that the research effort would require a variety of data-producing parameters not necessarily critical to training per se.

Pretests were necessary for training programs in all skills if it was to be possible to determine the actual effects of training. Without a measure of pretraining to skill level it would be impossible to conclude that training had taught anything. The skill may otherwise be in the child's repertoire prior to intervention.

Post-tests, identical in substance to pretests, were necessary to draw conclusions about training effectiveness.

Probe tests were necessary in some phases of programming to determine when a child had learned a class of skills. In some of the proposed programs a class of skills was to be taught by sequentially teaching the child specific exemplars of that class. For example, in teaching a child to discriminate between symbols—circles, squares, triangles, etc.—a match-to-sample paradigm was employed. The child was taught to match (discriminate) two symbols, then a third was added, and so on. If the child could learn only by rote he would have to be trained on every symbol to be used, but if he could learn the concept of match-to-sample by shape he would eventually be able to match new shapes without prior training, i.e., to generalize the shape-matching concept. Thus, for the purpose of pinpointing the time at which a child accomplished such generalizations, the child would be taught two exemplars and then probed to determine his performance on other exemplars of the same class. If a child performed successfully in the probe test one could conclude that he had generalized the concept (matched-to-sample) and needed no further training on that class of skills.

Generalization tests were required in some cases in addition to the probe tests during training on a skill. These tests, like probe tests, were intended to sample the child's behavior in extending a class of specifically taught skills to other members of the same class. For example, one of the phases of programming was designed to teach 10 nounlike responses to 10 pictures representing different noun concepts: boy, girl, man, woman, baby, etc. Training included only one stimulus picture per noun, and was followed by a post-test using these same 10 pictures as stimuli. When a child had completed the post-test, indicating that he had indeed learned to label these 10 pictures with the appropriate symbols, a generalization test was administered using different pictures of the same nouns. If a child completed the generalization test without error it could be concluded that he now had a concept which could be extended beyond one exemplar. He had apparently learned characteristics of ''man,'' for example, that he could use to correctly label ''man'' in a variety of different stimulus sets. These data would support conclusions about whether this training was teaching concepts or only simple rote responses. Not only would such information assist in program development, it would also be helpful in determining specific child characteristics relevant to prognosis and subsequent programming.

Response-by-response data were required to determine skill acquisition patterns. These patterns would serve as the basis for pointing out criterion levels, program weaknesses, and child characteristics that had to be considered in program revisions.

The data system required, after the above considerations, data from pretests, training, probe tests, post-tests, and generalization tests. It was concluded that appropriate data from each of these sources, for each class of skills to be taught, would eventually yield appropriate information about effectiveness, efficiency, and replicability of training in each of the classes of skills deemed necessary to language development.

DETERMINING NATURE OF DATA

The specific data to be collected in each of the abovementioned phases (pretest, training, etc.) included 1) discrete records of every response emitted to every stimulus presented, 2)

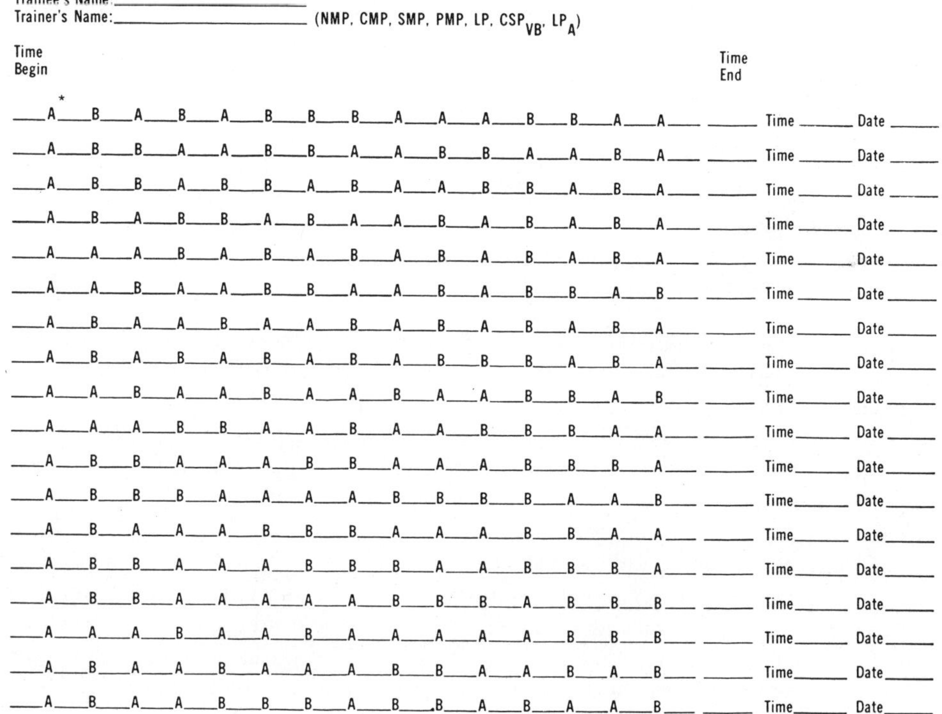

Trainee's Name: ____________
Trainer's Name: ____________ (NMP, CMP, SMP, PMP, LP, CSP_{VB}, LP_A)

Time Begin ... Time End

___A*___B___A___B___A___B___B___B___A___A___A___B___B___A___A___ ______ Time ______ Date ______
___A___B___B___A___A___B___B___A___A___B___B___A___A___B___A___ ______ Time ______ Date ______
___A___B___B___A___B___B___A___B___A___A___B___B___A___B___A___ ______ Time ______ Date ______
___A___B___A___B___B___A___B___A___A___B___A___B___A___B___A___ ______ Time ______ Date ______
___A___A___A___B___A___B___A___B___A___B___A___B___A___B___A___ ______ Time ______ Date ______
___A___A___B___A___A___B___B___A___A___B___A___B___B___A___B___ ______ Time ______ Date ______
___A___B___A___A___B___A___A___B___A___B___A___B___A___B___A___ ______ Time ______ Date ______
___A___B___A___B___A___B___A___B___A___B___B___B___A___B___A___ ______ Time ______ Date ______
___A___A___B___A___A___B___A___A___B___A___A___B___B___A___B___ ______ Time ______ Date ______
___A___A___A___B___B___A___A___B___A___A___B___B___B___A___A___ ______ Time ______ Date ______
___A___B___B___A___A___A___B___B___A___A___A___B___B___B___A___ ______ Time ______ Date ______
___A___B___B___B___A___A___A___A___B___B___B___B___A___A___B___ ______ Time ______ Date ______
___A___B___A___A___A___B___B___B___A___A___A___B___B___A___A___ ______ Time ______ Date ______
___A___B___B___A___A___A___B___B___B___A___A___B___B___B___A___ ______ Time ______ Date ______
___A___B___B___A___A___A___A___A___B___B___B___A___B___B___B___ ______ Time ______ Date ______
___A___A___A___B___A___A___B___A___A___A___A___A___B___B___B___ ______ Time ______ Date ______
___A___B___A___A___B___A___A___A___B___B___A___A___B___A___B___ ______ Time ______ Date ______
___A___B___A___A___B___B___B___A___B___B___A___B___A___A___B___ ______ Time ______ Date ______

*A and B designate the stimulus to be presented on that trial.

Figure 1. Single response record sheet.

Trainee's Name______________ Setting______________

Trainer's Name______________

Step	Begin Time	Stim.	Art_1	SN	VA	V	Prep	Art_2	OP	End Time	Trial	Elapsed Time
		A										
		B										
		A										
		B										
		A										
		B										
		B										
		B										
		A										
		A										
		A										
		B										
		B										
		A										
		A										
		B										
		B										
		A										

Figure 2. Chained response record sheet.

number of responses required for each step, 3) number of errors emitted during each step, 4) amount of elapsed training time required for each step, and 5) amount of time in each step during which stimuli were present. These times were recorded by beginning a clock at the presentation of each stimulus and stopping it when the response was completed. The total time on the clock could then be divided by number of responses to determine average response latency, or compared with total training time, to determine trainer speed and efficiency.

Three types of data recording sheets were designed. The single response record sheet (Figure 1) was used for recording responses in all tests and training where the task required the child to respond with only one symbol: a single word response or a match-to-sample task. The chained response record sheet (Figure 2) was used in tests and programs where sequential responses—word combinations or sentences—were required. The master record sheet (Figure 3) was used to summarize all data and to provide a readily accessible record of child progress.

A matrix outlining the major components of summarized data to be collected for each

Trainee's Name____________________ Trainer's Name____________________ Clinic Center________

Date Mo/Day/Yr	Program Step	Unprompted Responses	Errors	Percent Correct	Length of Session	Run Time*	Rate of Response**	Criterion Met	Comments

*Run time = time during which stimuli were available for child.
**Rate of response = run time divided by total responses (errors + unprompted).

Figure 3. Master record sheet.

Program Step	# Responses	# Errors	Training Time	Run Time
1. Pre-test				
2. Step 1 (training)				
3. Probe test				
4. Step 2 (training)				
5. Probe test				
6. Step 3 (training)				
7. Probe test				
8. Post-test				
9. Generalization test				

Figure 4. Matrix for summarized data.

phase of training is presented in Figure 4. Each phase of training received similar consideration in preparing appropriate data systems.

APPLICATION OF THE DATA SYSTEM

Determining Criterion Levels

After the actual administration of this set of paper programs had begun, one of the first major issues was to determine criterion levels. It was necessary, at each step in training, to establish some parameters of overt responding to determine that the child had completed that step of training. The commonly used procedure of intuitively assigning levels such as 9 or 10 or 39 or 40 responses correct was considered unacceptable since it was based on subjective researchers judgments rather than on child performance. Consequently, a simple statistical procedure for using child data as the basis for criterion levels was developed and tested.

The procedure to establish criterion levels was based on an assumption that every training task carries with it an inherent probability that a child will respond correctly. For example, if a two-choice task is presented to a child who has no previous knowledge of the skills required, the probabilities are 0.5 that the child will respond correctly. However, when sequential response data are tabulated it soon becomes obvious that the 0.5 probability does not mean that the child gets every other response correct. Rather, his data shows strings of correct responses, sometimes three or four responses in a row intermingled with similar strings of incorrect responses. He may get the first two trials correct, then miss one, have one correct, then miss three, averaging about 50% correct over a series of trials. If the correct responses are graphed they appear to fit a normal distribution curve. Thus, when the probability of a correct response is 0.5, a child is likely to have occasionally one, two, or three consecutive correct responses. He is less likely to have sequences of ten correct. It was hypothesized that it should be possible, using strings of correct responses as data, to determine statistical probabilities for response strings of various lengths, and to subsequently establish criterion levels that would in essence be statements of probability that a child had indeed learned a class of skills.

In this particular training the criterion levels were intended to indicate 100% correct responding and also to function as predictors that a child who performed at criterion on one day could return to the training environment within 24 hr and repeat the 100% correct performance. Thus, the initial data for determining criterion levels consisted of strings of consecutive correct responses through the following day in which a child made no errors. (The child was trained on a task until he had two consecutive sessions with no errors.) These data were collected for the first 10 children going through each program step; then all strings of consecutive correct responses before the last error, for all 10 children, were tabulated in a frequency distribution followed by calculation of the mean and standard deviation of strings, then the standard deviation was multiplied by 2.33 (the number of standard deviations between the mean and the 0.01 level of probability), and the product was added to the mean. The resulting number identified the length of a string of consecu-

	Procedure	Example
1.	Collect sequential response data until last error occurs.	√(correct), ×(incorrect) √√×√××√√√×√××√ ×√×√√√√×√×××√√ ×~~~
2.	Establish frequency distribution of strings of correct responses	# responses/string | frequency 1 | 卌 2 | 卌 卌 3 | 卌 卌 卌 4 | 卌 卌 5 | 卌 6 | 1
3.	Calculate Mean string length	a) $M = \frac{\text{Total correct responses}}{\text{Total strings}}$ b) $M = \frac{141}{46}$ c) $M = 3.07$
4.	Calculate Standard Deviation of strings	$SD = \sqrt{\frac{N\varepsilon X^2 - (\varepsilon X)^2}{NCN-1}} \rightarrow \frac{N\varepsilon X^2 - (\varepsilon X)^2}{N(CN-1)}$ SD = 1.24
5.	Multiply SD x 2.33 (fm .01 level of confidence)	DF x 2.33 = 2.89
6.	Add result in 5., above, to Mean	2.33 SD + M = 5.96
7.	Round result in 6., above, to next highest whole number. This is the criterion level.	6 consecutive correct responses.

Figure 5. Summary of procedures for calculating criterion levels.

tive correct responses that was likely to occur by chance no more than one in 100 times ($p = 0.01$). The procedures used for calculating criterion levels are summarized in Figure 5.

The criterion levels established from data of the first 10 subjects were then validated on subsequent children. Each child was trained until he could produce a string of consecutive correct responses as long as the calculated criterion level. Training was then stopped for the day, and the child was retested 23 to 24 hr later. The results showed that, in over 100 children tested, the criterion levels were accurate predictions of next day performance at a level very close to 99%. In other words, if a child met criterion on day I and was retested within 24 hr, the probabilities were at least 0.99 that he would score 100% correct on day II. The data showed deviations from the predicted results in less than one case per 100 tested.

The same procedures used to calculate criterion levels for skill acquisition were subsequently used to determine criterion levels for trainer/program failure. Strings of errors were treated in the same manner as strings of correct responses, and 0.10 probability levels were determined. These levels indicated points at which a child's performance deviated so far from the predicted that it was necessary to carefully examine his training and to determine procedural or child weaknesses that had to be compensated for if learning was to occur.

It should be made clear that these procedures are in no way restricted to application in this specific set of programs for language training. They are procedures that permit objective, statistical determination of criterion levels for any child, in any learning task where correct and incorrect responses can be sequentially recorded.

Furthermore, these procedures can be used for an individual child who spends considerable time on a training step. When sufficient strings of correct/incorrect responses have been recorded for one child, the correct strings can be tabulated, a mean and standard deviation calculated, and a criterion level determined for the child on that task.

It should also be mentioned that the same procedures for calculating criterion levels are applicable if more than 24-hr test/retest intervals are desired. Simply lengthen the test-retest intervals used in collecting the data on which calculations are based.

The most important aspect of this method of determining criterion levels is the assurance (provided to decisions) that a child has been taught the target behaviors. When such procedures are used and the teacher or researcher is asked, "How do you know that the child has learned the skill?" the response is simply " I do not *know* that he learned it, but I do know that the probabilities are at least 0.99 that he will emit 100% correct responding within 24 hr."

Use of Data to Revise Programs

Child data became the basis for all decisions about program revisions once the data for the "paper programs" became available. There is not space in this paper to begin to list all such revisions, but a few illustrative examples follow:

Revision of Noun Training Steps The paper program for teaching nouns was designed so that training began on one noun. The child had on the table in front of him two symbols, one representing "boy" and the other representing "horse." In the first step of training he was shown, on all trials, a stimulus picture of "boy" and was reinforced when he placed the symbol for "boy" on the response tray. When he met criterion for this behavior he received identical training for use of the symbol for "horse." He was shown the horse picture on every trial until he responded at criterion with the symbol for "horse." In the third step the stimulus pictures for "boy" and "horse" were presented in a random order so that on some trials the child would have to respond with the "horse" symbol and on others with the "boy" symbol. The data for the third step were rather surprising, as the error rate was at about the 50% level for nearly all children, indicating that responding was still at a chance level in spite of the first two steps. Subsequently, a group was run through the same training but with the first two steps omitted. These data were compared with the data of children who had gone through all three steps. It was discovered that children in both groups required approximately the same amount of training time and trials for step 3, and that steps 1 and 2 were needless expenditures of time. Those steps were eliminated from the final program. This example illustrates a case in which trainer intuition suggested a procedure that the data clearly indicated was inefficient.

Revision of a Pretest Procedure Some of the programs in this series are designed to do little more than teach a child to combine two or more behaviors that had previously been taught in isolation. The paper program procedures were designed so that the child was pretested on the skills to be taught and then, unless the pretest score was 100%, the child was placed directly into a rather extensive training program. However, many of the children made enough correct responses on the pretest that they were clearly not operating at a chance level. Therefore, a child's score on the pretest was evaluated before the child entered the actual training program. If he was responding above chance on the pretest, the pretest was rerun using reinforcement. If his score improved the test was run again, etc., until the child either failed to improve and was placed in the training program, or scored 100% and was able to move on to the next set of programs without having to go through that particular one. In one program revised in this manner, the mean training time from entry to completion of training was reduced from over 4 hr to 1 hr, 40 min. In another such program, training times were reduced from over 3 hr to only 45 min. This application of data resulted in a savings of over 4½ hr training time per child in these two programs alone.

Revision of Procedure for Teaching Chaining One of the paper programs was originally designed to teach a child to sequence eight symbols by color and number cues. A symbol with one red marker on its face was to go in the first slot of the horizontal response tray. A symbol with one orange marker was to go in the second slot, a green marker in the third slot, a dark blue marker in the fourth, a light blue marker in the fifth, a black marker in the sixth, two red markers in the seventh, and two orange markers in the eighth. This set of skills was taught by first teaching the child to fill the first slot, then the second slot, the third, and so on until he was correctly placing all eight symbols in their appropriate slots. This training was successful, but the data from the next phase of training in which this set of skills was combined with another set indicated an excessively high error rate in placing symbols in the last three slots of the tray. As a result, the sequencing program was revised to employ a backward chaining procedure in which the child was first taught to fill the last slot of the tray, then the last two slots, then the last three, etc. This procedure yielded data indicating that sequence training procedures required essentially the same amount of time regardless of the direction of the chaining. However, the data from the next program showed almost a total elimination of errors when the backward chaining procedure was used. This may have been because the child received extra practice on the last slots when the backward chaining procedure was used, and because the next program provided some support for appropriately filling the first slots. But in any case, error rates were almost totally eliminated and training effectiveness and efficiency were both markedly improved with the backward chaining procedure.

Revision of Number of Sequential Items to be Taught Data from the sequencing program discussed above yielded another interesting finding. Children averaged slightly over 4 hr to complete training on the eight-unit sequence, but nearly 2 of those 4 hr were spent on training of the eighth member. Since the program strategies did not absolutely require an eight-unit sequence, the sequence was reduced to seven units. The data from children run through these procedures yielded mean training times of 2 hr, 10 min, a savings of nearly 2 hr training time.

Revision of Stimuli Used The data indicating responses with specific symbols to specific stimulus pictures were invaluable in strengthening the training programs. It was soon discovered that children consistently made certain confused responses during training. They had unusual difficulty discriminating between two symbols in some cases, and between two pictures in others; the woman and boy pictures were particularly difficult. We tried to change training order and to manipulate other variables that might cause these specific failures, but the results remained consistent. Finally, the shapes of difficult symbols and the configurations of difficult pictures were changed, and the problems were eliminated. These revisions were of particular interest because the pictures and symbols had been very carefully selected prior to training, and the research staff had carefully selected shapes and pictures that were easily discriminated. The judgment of the research staff was obviously different from the children's, and only the data were an adequate indicator of appropriate stimuli for training.

Revisions of Specific Skills to be Taught The intent of this set of programs was to use the geometric symbols as a vehicle for teaching children the concepts and rules basic to language usage, and then to transfer these rules to a spoken response topography. The original paper program was designed to teach each of the skill classes listed earlier in this chapter. There were programs to teach declarative sentences, compound sentences, complex sentences, adjectives, adverbs, verb tense, plurality, and a variety of other linguistic functions. All of these aspects of language were taught to several children during the initial phases of the program development. However, as the focus of the research shifted from teaching nonspeech to transferring nonspeech language to spoken symbols, and a variety of speech training procedures were tested and studied, the data yielded another interesting finding. Children who were exposed to speech (see Carrier and Peak, 1975, for description of procedures) during nonspeech training did not require training on all of the varied linguistic structures before beginning to acquire and use speech. The data indicated that 73% of the children were using speech by the time they finished training on one sentence type. They were also acquiring new vocabulary and syntax outside of training, and had become viable candidates for more conventional speech and language training procedures. Of the remaining 27%, only one child failed to learn spoken responses and to qualify for speech and language training after training efforts were focused on spoken responses, and after completion of training on the first nonspeech sentence type. As a result of these findings it was possible to reduce the volume of the program by nearly 75% and to cut nonspeech training times by nearly half.

Use of Data to Determine Effectiveness

Program effectiveness was determined by the percentage of children who met predetermined criterion levels described earlier in this paper. During program development, a child's failure to meet criterion always resulted in program revisions. The end product program was effective with over 95% of the children with whom it had been used. This meant that over 95% of the children in this program reached a 100% correct level on each program step, and that 99% of those children emitted that same response the following day.

Early in the process of development the data indicated another weakness in the general program that greatly reduced the ultimate effectiveness. The criterion levels were reasonable assurances that the child would be able to perform at a 100% level if retested within 24 hr. However, in some programs retention for longer periods of time was desirable, but was not found to occur in all children. As a result, a subprogram was added to the series. The sole intent of the subprogram was to teach a child, by gradually increasing time intervals between retests, to retain the skills for longer periods of time. This subprogram increased retention over a 7-day interval from 56% of learned skills to 97%.

Use of Data to Determine Efficiency

Efficiency is always a relative variable, so the intent in studying the efficiency of this set of programs was essentially to establish a feasible efficiency level. This attempt became a minor problem as the efficiency data became available. The data indicated that the mean training time for children to progress through this set of programs—to go from nonverbal to the point of original seven-word spoken sentences—was slightly under 15 hr. Thus, overall efficiency was not as critical as were some of the efficiency-related revisions discussed earlier in this chapter.

Efficiency data, however, did serve a variety of other rather valuable functions. Comparisons between training times for skill classes taught one after another, but similar in nature, indicated that children learn similar skills at faster and faster rates as they progress through the training. The first two verbs take a mean training time of 100 min, the second takes 65 min, and the fifth takes a mean time of only 35 min. The first set of 10 nouns takes a mean time of 131 min, whereas the second set requires a mean time of 48 min. Such findings suggest that the child is not only learning the prescribed skills, but is also learning strategies for acquiring new language. He is learning to learn language.

The efficiency data have also been invaluable for others using the programs as indicators of the rate of progress to expect. They have become a functional component of the published program as they tell the trainer when to begin considering the possibility that training may not be going as it should, and that trouble-shooting should be considered.

Use of Data to Determine Replicability

The primary issue involved in studying replicability was to determine whether these programs, developed in the laboratory, would maintain both effectiveness and efficiency when used in clinics where conditions could not be so carefully controlled. The programs were given to clinicians in several centers for retarded children, and the data generated by these trainers were compared to the laboratory data. The clinical data, when viewed as a whole, were identical to the laboratory data. However, there were differences between some of the clinics; some progressed slower, and some faster. Study of this issue unveiled the fact that some of the children trained in clinics were slightly higher level than those serving as subjects in the laboratory, perhaps explaining the increased rate of skill acquisition. The children with slower acquisition rate were not markedly different from those in the laboratory work, but the data immediately showed that the trainers were deviating from the prescribed training procedures. Steps were skipped, criterion levels were not met, etc. The replicability data, in this case, suggested that additional care had to be taken in training the trainers.

SUMMARY

This paper presents some major steps involved in developing a data system as a basis for designing a set of language training programs. The procedures discussed here are not, for the most part, restricted in application to language programming, or to this specific set of programs. Rather, they are generally applicable to most program development efforts and are presented here primarily to illustrate their adaptability to language programming and research.

Although the strategies for designing and using a data system such as this one are not unique to this particular task, it should be made clear that task definition is extremely important if a data system is to be anywhere near maximally efficient. The system must meet the task requirements, and can do this in a comprehensive manner only if the task is carefully analyzed and considered as an integral part of the data system preparation.

It should be stressed that a data system can add tremendous power to a research endeavor of this type without requiring extensive statistical knowledge. In this case, much of the data management required little more than descriptive summaries, which in turn required little more than simple arithmetic. Most of the statistical tests employed used simple, normal curve statistics, and only a few cases called for other types of data treatment. The data management system discussed in this paper would not require any extensive knowledge of statistics per se.

REFERENCES

Carrier, J. K., Jr. 1973. Application of functional analysis and a non-speech response mode to teaching language. Parsons Research Center Report No. 7, February, Parsons, Kansas.

Carrier, J. K., Jr. 1974a. Application of functional analysis and a nonspeech response mode to teaching language. In: L. V. McReynolds (ed.), Developing Systematic Procedures for Training Children's Language. Asha Monogr. No. 18.

Carrier, J. K., Jr. 1974b. Nonspeech noun usage training with severely and profoundly retarded children. J. Speech Hear. Res. 17:510–517.

Carrier, J. K., Jr., LaCroix, Z., and Critcher, C. 1973. Use of nonspeech training to facilitate learning of spoken communication skills. Paper presented at the Spring Conference of the Oklahoma Speech and Hearing Association, April, Oklahoma City.

Carrier, J. K., Jr., and Peak, T. J. 1975. Non-SLIP (Non-speech Language Initiation Program. H & H Enterprises, Lawrence, Kansas.

Premack, D. 1970. A functional analysis of language. J. Exp. Anal. Behav. 14:107–125.

Premack, D. 1971. Language in chimpanzee? Science 172:808–822.

Schmidt, M. J., Carrier, J. K., Jr., and Parsons, S. 1971. Use of a non-speech mode for teaching language. Paper presented at convention of the American Speech and Hearing Association, Chicago.

Skinner, B. F. 1957. Verbal Behavior. Appleton-Century-Crofts, New York.

SUGGESTED READINGS

Bosley, S., and Carrier, J. K., Jr. 1973. Establishing linguistic behavior in severely retarded children. Paper presented at Region V, American Association on Mental Deficiency Convention, October, Wichita, Kansas.

Critcher, C., Carrier, J. K., Jr., and LaCroix, Z. 1973. Speech and language training using a non-speech response mode. Paper presented at the annual meeting of the American Speech & Hearing Association, October.

Glass, A., Gazzaniga, M., and Premack, D. 1973. Artificial language training in global aphasics. Neuropsychol. 11:95–103.

Hollis, J. H., and Carrier, J. K., Jr. 1974. Communication deficiencies from chimp to child. Educ. Considerations 1:6–11.

Huffman, L. L. 1973. An experimental analysis of the acquisition of *is* and *are* by deaf children using a non-speech symbol system. Unpublished doctoral dissertation, University of Kansas.

Kuntz, J. B. 1974. A nonvocal communication development program for severely retarded children. Unpublished doctoral dissertation, Kansas State University.

LaCroix, A., and Carrier, J. K., Jr. 1973. Clinical application of experimental language programs for severely and profoundly retarded children. Paper presented at the American Association on Mental Deficiency Convention, June, Atlanta.

Parsons, S., and Carrier, J. K., Jr. 1971. A proposed language program based on David Premack's program for Sarah, a chimpanzee. Paper presented at Spring Meeting of Oklahoma Speech and Hearing Association, April, Oklahoma City.

Peak, T. J., and Carrier, J. K., Jr. 1973. Establishing prelinguistic responses in severely retarded children. Paper presented at Region V, American Association on Mental Deficiency Convention, October, Wichita, Kansas.

Premack, A. J., and Premack, D. 1972. Teaching language to an ape. Sci. Am. 277:92–99.

Premack, D., and Schwartz, A. 1966. Preparations for discussing behaviorism with chimpanzee. In: F. Smith and G. A. Miller (eds.), The Genesis of Language. M.I.T. Press, Cambridge, Massachusetts.

1970. The education of Sarah. Time Mag., September 21:51–52.

1974. Teaching primates to speak. Phys. World, August, Vol. II, No. 8:50–57.

OBSERVATIONAL STUDIES OF GROUP PROCESSES

Introduction

Martha Perry

The two chapters of this section deal with the observation of social interactions of retarded and normally developing children. The approaches presented by Gottlieb and Porter et al. are quite different. Gottlieb (chapter 12) outlines a broad overview of conducting social adaptation research in an educational setting. His chapter emphasizes the importance of conceptualizing a framework for viewing social adaptation and filling in gaps in that framework before proceeding to detailed and sophisticated observational methodology. On the other hand, Porter et al. present in chapter 13 a study using such a methodology to describe and compare social preferences and interactions.

The overview presented by Gottlieb reviews both his own and others' research relating to the social adaptation of mentally retarded children in the schools. He points out a lack of such research and notes the unique properties of the schools as a social system necessitating separate conceptualizations. In the realm of social adaptation within schools several influences are considered important. First, the behaviors exhibited by the retarded children are crucial; but beyond that, those behaviors are reacted to by peers and teachers who themselves have unique characteristics, and all of these behaviors occur within a context or setting that varies. Gottlieb organized his research review to assess our knowledge about the influence of these various factors on social adaptation. The existing research focuses mostly on the role of a retarded child's observable behavior on social interaction. There seems to be a relative neglect of the role of peer group characteristics, teacher reactions, and setting influence. Gottlieb argues that because these various factors are so inextricably interrelated, a greater understanding of each should be sought before research moves toward more detailed observational methodology, research design sophistication, and expense.

The data-based chapter of Porter et al. presents an ethological study of social interaction of retarded and normally developing children in a free play setting. Its specific aims are descriptive, rather than designed to isolate the influence of conceptually developed factors as advocated by Gottlieb. In particular, the observations aimed at describing interpersonal distance, social performances, and interactions when both retarded and normally developing children were simultaneously present. His findings that nonretarded children interact most frequently with others like themselves rather than with retarded peers provides behavioral corroboration for some of the sociometric studies reviewed by Gottlieb.

These two chapters point out some differences in strategy in the study of social interactions. Both, of course, recognize and deal with the complexity of social interaction. One strategy, however, prefers to isolate and vary independently the elements that influence interaction before proceeding to naturalistic, observational studies of complex situations. The other strategy was the reverse; to observe and describe free and complex interactions, without the burden of detailed a priori expectations about specific behavior. The implications of these strategies recall the many historical and ongoing discussions of experimental (controlled) research compared to field (naturalistic) research. The resolution of issues relating to individual versus group data, the validity of data collected in experimental versus natural settings, data based on self-report or direct observation was no more clear-cut than usual. Another issue raised by Porter et al.'s observational study, the relative merits of live observation versus video recorded observation, is likewise not resolved. The issues highlighted by these two chapters are important and merit consideration so that we do not become so enamored with a single approach that we fail to consider the utility of multiple research approaches for understanding mental retardation. At the very least, we might benefit by keeping abreast of the work of others who approach social interaction phenomena from different directions.

chapter 12

Observing Social Adaptation in Schools

Jay Gottlieb

The present essay attempts to provide an organizing framework for studying educable mentally retarded (EMR) children's social adaptation in school. The need for such a framework is evidenced by the fact that investigations of EMR children's social adaptation have not reflected a unified conceptualization of the complex issues involved. Instead, researchers have produced a series of unrelated investigations on such topics as self-concept, attitudes, level of aspiration, curiosity-seeking behavior, paper-and-pencil indices of adjustment, and so forth. The diversity of these studies, coupled with the methodological inadequacies of many of them, has delayed both the theoretical development in this area and the practical applications that research might generate, and has resulted in a body of literature that defies meaningful generalization.

The need for a conceptual framework to study social adaptation is further mandated by the importance it has recently gained in decisions concerning the appropriate classification of children. The movement to avoid relying so heavily on traditional tests of intelligence has forced researchers and practitioners to search elsewhere for meaningful behavioral indications of mental retardation. Since adaptive behavior has long been included as an integral part of the definition of mental retardation (Grossman, 1973) it is not surprising that attention has turned toward it. However, there are difficulties in using the concept of adaptive behavior for school-related decisions. Unlike the intelligence test movement, which originally developed from the need to identify appropriate educational placements for slow-learning children, the study of adaptive behavior has not had its roots deeply embedded in the educational scene. Historically, adaptive behavior has focused on indices of self-help behavior, abilities that have greater relevance to institutional decision making than to public school programming. For example, the test of adaptive behavior sponsored by the American Association on Mental Deficiency was initially developed to assess skills of institutionalized retarded people, not skills of retarded children attending public schools. As a result of the historic emphasis on institution-relevant behavior, some recent attempts to apply information obtained from tests of adaptive behavior to educational decisions have actually contributed little to our understanding of appropriate educational practices for children classified as mentally retarded. This lack of contribution is not because the topic is inappropriate for inclusion in educationally relevant definitions of mental retardation, but because it is inappropriate to infer that tests designed to measure adaptive behavior in an institution, the home, or the community will provide information about behavior that is adaptive in school. Although there are obviously many elements of adaptive behavior that transcend a particular environment, the school social system is sufficiently unique to require its own configuration for what is and is not to be considered adaptive behavior. Until it is possible to catalog the elaborate nexus of behavior that comprises social adaptation in school, one is unlikely to employ the concept to its maximum advantage, such as in classification decisions or training practices.

This chapter is an attempt to begin this cataloging task. In the following sections are presented domains of behavior that could be included when considering social adaptation in school. Most of these behavioral domains are reviewed only briefly, with major attention paid to those domains that have received minimal attention in the literature on special education. Aspects of social adaptation that have been actively studied elsewhere are not emphasized here. The final section of the essay focuses on some general considerations for observing social adaptation processes in the classroom.

AN EDUCATIONAL PERSPECTIVE ON SOCIAL ADAPTATION

In the simplest sense, a child's social behavior is adaptive when he is able to interact successfully with other people in his educational environment. In other words, social adaptation refers to patterns of behavior that enable the retarded child to present himself to others in a positive light, and to achieve desired results from the encounter. This interpersonal orientation to the study of adaptive behavior in school is based on the assumption that the mentally retarded child's observable behavior is a primary determinant of successful adaptation. The mentally retarded child's observable repertoire of academic and nonacademic behavior attracts social consequences insofar as it influences the way he interacts with others, and the way others interact with him. The dynamic quality of interpersonal behavior that the retarded child exhibits signifies to others whether he is a person with whom they wish to interact, befriend, ignore, or reject. Put another way, the observable behavior of the EMR child is self-labeling: it labels him either as a competent, likable individual who is worthy of attention, or as an unworthy individual who is to be ignored or overtly rejected.

It is not sufficient to consider a mentally retarded child's behavior as socially adaptive solely on the basis of his own manifestations. Other participants in the social encounter must be considered when making such judgments, as must the social context in which the interaction occurs. A behavioral expression can be socially adaptive when directed toward one person but not another, and similarly, appropriate in one context but not another, even when directed toward the same individual. A simple illustration is the child who calls out to the teacher during a silent reading exercise and is greeted with a considerably different reaction than when he calls out during a free play period. Few would disagree that learning when to engage in certain behavior and when not to is itself a critical element of adaptive behavior.

It is because people react differently to similar behavior that they must be included as necessary to a retarded child's chances for successful social adaptation. Even if the EMR child's social behavior appears adaptive to a nonparticipant observer, it cannot be construed as adaptive if it is not interpreted as such by the people to whom it was directed. There are undoubtedly instances when a behavioral act is perceived as adaptive by one audience while simultaneously viewed otherwise by another audience, as when teacher and peers maintain different norms for acceptable behavior.

A mentally retarded child's behavior occurs in a variety of social environments, even within the relatively narrow range of environmental options imposed by the school organization. Depending on the particular structure and rules governing an individual school, retarded children may interact with nonretarded peers in regular classrooms, resource rooms, gymnasiums, lunchrooms, and corridors. Different behaviors are expected in different settings, and school personnel allow varying degrees of latitude for deviations from expected behavior in each: running may be acceptable in the gym, whispering in the corridors, and silence in the classroom. Each setting provides the mentally retarded child with a platform from which to display a different repertoire of behavior, one that is being scrutinized constantly by peers and teachers alike, who use it to form impressions of the retarded youngster. It is also likely that impressions formed by peers and teachers transfer somewhat across social settings so that impressions formed during class activities transfer to free play activities even though different skills are called for in each activity. The extent to which the mentally retarded child's behavioral repertoire is similar across situations and evokes similar responses from others across situations is currently an unanswered question.

The possibility that children can adapt differently to the many educational settings illustrates the complex, multidimensional nature of social adaptation. At least four sets of influences could shape the quality of EMR children's successful social adaptation in school: a) the retarded child's observable behavior, b) characteristics of the peer group, c) the observable reactions of the teacher who establishes and enforces norms of appropriate behavior for her class, and d) the social setting. To the extent that we examine singular and interactive effects of these influences, our knowledge of mentally retarded children's social adaptation in school will be greatly increased from its present state, in which we know that he is the victim of negative stereotypes and social rejection (Gottlieb, 1975a), but have only vague guesses as to why this is. A more detailed discussion of each set of influences follows.

BEHAVIOR AND CHARACTERISTICS OF THE MENTALLY RETARDED CHILD

Although there may be some general behavioral patterns common to many mentally retarded children, for the most part each EMR child is unique and behaves in idiosyncratic ways. The distinct stimulus cues that each child emits are constantly evaluated by others, who then use the information to form elaborate and durable portraits of him. The ease with which these portraits are constructed and the durability of their existence has been commented on by several authors, and has been experimentally validated (Kleck, Richardson, and Ronald, 1974).

Although there is a variety of ways to classify the general characteristics and behaviors of mentally retarded children that could affect the quality of their interpersonal performance, an elegant and useful framework was suggested by Richardson (1975) in his discussion of the ways mentally retarded people become identified. According to Richardson, people may be identified as mentally retarded on the basis of their behavior, appearance, or movement. His framework is employed in this discussion with a slight modification. From the present vantage, a retarded child's social participation in the everyday flow of events in his classroom is influenced by the quality of his *interactive behavior* and his *physical stimulus properties*. A few of the myriad ways that interactive behavior and physical appearance could affect the retarded pupil's social experiences are discussed below.

INTERACTIVE BEHAVIOR IN THE CLASSROOM

There is little doubt that the way one person behaves with another influences how he is perceived and reacted to by that other person (Gottlieb, 1975b). In question is which specific behavioral act, or series of acts, has the greatest impact on the ongoing flow of interaction. Surprisingly, very little research has been concerned with retarded children's overt behavioral interactions in the classroom. Most studies of EMR children's behavior have used rating scales to obtain measures of behavioral performance. In this way, two broad categories of retarded children's behavioral performance have been studied as they might influence other people's perceptions: low academic performance or general intellectual dysfunctioning (Dentler and Mackler, 1962) and perceived misbehavior (Gottlieb, 1975b, 1975c; Johnson, 1950).

It is immediately obvious, however, that general intellectual dysfunction or a general measure of misbehavior are very broad descriptors that lack the necessary specificity to describe particular overt acts that occur during a social encounter. The most effective way to understand the importance of cognitive dysfunction and misbehavior as contributors to social performance is to narrow the range of behaviors that are subsumed under each category and to identify the most salient individual acts that comprise the larger categories.

Overt Indices of Cognitive Dysfunction

It is superfluous to say that mentally retarded children exhibit poor cognitive performance. A more pressing concern is to describe observable patterns of cognitive dysfunction. Although there are many ways to organize a taxonomy of cognitive dysfunctions, for the present purposes it is useful to consider those aspects of behavior that are easily observed during a social encounter and are likely to be used by other participants to evaluate the desirability of the EMR individual. For the sake of simplicity, we consider retarded children's verbal and nonverbal communication skills as overt indices of cognitive dysfunction. This compact taxonomy is presented to illustrate the potential importance of these categories as influencers on retarded children's social adaptation in class. Although considerable research has been reported on verbal communication, such as language, very little research has dealt with the social consequences of language in the classroom or elsewhere.

Verbal Communication Skills One of the central axioms of social encounters is that people want to present themselves in the most favorable light possible. This is often achieved through their facility with verbal communication skills. People communicate for many reasons: to transmit information and feelings, and to evoke approving responses from others (Argyle, 1969). Unfortunately, mentally retarded people are deficient in verbal communication skills to the degree that poor interpersonal communication abilities are one of the defining characteristics of mental retardation (Grossman, 1973). Deficiencies in speech skills, such as in levels of complexity and articulation, as well as in comprehension skills, are clear signs that a person is functioning below an expected norm and is somehow "different" from other people.

Mentally retarded children's verbal communication abilities are deficient in a number of ways that could adversely affect their social encounters. They typically have higher incidences of speech pathologies than nonretarded children (Spradlin, 1963), make more grammatical errors (Carlton and Carlton, 1945), have a more limited vocabulary (Harrison, Budoff, and Greenberg, 1975) and generally have delayed language acquisition. Furthermore, retarded children have a variety of communication deficits involving the use of linguistic codes, and may not be aware that variants of these codes are employed in different social settings. For example, although it may be acceptable to use the vernacular when speaking to friends, it may not be with the teacher. To present himself as a competent individual worthy of acceptance, the retarded child may have to demonstrate that he is competent in the use of linguistic codes and that he is able to use codes appropriately in many social settings.

The retarded child's social interactions are likely to be affected not only by the quality of his verbal skills but also by the quantity of his verbal dialogue. Length of verbal communication has been found to be positively related to liking. Individuals who communicate more may also be liked more, and in turn, reciprocate the liking response to others (Berscheid and Walster, 1969), thereby completing a mutually rewarding encounter. On the other hand, individuals whose verbal exchanges are restricted in quantity or variety may contribute to a mutually disagreeable set of verbal interactions.

The point emphasized here is that a mentally retarded child's verbal facility has consequences beyond the role of verbal learning and concept formation skills. Verbal communication skills are likely to exert strong influence on the EMR pupil's social interaction with his peers and research is needed to increase our understanding of the dynamics of these influences. The impact of both the quality and the quantity of the retarded child's verbal dialogue requires clarification.

Nonverbal Communication Skills There are many ways other than verbal dialogue that people can present themselves to others. During social interaction between two or more people, a number of nonverbal signals occur in parallel with verbal cues, and taken together, represent the totality of the communication. It is conceivable, however, that nonverbal cues alone, especially inappropriate cues, are salient and communicate sufficient information for others to decide how much they value the retarded person.

There are a number of nonverbal interactive behaviors that both mentally retarded and normal children could exhibit that would be self-labeling when they are inappropriate.

For example, there are culturally prescribed, though not formally codified, rules governing the appropriate use of hand and facial gestures, bodily posture, interpersonal space, eye gazing, nonverbal aspects of speech such as intonation, speed, and so forth, as well as positive reinforcers such as nodding approval. Mehrabian (1971) demonstrated how variations in one participant's nonverbal behavior toward another influenced the latter's verbal and nonverbal behavior.

A number of questions arise when attempting to apply our knowledge of nonverbal aspects of behavior to mental retardation. One concerns whether the range and appropriateness of EMR children's nonverbal behavior is equivalent to their non-EMR peers'. Although very little research effort has been directed toward nonverbal aspects of EMR children's behavior and few definitive answers are available, the likelihood is that mentally retarded children are not so competent as their nonretarded peers at expressing or interpreting certain nonverbal affective behavior.

At issue is whether the mentally retarded child realizes the function that nonverbal behavior serves; that the nonverbal messages he emits are interpreted by others as true reflections of the way that he feels. People interpret a retarded child's frown as an indication that he is sad or angry, and his smile as an indication that he is happy. However, there is little evidence to the veridicality of the EMR child's nonverbal behavior and the message he wishes to communicate. If the retarded child's nonverbal expressions are not veridical with the intent of his communication his social interactions will undoubtedly suffer. As an example, the child who does not adopt an appropriate facial expression to indicate that he is sorry for his past infractions is likely to displease his teacher and exacerbate the situation.

Nonretarded children may make other assumptions regarding the behavior of an EMR pupil. For instance, frowning at the EMR child will communicate anger with him. Put another way, non-EMR peers may expect the retarded child to interpret properly the meaning they attach to their own (non-EMR) behavior. Again, there is little available evidence to indicate whether this assumption is correct. Research is necessary to indicate whether EMR children are aware of the reciprocal relationship involved between their own nonverbal behavior and reactions of others. If they are not aware it could explain in part why retarded children are thought to misbehave often. They may be considered as behavior problems because they violate expectations of the people with whom they interact. More will be said on the perceived misbehavior of retarded children as we consider the second global category of behavior that has appeared in the research literature.

Overt Indices of Misbehavior

The second major category of behavior that has been studied as it relates to the way mentally retarded children interact with others is the antisocial/aggressive behavior they are perceived to exhibit. Since the retarded child's social adaptation in school is likely to be influenced in large part by the extent of his social acceptance or lack of rejection, a child who misbehaves is not likely to be socially acceptable to his peers and consequently is not likely to adapt socially to the demands of the classroom group.

Various investigators have suggested that a retarded child's social functioning suffers because he misbehaves (Baldwin, 1958; Johnson, 1950). Although it is possible that mentally retarded children do engage in excesses of antisocial behavior, the studies by Johnson and Baldwin cannot legitimately be used as evidence that they do. The research paradigm employed by these investigators involved obtaining a sociometric ranking of retarded and nonretarded children, and sometime afterward asking the nonretarded respondents the reason for their sociometric choice. There are several limitations with this approach. The major difficulty is that the nonretarded respondents may have felt obligated to justify their sociometric rejection of the retarded children thereby maintaining that they engaged in antisocial behavior.

An illustration of the complex nature of relationships between perceived misbehavior and social status is evident in a study by Gottlieb (1975b). The study examined correlates of social acceptance and rejection of 324 EMR children who attended one of 152 schools. The results showed a significant correlation between teachers' and peers' ratings of EMR children's perceived misbehavior and the EMR children's social rejection scores, but no significant correlation between teachers' and peers' ratings and the children's social acceptance scores. Perceived cognitive ability was found to relate significantly to social acceptance. These data suggest that a) social acceptance and social rejection are not two ends of a single continuum but may represent two distinct continua, b) attempts to decrease retarded children's social rejection should concentrate on reducing their perceived misbehavior whereas attempts to increase the social acceptance of retarded children should concentrate on improving their perceived academic competence, and c) greater attention should be paid to the precise acts by retarded children that are perceived as misbehavior by their nonretarded peers. From this perspective some specificity can be gained by examining two categories of misbehavior: a) inappropriate or bizarre behavior and b) aggressive behavior directed toward another person. The relative contribution of each of the two categories may be worth examining as contributors to a retarded child's social rejection and implicitly to his failure to adapt to the social demands of his environment.

Inappropriate or Bizarre Behavior In the absence of an empirically validated set of behaviors that has been found to be perceived negatively by peers, it is difficult to develop such a set in the abstract. However, Bonney and Powell's (1953) data on differences in social behavior between sociometrically high and low children offer some clues. One primary behavior pattern that differentiated these two groups was "nonconforming behavior that is not directed against any one child" (p. 487). Included in this category of behavior were making noises, running across the room, falling on the floor, and reading or talking aloud. On the other hand, the behavioral category of bodily self-contact (nail biting, sucking fingers, twisting clothes) failed to differentiate between the two groups of children. The behaviors that did not differentiate sociometrically high and low accepted children were not so noticeable as the behavior that did discriminate between them. A general hypothesis that could be advanced from the data of Bonney and Powell is that the effect of inappropriate behavior on the evaluations of others is directly related to the obtrusiveness of the behavior, that is, making noise is more obtrusive than bodily self-contact. Behavior that is highly visible or audible and violates other people's standards for acceptability would therefore, have the greatest effect on the child's social status.

In 1975, a study was conducted that was not a direct test of the obtrusiveness hypothesis, but did examine the effect of a highly visible antisocial behavior on the attitudes of nonhandicapped peers (Gottlieb, 1975c). Two video tapes were developed showing a child playing with clay. On the first tape an actor displayed appropriate behavior, molding the clay while seated behind a school desk. On the second, the same actor displayed antisocial behavior, throwing the clay on the floor and stomping on it. Subjects viewed one of the two video tapes. Half the subjects who viewed the actor in each video tape were told that he was a mentally retarded boy in a special class, whereas the remaining half were told that the boy was in a fifth grade class. Thus, four treatments were established. Subjects could have viewed an actor who was depicted as a) normal and displaying appropriate behavior, b) normal and displaying inappropriate behavior, c) retarded and displaying appropriate behavior, or d) retarded and displaying inappropriate behavior. The results of the study indicated that the behavior displayed by the actor was the most significant determinant of attitudes toward him. The actor received less favorable attitudes when he displayed aggressive behavior than when he displayed appropriate behavior. He received the least favorable attitude scores when he was labeled mentally retarded and he engaged in inappropriate behavior. The study indicates that when a retarded child displays inappropriate, socially aggressive behavior that is highly obtrusive he is rejected by his peers. However, to reiterate, the experiment was not a direct test of the obtrusiveness hypothesis and it remains to be demonstrated whether a display of behavior that is either more or less obtrusive would result in a corresponding level of attitude favorability directed toward the transgressor.

Aggressive Behavior Directed Toward Another Person It is probably safe to assume that aggressive behavior directed toward another person is more threatening and probably more obtrusive than inappropriate behavior directed toward self or an object. Little research has been conducted regarding the extent to which mentally retarded children actually exhibit aggressive behavior toward their peers, although teachers and peers did report in one study that EMR children do manifest more misbehavior than normal children (Gottlieb, 1975b).

In a study involving direct observation of the ongoing behavior of retarded and nonretarded children, no significant differences emerged in the behavior displayed by retarded children in regular classes, low IQ children not identified as mentally retarded, or mentally typical children, although integrated EMR children engaged in significantly more prosocial behavior than segregated EMR children (Gampel, Gottlieb, and Harrison, 1974). In a parallel study, Gottlieb and Budoff (1973a) observed that exhibition of verbally expressive behavior correlated significantly with social status. That is, EMR children who were verbally aggressive were rejected more frequently than EMR children who were not, regardless of whether they were enrolled in segregated classes or regular grades. Significant relationships between physically aggressive behavior and social status were not found.

Although observations of ongoing behavior may provide a more valid picture of EMR children's behavior than can be obtained from retrospective judgments of their behavior, that method has its shortcomings. Observational data collection by nonparticipant observers typically occurs over a brief time frame, and the observer has little way of knowing the pattern of behavior displayed by the target child at times when he is not being observed. It is entirely conceivable that the EMR child could have engaged in a single instance of aggressive behavior sometime in the past and that his behavior was so salient that it tainted his reputation among his peers for a long time after the behavior actually occurred. Thus, attempts to relate ongoing observed behavior to other variables such as social status frequently result in considerable amounts of unexplained variance in the criterion. Greater predictive power in a criterion could probably be attained by a) experimentally manipulating variables that occur in the classroom, b) collecting introspective data that could be used to provide background information to interpret the observed behavior, and c) continuous monitoring of relevant behaviors over an extended period of time.

In summary, the available data suggest that teacher and peer perceptions of EMR children's misbehavior adversely affect the degree to which they are socially accepted. The assumption is being made here that lack of acceptance adversely affects the retarded child's social functioning in school. However, misbehavior alone is not likely to explain entirely the mentally retarded child's generally poor social adaptation, since the data indicate that he does not typically engage in more misbehavior than his nonhandicapped peers. The relative contribution of the retarded child's cognitive abilities and his behavioral manifestations to social adaptation remains unknown.

Physical Stimulus Properties

A considerable amount of research stresses the importance of physical appearance for social acceptance and interpersonal behavior. For example, physical appearance has been found to relate to interpersonal attraction among preschoolers (Dion, Berscheid, and Walster, 1972) and school age children (Cavior and Dokecki, 1973; Kleck, Richardson, and Ronald, 1974). Similarly, physical appearance has been found to influence interpersonal behavior. Kleck, Ono, and Hastorf (1966) found that individuals tended to be more emotionally aroused and terminated an encounter more abruptly when interacting with a physically stigmatized person than with a nonstigmatized person. Also, Kleck and Rubenstein (1975) reported that attractive people were more frequently engaged in direct eye contact, smiled at, and sought out for social interactions.

Most of the research relating appearance to interpersonal acceptance or behavior has been concerned with facial appearance. However, other physical appearance attributes, such as motor coordination, dress, and neatness may also have relevance for mentally retarded children's social adaptation to school. Malpass' (1963) review of the research on motor skills in mentally retarded people concluded that there is a low positive correlation between motor and mental ability scores; however, a relevant question is whether the severity of motor dysfunction is sufficiently visible to others that it impairs the social relationships of EMR children. It is therefore important to determine the incidence of visible motor impairment in a population of EMR school children. Both Richardson (1975) and Kleck (1975) have suggested that appearance factors affect the retarded individual's social functioning, primarily by influencing the ways others react to them. That suggestion is supported by recent laboratory results of Siperstein and Gottlieb (1977), who found that physical appearance affected subjects' ratings of a child. That is, a stigmatized child was rated less favorably than a nonstigmatized child when both performed identically on an academic task. From the perspective of EMR youngsters in school, however, where incidence of blatant physical stigmata is probably not as great as it is for more substantially retarded persons, the salient aspects of their appearance that are evaluated negatively by their peers or teachers must be identified. To date, few data are available on this topic.

As indicated earlier in the essay, the characteristics and behavior displayed by the retarded child are not the sole determinants of his social adaptation; the characteristics of the people with whom he interacts must also be considered.

CHARACTERISTICS OF THE PEER GROUP

Virtually all of the literature about EMR children's social functioning in school has been obtained from social ratings or from direct observations. Unquestionably, the majority of research has been of the social rating variety. The typical research paradigm in social rating studies has been to ask peers to state their preferences for each of their classmates. Two general limitations of this approach have precluded meaningful synthesis of this data base: the first stems from an absence of information regarding characteristics of the children who rate their EMR peers, the second involves the data collection procedures that have been employed throughout this literature.

Characteristics of Children Who Rate EMR Children

Sociometric and attitudinal studies of EMR children require respondents to express how much they like or dislike retarded children in general, or a specific retarded child. Often one knows little about the characteristics of children who rate their EMR peers. One does not know their sex, prior experience with retarded children, or other characteristics that might influence their responses. One's ignorance regarding the effects of rater characteristics on judgments of EMR children is especially obvious in attempts to intervene in order to improve the social acceptance of retarded children. Probably because of this ignorance these attempts have uniformly failed to achieve durable improvements in the social status of EMR children. For example, both Rucker and Vincenzo (1970) and Lilly (1971) implicitly assumed that an EMR child would become better accepted by his non-EMR peers if he and a normal child were paired together on a school-related task. If, for the sake of argument, the investigators unknowingly required EMR children to work together with non-EMR children who harbored an initial dislike for them, a likely outcome of the interaction would be for the non-EMR children to increase their dislike of the retarded pupils, perhaps as a means to justify their initial dislike. Thus, in the absence of information about characteristics of children who rate or interact with EMR pupils, one runs the risk of structuring an intervention that could have an opposite effect to the one anticipated.

Unfortunately, the meager amount of research that has examined the effects of rater characteristics on judgments of EMR children has resulted in equivocal findings. To illustrate, Gottlieb (1969) found that well adjusted children were more likely than poorly adjusted children to express favorable attitudes toward retarded peers. Gottlieb was unable, however, to replicate the finding in a subsequent investigation (Gottlieb, Cohen, and Goldstein, 1974), although the data were in the predicted direction. Other examples of the inconclusive nature of research findings regarding the effect of rater characteristics are the studies by Monroe and Howe (1971) and Bruininks, Rynders, and Gross (1974). Monroe and Howe found that middle class adolescents were more accepting of EMR individuals than lower class adolescents. Bruininks et al., on the other hand, found the opposite; inner city children were more accepting than suburban children of EMR pupils. Finally, some studies have reported that girls express more favorable attitudes than boys toward EMR children (Siperstein and Gottlieb, 1977), whereas other investigations have reported no significant differences between boys and girls in their ratings of EMR children (Willey and McCandless, 1973).

Individual Ratings Versus Group Consensus

Without exception, studies on EMR children's social status have required respondents to state their like or dislike for retarded children on an individual basis; that is, respondents were instructed to provide their own rating without reference to their neighbors'. This methodological approach to measurement of social choice is seriously limited. In the everyday classroom routine, one child's behavior toward another is seldom exhibited on a one-to-one basis without the approval or support of other class members. This is simply another way of stating that the classroom as a group exerts various pressures on individual members to behave in certain ways and exerts sanctions against those who violate established and accepted norms. The assumption that individual ratings of EMR pupils represent a valid measure of interpersonal feelings that are likely to translate into observable behavior must be seriously questioned in the face of considerable data indicating that the group per se could influence attraction patterns among individual members (Schmuck and Schmuck, 1975).

To determine whether individual attitudes toward retarded children are similar to attitudes that occur in groups, a study was conducted to examine the effects of forced consensus (Siperstein, Bak, and Gottlieb, 1977). The rationale of this investigation was that individual ratings of EMR children probably present an unrealistically favorable portrait partly because the non-EMR respondents do not wish to express socially undesirable opinions about retarded children. If the respondents were made aware that other children also feel negatively toward the retarded classmates, they might be less inclined to inhibit their negative feelings and would respond accordingly. The expectation that retarded children are less well accepted than the sociometric data generally indicate came from several sources. First, daily observations of EMR children in regular classes did not depict as favorable a picture as the research data reported; second, other data that were not collected with paper and pencil instruments indicated that EMR children are seldom selected as partners in game situations (Gottlieb and Davis, 1973).

Thus, our hypothesis was that group rating of an EMR pupil would be less favorable than individual ratings, but that no significant difference between group and individual ratings would emerge for the mentally typical child. The method used to test the hypothesis was similar to the one described previously to study the impact of aggressive behavior on attitudes (Gottlieb, 1975c). Respondents listened to one of two audio tapes and were shown a photograph that they were told was the boy they were listening to on the audio tape. In one tape the target actor was presented as a competent speller of average physical appearance. The second tape portrayed an incompetent speller who was shown in a photograph to be a physically stigmatized individual with Down's syndrome. After listening to the tape and viewing the photograph, subjects' attitudes were assessed three times; individually, in groups of four where the group had to reach consensus regarding their attitudes, and again individually. The results of the study confirmed the hypothesis. There was a significant decrement in attitude favorability from the initial rating to the consensus, but only for the subjects who viewed the incompetent, stigmatized actor. Subjects who viewed the competent, normally appearing actor did not change their attitudes as a function of group discussion. Interestingly, the drop in attitude favorability from the initial testing to the consensus testing was maintained during the postconsensus trial.

The results of the above investigation (Siperstein et al., 1977) illustrate the limitations of the sociometric and attitudinal data that have been obtained to assess social status of retarded children. The Siperstein et al. data suggest that the sociometric and attitudinal literature, which already indicates that mentally retarded children occupy an inferior position in the social hierarchy of their classroom peer group, has presented an overestimate of their true social position. Collective ratings of EMR children may be better indicators of ongoing classroom practices than individual ratings because the actions of a single individual toward a retarded child are observable by other children who often support ''scapegoating'' behavior toward the EMR child.

The investigation by Siperstein et al. indicates the need to examine the effect of group properties on attitudes toward retarded children that could affect their successful social adaptation. Although it is intuitively apparent that the retarded child is not likely to fit in well with every classroom group, we have only vague notions about the characteristics of classroom peer groups that will maximize the probability for successful integration. Group characteristics such as degree of cohesiveness, nature of established norms, communication patterns, and quality of peer leadership could all have an influential effect in determining whether a retarded child is likely to be an integral member of his classroom unit. Few studies have examined these issues, especially as they relate to the mainstreaming of EMR pupils in the regular grades.

It is suspected, although there is no evidence, that typical research findings on group structures of normal children may not apply when a mentally retarded child is enrolled in the group. For example, Schmuck and Schmuck (1975) review evidence regarding the beneficial effect of group cohesiveness on classroom productivity, depending on the group's norms. These authors define cohesiveness as the condition that exists when social choices are dispersed among all members of the class and are not concentrated among a few. They contend that the more clearly a classroom group defines its popular and unpopular members, the less cohesive it is likely to be and the less it will work as a functional unit. Since retarded children are known to be assigned to a clearly articulated, unpopular position in the group, does this imply that their presence reduces the cohesiveness of the group? As another example, is the EMR child likely to adapt socially to the cohesive classroom that has strongly ingrained norms against academic learning, as is often the case in inner city classes? If this is so, the benefits of successful social adaptation must be weighed against the likelihood that the child will not progress academically.

In short, it is time for educators to consider the characteristics of the classrooms into which they send retarded children to be mainstreamed. Although education administrators undoubtedly do employ some criteria when making these decisions, they have little empirical evidence on which to rely. A mentally retarded child's successful social adaptation is likely to be strongly influenced by his peers, but under what conditions? Until we gain some understanding and answers to this last question, we are unlikely to speak knowledgably about the EMR child's social adaptation in school settings.

THE CLASSROOM TEACHER AND SOCIAL ADAPTATION

EMR children's social adaptation is likely to be influenced not only by their peers but also by their teachers' reactions. The teacher, being the most influential member of the classroom group, is able to influence the retarded child's behavior directly through the many reinforcers and sanctions she controls, and is able to influence the retarded child's behavior indirectly by the controls she exerts over the peer group. For example, Flanders and Havumaki (1960) found that students consistently praised by their instructors had higher social status from peers than students who were not praised. In a study more directly related to EMR children, significant relationships between teacher and peer perceptions of EMR children's behavior were found, with teacher ratings explaining more variance in the social status criterion, even though the criteria were obtained from peer ratings (Gottlieb, 1975b).

The importance of teacher influence on the retarded child's social adaptation is beyond question. In greater doubt are teacher behaviors that convey attitudes to the children. Considerable research has been directed toward this issue, with the work of Good and Brophy (1972) and their associates among the more recent. The teacher expectancy phenomenon is not discussed in this section; instead a hypothesis is offered as to why teachers feel the way they do about having handicapped children in the classroom; that is, negatively (Shotel, Iano, and McGettigan, 1972).

If one begins with the general proposition that people need to feel competent (White, 1959), then a situation that threatens their sense of competence is likely to be viewed with alarm. Those who measure their own competence as teachers by the achievement gains posted by their students would be especially susceptible to having their sense of competence threatened by the presence of a retarded child—a child who not only learns at a very slow pace, but may be perceived as requiring so much of the teacher's time that he adversely affects the educational performance of other class members. The threat of being unable to teach a child may be especially worrisome at a time when it is fashionable to place the entire onus of poor academic performance on the teachers. Thus, the prediction could be advanced that teachers with a known history of successful teaching experience, and a more secure knowledge of their own competence, that is, those who perceive their teaching abilities as instrumental in improving children's academic performance, would be less adverse to the presence of a retarded child in their classroom. This prediction should be more likely to obtain for teachers who are apt to attribute the child's performance to their own abilities than to a variety of child attributes that are known to be associated with academic performance.

No studies have been conducted, to my knowledge, on the reasons why teachers harbor certain attitudes toward retarded children; however, as the previously cited data indicate, their attitudes do affect the child's social functioning in class.

THE ENVIRONMENTAL SETTING AND SOCIAL ADAPTATION

The effects of various environmental conditions on EMR children's school performance have received scant attention in the literature. It is a gross oversimplification to suggest that EMRs behave or are reacted to in a fixed way regardless of the environmental circumstances in which the interactions occur. The main thesis of Mercer's (1973) work is that children behave differently in different environments, that many children who display maladaptive behavior in school do not exhibit maladaptive behavior in the home or community. Mercer cogently argues that only children who display maladaptive behavior in all situational contexts should be classified as mentally retarded. Other data are also available which indicate that peer judgments of retarded children vary as a function of the situational context. Gottlieb (1971) reported that attitudes toward retarded children in class were less favorable than to retarded children at play. Gottlieb attributed these findings to the fact that mental retardation is defined in terms of academic incompetence and not athletic ineptness, and that differing attitudes reflect the retarded children's relative abilities in academics and athletics.

Environmental variations could affect the EMR child's social adaptation to school in a number of ways. One way of organizing these possible variations is to consider the nature of academic demand placed on the child as a contributing factor, and the degree of structure imposed by the environment as a second factor.

The Nature of the Academic Demand

At a time when Congress has legislated that all handicapped children be educated in the least restrictive environment (Public Law 92-142), the most important and difficult decisions to be made regard what and how to teach the child. When the smoke from sociopolitical issues of culture-fair testing and due process clears, teachers are left standing alone to choose and implement an *educational* program for their EMR charge.

Perhaps the most immediate decision to be made is what level of academic achievement should be expected of the retarded child in the regular class. The potential difficulty inherent in the decision stems from two sources. If the material is too difficult, the EMR pupil is likely to become frustrated and angry, and thus misbehave. On the other hand, if the EMR pupil is asked to perform at a level commensurate with his abilities, which can often be 3 to 4 years below the modal performance of his classmates, he may be embarrassed to participate in the academic work because his materials are too childish. This, too, can result in frustration, anger, and misbehavior. There is a possibility, then, that the retarded child in a regular class will become frustrated and angry and will misbehave regardless of the academic appropriateness or inappropriateness of his learning materials.

Given the rapidity with which mainstreaming programs have developed, how have schools coped with the problem of identifying the appropriate level of academic demand to place on their retarded pupils? Data from two large scale studies indicate that retarded children are being integrated primarily into low track regular classes where the majority of children read below grade level (Yoshida, MacMillan, and Meyers, 1976), and are integrated into classes which are overrepresented with children of their own racial group (Gottlieb, Agard, Kaufman, and Semmel, 1976).

There is currently little information available regarding the impact of variations in academic demand on retarded children's social performance. In his influential critique of special classes, one of Dunn's (1968) arguments was that retarded children could be maintained in regular classes because general education has developed a number of individualized curricula which would allow retarded children to work at their own appropriate level. Regardless of whether Dunn's assertion regarding the ability of regular educators to accommodate the academic needs of EMR children is correct, few would argue that retarded children in regular classes would benefit from academic instruction geared to their own ability level. However, when the abilities of a retarded child are seriously below those of his classmates the situation carries potential risk of adverse social consequences to the child, and someone must decide on the relative merits of academic appropriateness and social inappropriateness.

Degree of Structure Imposed by the School

Teachers vary considerably in the freedom they allow children to move about the classroom, talk to friends, do individual as opposed to group work, and so forth. These environmental variations could influence the retarded child's behavior and, in turn, the way he is perceived by others. To illustrate, in a classroom where the teacher imposes a rows-by-columns seating arrangement, enforces strict rules against movement and talking, and encourages individual seat work, the EMR child is likely to exhibit a more restricted range of behavior than in a classroom where the teacher allows great latitude in movement, talking, etc. If the child has freedom to display a wide range of behavior and the behavior violates the norms or expectations of his classmates, probability is increased that his social functioning will be adversely affected and social rejection is a possible consequence.

In a series of investigations, the proposed relationship of behavioral freedom and social rejection has been studied. In the first of these studies (Goodman, Gottlieb, and Harrison, 1972), the social acceptance of EMR children integrated in regular classes of a nongraded elementary school was compared with the social status of EMR children who remained segregated in the same school. The results indicated that nonretarded male judges rejected the integrated EMR children significantly more than the segregated children. No significant differences were obtained in females' judgments of the integrated and segregated EMR children. The finding that boys were significantly more rejecting of integrated than segregated EMR children was contrary to the initial prediction that the study was designed to test. The prediction that the integrated EMR children would be better accepted was based on the assumption that integration would promote greater contact between EMR and normal children, reduce the strangeness between the two groups, and result in more favorable attitudes toward the retarded. The fact that the initial prediction was not supported generated the second prediction that acceptance was contingent on EMR children's manifest behavior and EMR children would be least accepted under circumstances in which they have greatest opportunity to display a wide repertoire of behavior, which presumably would not conform to the levels expected by their non-retarded classmates.

The second prediction was tested in two schools that had the same academic curriculum but differed greatly in the physical structure of the school buildings (Gottlieb and Budoff, 1973b). One school was the traditional "egg-crate" school in which EMR children were enrolled in regular classrooms of about 25 to 30 children. The second school contained no interior walls, allowed substantial freedom for children to move and run about the entire school building, and enabled the EMR children's behavior to be witnessed by a substantial number of children in the school. The results supported the second prediction, that is, EMR children in the school without interior walls were rejected significantly more frequently than comparable EMR children who were enrolled in a traditional classroom structure that restricted their behavioral repertoire.

The second study was replicated in a more affluent community by Gottlieb, et al. (1974). In this study attitude rating scales were used rather than the sociometric techniques used in the previous studies. Again, the results indicated that EMR children were the recipients of least favorable attitudes when they were in educational environments where their behavior was most visible to their peers.

These results support the proposition that EMR children's social acceptance, and by extension their social adaptation, is inferior to their normal peers', especially in environmental circumstances where they are able to display a wide range of behavior that does not conform to the standards imposed by the peer group. Such data suggest that the social adaptation of the mainstreamed retarded child might be facilitated if he were alerted to the behavioral expectations of the children in his class and instructed in ways to adhere to these standards. This instruction should occur before the EMR child's placement in the regular class because, as it has been stated previously, children's first impressions of other children are durable and resistant to change. If the retarded child is seen by his classmates as unable to function socially at an acceptable level, he is unlikely to effect a proper social adaptation.

Although the physical structure of the school building itself imposes certain possibilities for behavior expression, environments can also vary in other ways. The teacher can structure the academic environment so that children work either individually, cooperatively, or competitively. Most frequently, teachers require children to work individually, usually by talking to the group as a whole. In fact, Adams' (1971) data indicate that regular class teachers spend approximately 68% of the time lecturing to the group as a whole. Similar findings were reported by Agard (1975) who studied instructional patterns in regular classes and observed that approximately 76% of the instructional activities in regular classes occurred in large groups. Agard's data were collected by naturalistic observations and indicate that most children, including retarded children, work individually, or at least not directly with their peers.

Whereas the major portion of EMR pupils' experiences in class occurs during individual work episodes, the available research data suggest that cooperative social and work arrangements are the most likely to have a positive effect on children. In his review of the literature, Slavin (1975) stated that cooperative reward structures have more positive effects on social outcomes than do either competitive or individual reward structures. However, Slavin also indicated that purely cooperative reward structures have not been shown to be superior to competitive or individual reward structures in producing gains in cognitive learning. The research cited by Slavin, however, was conducted on intellectually typical children, and it remains an open question whether similar findings would obtain for mentally retarded children.

There is some evidence that a variant of cooperative structure does promote academic gains among mentally retarded children. Jenkins, Mayhall, Peschka, and Jenkins (1974) reported that peer tutoring was more effective than teacher-led small groups in improving the academic performance of learning disabled and mentally retarded children. However, these investigators did not examine the effects of peer tutoring on the social adaptation of EMR children. Most research on peer tutoring has concentrated on academic outcomes to the exclusion of social outcomes. One of the more important research questions at present concerns the relative effects of cooperative and individual work arrangements on the social performance of EMR children.

If one is to understand the dynamics of social adaptation in school, some of the research questions that were raised in this essay, including the relative effects of cooperative and individual work arrangements on the social performance of EMR children, require answers. From the present perspective, the most effective way to investigate these questions is with observational procedures supplemented with interview or questionnaire data.

OBSERVING SOCIAL ADAPTATION

Historically, studies that have examined the nature of retarded children's social adaptation or social adjustment have relied heavily on paper and pencil indices of behavior. These questionnaires are economical to administer and provide easily scorable data. However, there are a number of difficulties in relying exclusively on paper and pencil questionnaires when drawing conclusions about social adaptation. First, information that is obtained from paper and pencil questionnaires to which the *retarded child* must respond are often of dubious value. Often, the retarded child has difficulty understanding the directions or the content of the questionnaire, regardless of the pains the investigator takes to minimize the complexity of the task. Second, *nonretarded peers,* who are not likely to have difficulty understanding the directions to the task, are often motivated not to respond as they truly feel. The social desirability bias, in which children respond with socially desirable answers rather than with their "real" feelings, was demonstrated in a recent study that dealt with attitudes toward mentally retarded and physically stigmatized children (Siperstein et al., 1977). Finally, *classroom teachers* also have a stake in providing a socially approved set of responses lest they appear incompetent or out of vogue in their educational philosophy.

These limitations do not imply that verbal questionnaire data are inappropriate or unlikely to be of value. Information obtained from interviews provides clues as to the degree of veridicality among indices of direct observation, perceptions of teachers and peers, or self-reports of the same event. Discrepancies among these indices alert us to probe for the causes of the lack of veridicality.

Not only do measures obtained by direct observation allow the investigator to determine the veridicality of these measures obtained from questionnaires, there are a number of other benefits provided by direct observation. Many of these advantages were cited by Brandt (1975). Expanding slightly on Brandt's discussion, the advantages of direct observations can be grouped into four categories: a) identification and measurement of dimensions of educational programs or processes, b) identification and measurement of student outcomes or products, c) identification of linkages between process and products, and d) identification and measurement of the frequency and intensity of variations in processes or products.

Identification and Measurement of the Educational Treatment

The dimensions of classroom processes concern the everyday events that occur in the classroom. From a research perspective, these dimensions define the educational treatment. In the past, research in special education has typically failed to specify the treatment with any degree of precision, mainly because investigators omitted observational data from their data collection options. The failure of research in special education to define educational treatments is not a new concern, having been voiced by Kirk (1964) in his critique of the "efficacy" research. Unfortunately, few attempts to correct this gap have appeared in the years since Kirk first voiced this concern.

The value of using observational indices of classroom processes to identify educational (research) treatments was nowhere more prominent than in the recent monograph on Follow Through classrooms (Stallings, 1975). The investigator was able to demonstrate how ongoing classroom processes, including teacher praise and teacher academic demands, contributed significant amounts of the variance in pupils' achievement. In fact, the author concluded that "observed classroom procedures contributed as much to the explanation of (achievement) test score differences as did the initial ability of children" (p. 104). In short, observational methods allow for the description and measurement of the educational treatment.

Identification of Outcome Measures

Educational research with mentally retarded children has traditionally placed considerable emphasis on social outcomes. In fact, as has been discussed previously, mental retardation is defined in terms of intellectual deficiency *and* deficiency in adaptive behavior, including social functioning. Since social adaptation is contingent on an individual's interactions with others it appears reasonable to suggest that measures of the adequacy of a retarded child's social adaptation should be based on the extent to which he demonstrates proficiency in his interpersonal dealings. The only way to determine the adequacy of these interpersonal competencies is to observe them. Reports of teachers, peers, or the retarded children themselves only provide estimates of how they perceive the overt behavior displayed by the retarded pupil, and the validity of the perceptions could ultimately be determined by comparing them to measures of direct observation.

Furthermore, direct observation is ideally suited to measuring variables that comprise the adaptation process, such as those raised in this chapter. To illustrate, recognition of facial affect, correct use of interpersonal space, providing verbal reinforcement to peers, etc. are best measured by observation rather than by questionnaires or oral interviews.

Process-Product Linkages

The catalogue of behavioral domains that comprise social adaptation in school requires a mechanism to study the causal effect of some behaviors on others. For example, it has been indicated that children's behavior in school is undoubtedly influenced by the reactions of peers. This implied that when a mentally retarded child exhibits certain behaviors, the reactions of his peers will influence his subsequent behavior. The sequential nature of classroom behaviors requires a vehicle that enables the researcher to study the effect of one behavioral expression on another.

Observational methods are ideally suited to such analyses, as Bakeman has indicated elsewhere in this volume. One virtue in this approach is that by examining independent and dependent variables that occur in temporal proximity to each other, the predictive power of the independent variables is likely to be increased. Previous classroom research in special education, and regular education as well, has typically explained only minimal amounts of variance in the criterion measure, mainly because the specific independent variable(s) that were supposed to influence the criterion were either unknown, not controlled, or so temporally removed from the criterion that their effects became diluted.

Variations in Processes and Outcome

One of the major values of direct observation, especially with regard to recently mainstreamed children, is that behavior can be measured continuously. Because different degrees of exposure to education treatments affect self-concept (Schurr, Towne, and Joiner, 1972) and social status, it is important to document not only the sequential but also the longitudinal changes in processes that might contribute to changes in pupils' outcomes. To date, no such documentation exists in the area of special education. All available research has treated pupils' outcomes as static one-shot measures (i.e., the outcome measures were collected most often at one point in time) or else data were collected on two or three occasions (e.g., Budoff and Gottlieb, 1976). Measures of direct observation enable continuous, repeated measurements of both process and outcome variables, and enable more precise examination of the effects of variations of processes or changes in outcomes.

Closely related to the issue of variations in process behavior is the concern with the frequency with which a behavior occurs. In direct observation procedures, such as time sampling, frequencies of behavior are aggregated across time segments within a behavioral category. This technique produces a summary score that may not accurately reflect the importance of behavior that occurs with low frequency, but could critically influence social adaptation. In other words, certain low frequency behavior may be so salient as to have a lingering effect on the perceptions and behaviors of others and in turn lead to poor social adaptation by the retarded child. Observational research could be designed to capture these critical low frequency behavioral events that occur naturally in the ongoing classroom.

Limitations of Observational Research

A major limitation of observational research is that the observer has little way of knowing the historical context in which ongoing behavior occurs. The cumulative history of experiences between two participants to an observed interaction undoubtedly influences the quality of that interaction. An initiatory response that seems neutral or positive to an observer may be interpreted very differently by the person to whom it was directed, depending on the past history of interactions between the interactors. As a result, observational data are time delimited, and may not correlate highly with behaviors that are not so time bound, such as sociometric ratings. This limitation of observation data is especially important when observing mentally retarded children (or any nonaccepted children), most of whom have known histories of unacceptable or inappropriate behavior. The behavior that a child exhibits during an observation period may be interpreted by the target in the context of the child's past behaviors in the same or similar situations. The failure to account for past experiences between the interactors may help to explain why the few studies that attempted to relate indices of observed behavior to social status (e.g., Gottman, Gonso, and Rasmussen, 1975) found only low positive relationships. That is, the apparently positive behaviors that are being observed are viewed by the target as suspect because of a known history of unpleasant interactions with the initiator, influencing the target child to respond accordingly.

Because of this limitation in the inferences that can be drawn from observational data, a useful strategy may be to supplement behavioral observations with interview-type data which would provide the researcher with some basis to interpret his observations. By questioning children about their prior experiences with a particular child, the observer can gain additional insights into the historical aspects of the relationship that he otherwise could not obtain.

SUMMARY AND CONCLUSIONS

In this essay, it was attempted to develop a framework from which to study EMR children's social adaptation in school. The factors that could affect social adaptation were discussed, including the retarded child's behavior and characteristics, the characteristics of the peer group, the influence of the classroom teachers with whom the child comes in contact, and the environmental context in which his interactions occur. The various elements that comprise the framework are presented in Figure 1.

Because variations occur in each element that comprises social adaptation, it is not an invariant phenomenon. It may not be unusual for a child to adapt to the demands of the academic environment one year but not the next. Similarly, a child may adapt socially to one classroom but not another, even during the same day.

Social adaptation as presented here is composed of many elements, and variations in each are to be expected. Also, the covariation of the elements seriously complicates

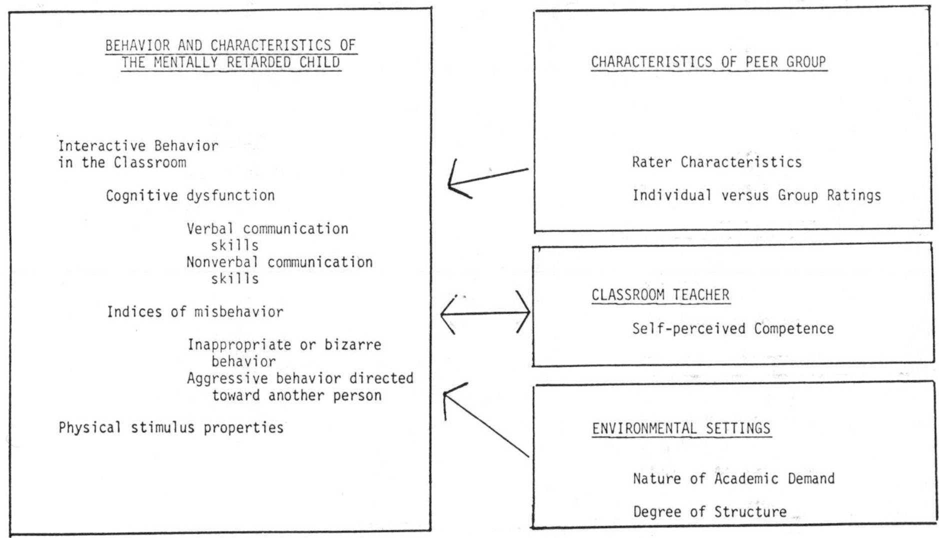

Figure 1. Domains of variables comprising social adaptation. Directions of arrows indicate directions of influence.

attempts to study social adaptation, and conclusions that a mentally retarded child is or is not adapting simply as a function of a single element are probably overly simplistic. There is little doubt that some elements of the catalogue presented here exert a reciprocal influence on the others. A meaningful statement vis-à-vis a retarded child's social adaptation would have to specify the circumstances in which he is or is not adapting, and give some indication why he is or is not. It seems highly unlikely that a single score obtained from a paper-and-pencil instrument will be able to capture the complexities of a child's social adaptation. The most profitable information regarding social adaptation is likely to be produced by detailed observations, by his peers and teachers, of the child during differing class activities.

The framework that was suggested here indicates the many areas where our knowledge of social adaptation is seriously limited. A number of researchable questions were raised, answers to which would substantially improve our knowledge of retarded children's behavior. Few studies have examined the impact of a retarded child's communication skills on the perceptions of his peers or teachers. What specific features of his verbal or nonverbal skills are reacted to negatively by the people with whom he interacts? Also, what are the relative contributions of cognitive and social deficits to the mentally retarded child's social adaptation? In one study, it was found that cognitive deficits affect the retarded child's social acceptance whereas social deficits affect his level of social rejection (Gottlieb, 1975b). What implications does this phenomenon have for training EMR children to render them more capable of successfully interacting with their peers? A related question is whether it is more debilitating to a child to be socially rejected by his peers or completely ignored. The traditional way of scoring sociometric instruments assigns a higher score, that is, a more favorable score, if the child is ignored than if he is rejected. Is this scoring system mirrored in its impact on the child? Is being rejected more debilitating than being ignored? Also, do EMR children display motoric problems that are so obvious that it affects their social adaptation? If so, what is the incidence of these problems and how do they interact with other attributes, such as verbal skills?

A host of unanswered questions revolve around the effects of peer group composition on the EMR pupil's social adaptation. Issues regarding cohesiveness, norms, peers' socioeconomic status relative to the EMR child's, and the extent to which his classmates were informed about his arrival into their class could all affect the EMR child's social adaptation.

Similarly, little information is available regarding the characteristics of classroom teachers that will maximize the probability of the child adapting to the social and academic demands of his class. The teacher's influence is so pervasive that she is capable of seriously affecting the social adaptation of all children, including those with histories of successful prior experiences in school. How much more important is she to the retarded child whose history has been filled with negative school experiences? What interpersonal sensitivities must the regular class teacher possess to facilitate the social adaptation of the EMR child?

Furthermore, research evidence suggests that different environmental structures could affect children's social performance. Unfortunately, there is a long distance between the experimental laboratory and the classroom. Although cooperative work structures seem to improve children's social performance, other data indicate that the vast majority of teachers still use large group lectures to convey information. The many possible varieties of group instruction that can be implemented in the classroom to improve the social performance of all children are seldom used. Such data make one wonder about the daily educational programs to which mainstreamed children are being subjected.

The final point concerns the need to validate the set of behaviors presented here, or any set of behaviors that are thought to be important for mentally retarded children's behavioral repertiore. All too often a researcher studies particular behaviors with too little rationale. One of the main needs at present is to validate behaviors that are selected for study. There are a number of ways to validate behaviors, such as relating them to sociometric status scores, determining that teachers believe them to be important for children's success in class, or observing the overt responses that the target person displays as a result of behavior exhibited by the initiator. To illustrate this last method, the behaviors that a mentally retarded child exhibits would be validated by observing whether there is a systematic pattern of responses displayed by teachers or peers that directly (or indirectly) follow the expression of a particular behavior. We will be in a position to improve the social adaptation of mentally retarded children only when we know which of their behaviors are responsible for poor levels of adaptation.

ACKNOWLEDGMENTS

The comments of a number of colleagues greatly improved this manuscript. These include Drs. Louise Corman, Samuel L. Guskin, James L. Hamilton, Donald L. MacMillan, Nancy Safer, Gary N. Siperstein, and Roland K. Yoshida. Any faults rest solely with the author.

REFERENCES

Adams, R. S. 1971. A sociological approach to classroom research. In: I. Westbury and A. A. Bellack (eds.), Research into Classroom Processes: Recent Developments and Next Steps. Teachers College Bureau of Publications, Columbia University, New York.

Agard, J. A. 1975. The classroom ecological structure: an approach to the specification of the treatment problem. Paper presented at annual meeting of the American Educational Research Association, Washington, D.C.

Argyle, M. 1969. Social Interaction. Methuen & Co. Ltd., London.

Baldwin, W. K. 1958. The social position of the educable mentally retarded child in the regular grades in the public schools. Except. Child. 25:106–108, 112.

Berscheid, E., and Walster, E. 1969. Interpersonal Attraction. Addison-Wesley Publishing Company Inc., Reading, Massachusetts.

Bonney, M. E., and Powell, J. 1953. Differences in social behavior between sociometrically high and sociometrically low children. J. Educ. Res. 46:481–496.

Brandt, R. M. 1975. An historical overview of systematic approaches to observation in school settings. In: R. A. Weinberg and F. H. Wood (eds.), Observation of Pupils and Teachers in Mainstream and Special Education Settings. Leadership Training Institution/Special Education, University of Minnesota, Minneapolis.

Bruininks, R. H., Rynders, J. E., and Gross, J. C. 1974. Social acceptance of mildly retarded pupils in resource rooms and regular classes. Am. J. Ment. Defic. 78:377–383.

Budoff, M., and Gottlieb, J. 1976. Special class EMR children mainstreamed: a study of an aptitude (learning potential) × treatment interaction. Am. J. Ment. Defic. 81:1–11.

Carlton, T., and Carlton, L. E. 1945. Oral English errors of normal children and of mental defectives. Elementary School J. 45:340–348.

Cavior, N., and Dokecki, P. R. 1973. Physical attractiveness, perceived attitude similarity, and academic achievement as contributers to interpersonal attraction among adolescents. Dev. Psychol. 9:44–54.

Dentler, R. A., and Mackler, B. 1962. Ability and sociometric status among normal and retarded children: a review of the literature. Psychol. Bull. 59:273–283.

Dion, K., Berscheid, E., and Walster, E. 1972. What is beautiful is good. J. Pers. Soc. Psychol. 24:285–290.

Dunn, L. M. 1968. Special education for the mildly retarded—is much of it justifiable? Except. Child. 34:5–22.

Flanders, N., and Havumaki, S. 1960. The effect of teacher-pupil contacts involving praise on the sociometric choices of students. J. Educ. Psychol. 51:65–68.

Gampel, D. H., Gottlieb, J., and Harrison, R. H. 1974. A comparison of the classroom behaviors of special class EMR, integrated EMR, low IQ, and nonretarded children. Am. J. Ment. Defic. 79:16–21.

Good, T., and Brophy, J. 1972. Behavioral expression of teacher attitudes. J. Educ. Psychol. 63:617–624.

Goodman, H., Gottlieb, J., and Harrison, R. H. 1972. Social acceptance of EMR's integrated into a nongraded elementary school. Am. J. Ment. Defic. 76:412–417.

Gottlieb, J. 1969. Attitudes toward retarded children: effects of evaluator's psychological adjustment and age. Scand. J. Educ. Res. 13:170–182.

Gottlieb, J. 1971. Attitudes of Norwegian children toward the retarded in relation to sex and situation context. Am. J. Ment. Defic. 75:635–639.

Gottlieb, J. 1975a. Public, peer, and professional attitudes toward mentally retarded persons. In: M. J. Begab and S. A. Richardson (eds.), The Mentally Retarded and Society: A Social Science Perspective. University Park Press, Baltimore.

Gottlieb, J. 1975b. Predictors of social status among mainstreamed mentally retarded pupils. Paper presented at the meeting of the American Association on Mental Deficiency, Portland, Oregon.

Gottlieb, J. 1975c. Attitudes toward retarded children: Effects of labeling and behavioral aggressiveness. J. Educ. Psychol. 67:581–585.

Gottlieb, J., Agard, J. A., Kaufman, M. J., and Semmel, M. I. 1976. Retarded children mainstreamed: practices as they affect minority group children. In: R. L. Jones (ed.), Mainstreaming and the Minority Child. Leadership Training Institute/Special Education, University of Minnesota, Minneapolis.

Gottlieb, J., and Baker, J. L. 1975. The relationship between amount of integration and the sociometric status of retarded children. Paper presented at the annual meeting of the American Education Research Association, New York.

Gottlieb, J., and Budoff, M. 1973a. Classroom behavior and social status. Unpublished manuscript. differing in architecture. Am. J. Ment. Defic. 78:15–19.

Gottlieb, J., Cohen, L., and Goldstein, L. 1974. Social contact and personal adjustment as variables relating to attitudes toward EMR children. Train. School Bull. 71:9–16.

Gottlieb, J., and Davis, J. E. 1973. Social acceptance of EMRs during overt behavioral interaction. Am. J. Ment. Defic. 78:141–143.

Gottman, J., Gonso, J., and Rasmussen, R. 1975. Social interaction, social competence, and friendship in children. Child Dev. 46:709–718.

Grossman, H. J. (ed.). 1973. Manual on Terminology and Classification in Mental Retardation. American Association on Mental Deficiency,

Harrison, R. H., Budoff, M., and Greenberg, G. 1975. Differences between EMR and nonretarded children in fluency and quality of verbal associations. Am. J. Ment. Defic. 79:583–591.

Jenkins, J. R., Mayhall, W. F., Peschka, C. M., and Jenkins, L. M. 1974. Comparing small group and tutorial instruction in resource rooms. Except. Child 40:245–250.

Johnson, G. O. 1950. A study of the social position of mentally handicapped children in the regular grades. Am. J. Ment. Defic. 55:60–89.

Kirk, S. A. 1964. Research in education. In: H. A. Stevens and R. Heber (eds.), Mental Retardation. University of Chicago Press, Chicago.

Kleck, R. 1975. Issues in social effectiveness. In: M. J. Begab and S. A. Richardson (eds.), The Mentally Retarded and Society: A Social Science Perspective. University Park Press, Baltimore.

Kleck, R., Ono, H., and Hastorf, A. H. 1966. The effects of physical deviance upon face-to-face interaction. Hum. Rel. 19:425–436.

Kleck, R., Richardson, S. A., and Ronald, L. 1974. Physical appearance cues and interpersonal attraction in children. Child Dev. 45:305–310.

Kleck, R., and Rubenstein, C. 1975. Physical attractiveness, perceived attitude similarity, and attraction in an opposite-sex encounter. J. Person. Soc. Psychol. 31:107–114.

Lilly, M. S. 1971. Improving social acceptance of low sociometric status, low achieving students. Except. Child. 37:341–348.

Malpass, L. F. 1963. Motor skills in mental deficiency. In: N. R. Ellis (ed.), Handbook of Mental Deficiency. McGraw-Hill Book Company, New York.

Mehrabian, A. 1971. Verbal and nonverbal interaction of strangers in a waiting situation. J. Exp. Res. Person. 5:127–138.

Mercer, J. R. 1973. Labeling the Mentally Retarded. University of California Press, Los Angeles.

Monroe, J. D., and Howe, C. E. 1971. The effects of integration and social class on the acceptance of retarded adolescents. Educ. Train. Ment. Retarded 6:20–24.

Richardson, S. A. 1975. Reaction to mental subnormality. In: M. J. Begab and S. A. Richardson (eds.), The Mentally Retarded and Society: A Social Science Perspective. University Park Press, Baltimore.

Rucker, C. N., and Vincenzo, F. M. 1970. Maintaining social acceptance gains made by mentally retarded children. Except. Child. 36:679–680.

Schmuck, R. A., and Schmuck, P. A. 1975. Group Processes in the Classroom. Wm. C. Brown Co., Dubuque.

Schurr, K. T., Towne, R. C., and Joiner, L. M. 1972. Trends in self-concept of ability over 2 years of special class placement. J. Spec. Educ. 6:161–165.

Shotel, J. R., Iano, R. P., and McGettigan, J. F. 1972. Teacher attitudes associated with the integration of handicapped children. Except Child. 38:677–683.

Siperstein, G. N., Bak, J. J., and Gottlieb, J. 1977. Effects of group discussion on children's attitudes toward handicapped peers. J. Educ. Res. 70:131–134.

Siperstein, G. N., and Gottlieb, J. 1977. Physical appearance and academic performance as factors affecting children's attitudes toward handicapped peers. Am. J. Ment. Defic. 81:455–462.

Slavin, R. E. 1975. Teams-games-tournaments: a student team approach to teaching adolescents with special emotional and behavior needs. Unpublished manuscript, Johns Hopkins University.

Spradlin, J. E. 1963. Language and communication of mental defectives. In: N. R. Ellis (ed.), Handbook of Mental Deficiency. McGraw-Hill Book Company, New York.

Stallings, J. 1975. Implementation and child effects of teaching practices in follow through classrooms. Monogr. Soc. Res. Child Dev. 40, Serial No. 163.

White, R. W. 1959. Motivation reconsidered: the concept of competence. Psychol. Rev. 66:297–333.

Willey, N. R., and McCandless, B. R. 1973. Social stereotypes for normal educable mentally retarded, and orthopedically handicapped children. J. Spec. Educ. 7:283–288.

Yoshida, R. K., MacMillan, D. L., and Meyers, C. E. 1976. The decertification of minority group EMR students in California: its historical background and an assessment of student achievement and adjustment. In: R. L. Jones (ed.), Mainstreaming and the Minority Child. Leadership Training Institute/Special Education, University of Minnesota, Minneapolis.

chapter 13

Social Interactions in Heterogeneous Groups of Retarded and Normally Developing Children: An Observational Study

Richard H. Porter, Barbara Ramsey, Ann Tremblay, Maria Iaccobo, and Susan Crawley

The social behavior of retarded and normally developing children was observed and recorded in a free play situation in which members of both groups were simultaneously present. The normally developing children were found to maintain the closest mean proximity to another normally developing child, and to engage in several categories of social behavior with other normally developing children significantly more often than with retarded children. The retarded children, on the other hand, displayed no consistent preferences for retarded versus normally developing peers as measured by either mean proximity or frequency of social interactions. Few differences were found between the two subpopulations of children on mean frequencies of occurrence of the various categories of social behavior.

Most sexually reproducing species with internal fertilization require at least temporary social contact, and all mammalian infants are dependent upon maternal care for some time postnatally, so that these species could not survive without some form of species-specific social behavior. It is therefore not surprising that social behavior has been a favorite area of ethological research. The question of space utilization is closely interrelated with that of social behavior since the manner in which a species exploits its physical environment is often a function of its social organization, which itself is greatly influenced by ecological factors (cf. Crook, 1970; Wilson, 1975).

This research was supported by Grants HD-00973, HD-07054, and HD-00043 from the National Institute of Child Health and Human Development, and by Biomedical Sciences Support Grant FR-RR07087 from the General Support Branch, Division of Research Resources, Bureau of Health Professions, Education, and Manpower Training, National Institutes of Health.

In the study reported here, an ethological approach was adopted in an attempt to ascertain gross similarities or differences in the social behavior of retarded versus normally developing children when observed in a free play situation in which members of both groups were simultaneously present. Since social behavior plays such a critical role in human development, the effect of retardation on social interaction constitutes an important area of inquiry. With the recent interest in "normalization" (Wolfensburger, 1972), the natural habitat of retarded children is no longer necessarily a segregated institution. In many communities, normal children and adults are an integral part of the retarded child's environment. An ethological description of the social behavior of retarded children in the context of an environment including normal children is therefore in order. Accordingly, the specific aims of the project were twofold: 1) to describe and compare interpersonal distance in the retarded and nonretarded children; and 2) to describe and compare the social preferences and interactions of the two subpopulations.

INTERPERSONAL DISTANCE

Consistent patterns of spatial distribution by conspecifics have now been reported within a number of species (see review by Wilson, 1975). In his seminal work on spacing behavior, Hediger (1950) pointed out that members of many noncontact species tend to maintain a relatively fixed distance between one another, i.e., a species-typical "individual distance." Extensive data supporting a similar type of spacing behavior in human adults have been reported in studies of proxemics (Hall, 1966) and personal space (Sommer, 1969). Observations of spacing behavior in children have focused primarily upon interindividual spacing by dyads. King (1966) reported that the approach distance for pairs of children was affected by the proportion of "unfriendly" social interactions previously directed toward each other in an earlier free play session. Related research (Baxter, 1970) indicated that the interindividual spacing of pairs of 5 to 10-year-olds varied according to ethnic membership, sex, and indoor or outdoor setting.

Recently, investigators have begun to examine interpersonal spacing in established groups of children. McGrew (1975) applied the "nearest neighbor" technique to the dispersion of 20 preschool children in a classroom. The results indicated that pairs of children in closest proximity to one another tended to be of similar sex and age. No significant relationships between pairings and socioeconomic status, IQ, birth order, number of siblings, height, weight, or amount of nursery school experience were discovered. In investigating the social structure of an established preschool group, however, Hudson, McGrew, and McGrew (1970) found that sex and length of time in the nursery school were the most important factors influencing the social spacing behavior of the children.

Since recent research has emphasized the importance of territoriality among institutionalized severely retarded boys (Paluck and Esser, 1971a, b; Paluck, 1971), it was deemed worthwhile to investigate space utilization by retarded children (compared with normally developing children) outside of an institutional setting. Such basic knowledge might allow for the facilitation of social interactions within such groups, and thereby indirectly influence the effectiveness of various intervention programs.

SOCIAL PREFERENCES AND INTERACTIONS

Pratt and Sackett (1967) have reported that monkeys reared in total isolation, partial isolation, or peer groups subsequently preferred like-raised conspecifics in social preference tests. It was concluded that the preference for like-raised agemates may have been, at least partially, a function of an avoidance of monkeys from conditions other than the subjects' own because the animals could not interpret the "cues contained in the social behavior and countenance of the other two types of monkeys." These results from studies of nonhuman primates raise the question of whether children who are likely to differ in their abilities to interpret social cues and situations (i.e., retarded versus normally developing children) will actually interact with one another when placed in heterogeneous groups, or whether the children will interact only with similar peers. Of further interest, if the children of each subpopulation do engage in social interactions (regardless of social preferences), do the forms or frequencies of social behavior differ as a function of whether the children in question are retarded or nonretarded?

As for several recent ethological studies of human behavior, the theoretical concepts and specific research questions for the present study were adopted from the animal behavior literature. Thus, although one cannot indiscriminately generalize from data based on nonhuman species when attempting to understand human behavior, such data may serve as a basis for investigating whether similar or analogous phenomena do exist in humans. Furthermore, observational methodology and statistical techniques developed by animal behaviorists can be applied across species including *Homo sapiens*. It is therefore not surprising that several of the leaders of the embryonic science of "human ethology" began their research careers by studying the behavior of nonhuman species (e.g., Blurton-Jones, 1972a; Tinbergen and Tinbergen, 1972; Eibl-Eibesfeldt, 1975).

METHODS

Subjects

The subjects were 27 children 18 to 64 months old, from the Infant, Toddler, and Preschool Research and Intervention Project of the John F. Kennedy Center for Research on Education and Human Development. Twelve of these children (five females and seven males) were identified as *retarded* (mean IQ = 55) on the basis of developmental assessments (i.e., Bayley Scales, Denver Developmental Scale), psychometric tests (Stanford Binet), and various behavioral criteria (cf. Bricker and Bricker, 1971), and the remaining 15 children (10 males and five females) were project children characterized as *normally developing* (based upon these same measuring instruments), with a mean IQ of 106. The children were assigned to six groups of four children each, and one group containing three children. Each group was a heterogeneous mixture of retarded and normally developing children, with at least one child from each of these two subpopulations present in each. Within a given quad (or triad), the retarded and nonretarded children were age matched as closely as possible (mean chronological age = 46 months for the retarded and 36 months for the nonretarded children).

Procedure

On Monday to Thursday of each week, each group was removed separately from the classroom and placed in a small observation room for a 30-min session. The original purpose of these ''miniclasses'' was to enable practicum students in child development to observe and interact with small groups of children. During the first 5 min (or, in 16 instances, the first 10 min) of these 30-min sessions, the children were allowed to play freely with minimal intervention on the part of the single practicum student also present in the room. It was during these free play sessions that data were collected for the present study. In this manner, 105 free play sessions were observed and recorded, with the number of observation sessions per group ranging from 12 to 18.

The playroom measured 12 × 16 feet (see Figure 1 for floor plan). One-way mirrors along one of the long walls gave a complete view of this room from an adjacent observation booth. To facilitate an assessment of interindividual proximity, the floor of the room was marked off into a checkerboard grid pattern (2 feet on each side) by two series of parallel tape strips intersecting at right angles. A video tape camera was situated at the entrance to the room so that the entire room could be covered by rotating the camera on the

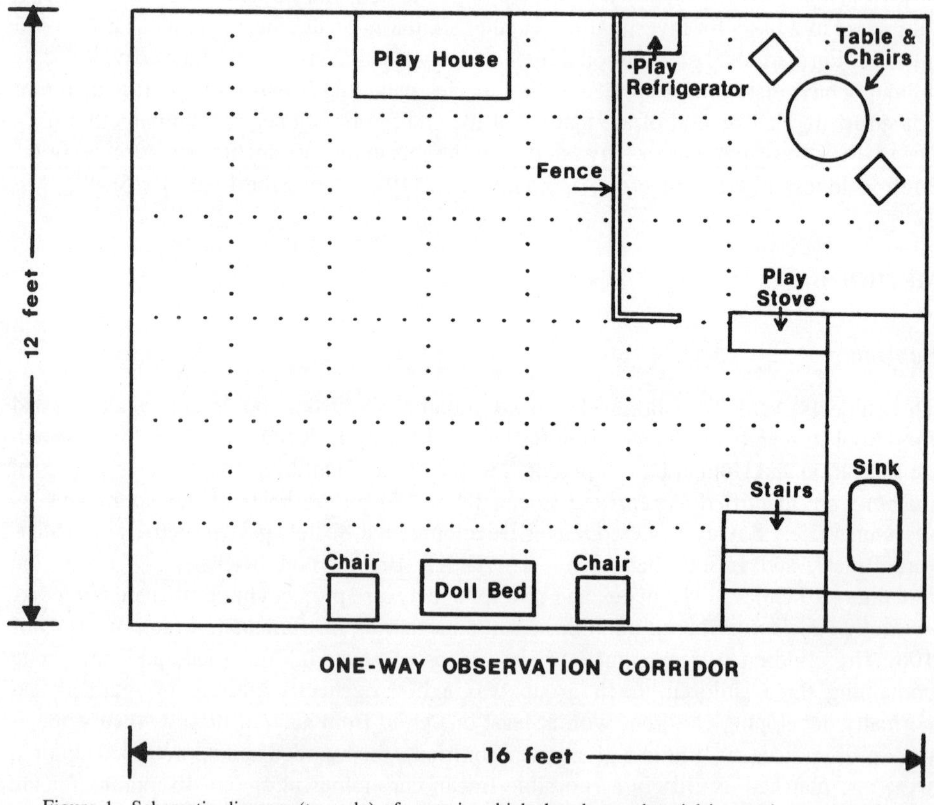

Figure 1. Schematic diagram (to scale) of room in which the observed social interactions occurred.

tripod. Microphones were suspended from the ceiling for simultaneous video and audio recording.

Data collection began as soon as all of the children in a particular group who were present at school that day had entered the test room. Because of frequent absences (mean number of absences = 3.67 for nonretarded and 2.75 for retarded children), many of the sessions had less than the full complement of children assigned to that group. However, all of the sessions from which data were collected had at least two children present. During the data collection period, the children were free to engage in unstructured free play. The practicum student was instructed to remain seated on the stairs (see Figure 1) and *not* initiate any interactions with the children unless an emergency or crisis (e.g., physical fighting) ensued. The adult student was further instructed to respond accordingly when a child made an attempt to interact with her, but to try to terminate such interactions as quickly as possible.

Interpersonal Proximity

At 15-sec intervals throughout each session, a tape-recorded tone sounded in the observation room. At that instant, the observer recorded the position of each child by marking their and the practicum student's respective symbols on a schematic scale diagram of the room and grid floor. During each session, one of the children of that group was designated as the "target," and his/her position was always the first to be recorded at the sounding of the tone.

The first step of the data reduction and analysis was to measure the distances (to the nearest foot) from the target child to each of the other children with an appropriately calibrated ruler for each of the 20 observations within a 5-min session. Next, the mean distances between the target child and all of the other children combined were calculated for each session.

For each week of observations, each child was assigned as the target for his/her group during at least one observation period. However, because of frequent absences and the fact that one group had three children instead of four, not all children were targeted the same number of times for the entire study. In all, 108 5-min free-play sessions were observed and analyzed, with each child serving as the target two to seven times.

Social Interactions

Unlike the measures of interpersonal proximity, which were recorded "live," social interaction data were obtained from audio-video tape recordings of the same free play sessions described above. During each session, one of the children was randomly designated as the target (not necessarily the same child as targeted for the interpersonal proximity measures for that session) upon whom the video tape camera was focused throughout that session.

Video tapes of all the free play sessions were observed and coded by the same two observers working in unison (i.e., they came to an agreement on each item of data scored). Following an initial observation period, a number of behavioral categories were established (see Appendix) and a behavioral coding technique was developed to aid in data collection. Whenever the target child engaged in any of the social interactions described in the appendix, that item was recorded along with the identity of the individual with whom the interaction took place. Such data were recorded only when the target child was interacting with a single identifiable peer. Records were also kept as to whether the target child was the initiator or recipient of a behavioral interaction, or whether there was no obvious initiator or recipient (in which case the two participants were scored as engaging *simultaneously* in a particular behavior). The data therefore included frequency counts of the various social behaviors (as defined in Appendix) engaged in by the target children, the identity of the other child with whom the targets interacted in each instance, and, when possible, the identities of the initiator and recipient of each of these interactions.

Reliability Check

Four months after all the tapes had been scored in the above manner, the original two observers checked their "intrarater" reliability by rescoring nine randomly selected sessions. To calculate the degree of concordance (see Smith and Connolly, 1972) between the frequency as originally scored and the reliability check for each behavioral category that had a non-zero frequency (on *either* the original scoring or the rescoring), the frequency of agreements was divided by the frequency of agreements plus disagreements. These reliability data (Appendix) indicate a generally high rate of agreement for the various behavior categories even after an intervening period of 4 months between the original and second scoring of the tapes. Those categories that had a low (but non-zero) frequency (i.e., less than three occurrences over the nine check sessions) are identified with an asterisk in the appendix. It should be noted that all instances of zero concordance scores seem to be a function of the extremely low frequencies of the respective behavior categories (i.e., a total of only one occurrence over the nine sessions in each instance).

Finally, since the two observers worked together and therefore "agreed" on all of the video tape data scored, a measure of interrater reliability would have been meaningless (i.e., this method of data collection is analogous to that involving only a single observer as far as interrater reliability is concerned).

RESULTS

Interindividual Proximity

The overall mean distance between the target children and the other children within the group did not differ significantly for the retarded versus nonretarded target children. The mean distance maintained between the retarded target children and all other children in their group was 5.0 feet compared with a mean of 4.7 feet for the nonretarded children. Likewise, a similar series of comparisons revealed no significant difference between boys and girls (collapsed across retarded and nonretarded) on their overall mean distance from the other group members (mean distance = 4.9 feet for boys, 4.6 feet for girls).

Proximity "Preferences"

Rank "preferences" for group peers based upon mean distance were obtained for each target child. These measures were determined by calculating the mean distances between the target child and each of the other members of his/her group (across all sessions in which that individual was targeted) and ranking these means from the smallest (rank = 1), through the largest (rank = 2 or 3 depending upon the number of children assigned to the group). In effect, these rank proximity preferences indicated the rank order of the mean distances maintained between a target child and the other children in the group. Thus, within a four-child group, the child who was nearest (on average) to the target would be ranked as 1, the furthest child from the target (on average) ranked 3, and the intermediate child on the mean distance measure ranked 2.

For statistical purposes, the rank preferences of the 15 nonretarded children for retarded versus nonretarded peers were tested by comparing the frequencies of occurrence of each subpopulation in each of the distance ranks against the frequencies expected by chance given the composition of the groups. For example, did nonretarded peers have the lowest mean distance (rank preference = 1) from the nonretarded target children more often than expected by chance alone? The actual statistical test consisted of computing a Z score based upon the difference between the obtained number of retarded and nonretarded peers versus the number expected by chance alone for each rank. A comparable series of statistical comparisons was made for the rank preferences of the 12 retarded target children for retarded versus normally developing peers; and finally, a similar series of tests was conducted to ascertain rank proximity preferences of both the male and female target children for peers of either sex.

The results of these analyses (summarized in Table 1 and 2) revealed that the nonretarded target children maintained the closest proximity (mean distance rank 1) to another nonretarded child significantly more often than to a retarded child ($Z = 2.11, p < 0.05$, two-tailed test). On the other hand, retarded children were found to be the furthest peer (based on average distance) from the nonretarded target children in four-child groups (i.e., proximity rank 3) significantly more often than expected by chance ($Z = 2.65, p < 0.005$). Thus, the nonretarded target children tended to have another nonretarded child as

Table 1. Number of retarded and nonretarded children in each mean distance preference rank for the *nonretarded* target children.

	Rank preference		
Subjects	1 (nearest)	2	3 (farthest)
Number of nonretarded children	11 $Z = 2.11$ $p < 0.05$	7 $Z = 0.03$ n.s.[a]	0 $Z = 2.65$ $p < 0.005$
Number of retarded children	4	8	12

[a]n.s. = not significant.

Table 2. Number of retarded and nonretarded children in each mean distance preference rank for the *retarded* target children.

Subjects	Rank preference 1 (nearest)	2	3 (farthest)
Number of nonretarded children	6 $Z = 0.11$ n.s.[a]	6 $Z = 0.11$ n.s.	8 $Z = 0.54$ n.s.
Number of retarded children	4	4	2

[a]n.s. = not significant.

their nearest neighbor, while maintaining the greatest distance from a retarded peer. The frequencies of retarded versus nonretarded peers in proximity rank 2 did not differ for the nonretarded target children.

The retarded target children showed no significant preferences for retarded versus nonretarded peers in any of the three proximity preference ranks. In other words, the retarded target children seemed to be indiscriminate in regard to their proximity to retarded versus nonretarded children.

The analysis of rank proximity preferences by sex revealed no consistent patterns of preference for either the male or female target children. That is, for each proximity rank, the frequencies of male and female peers did not differ significantly.

SOCIAL INTERACTIONS

Mean Frequencies

For each child, the mean frequencies of occurrence (i.e., over the session during which that child was targeted) of all of the behavior categories listed in the appendix were calculated. Separate mean frequencies were obtained for each category as a function of whether the *target child* was the recipient or the initiator of that behavioral category, or whether the interaction was a simultaneous event involving the target child and a peer with no readily identifiable initiator or recipient. Finally, separate mean frequencies of all behavioral categories were calculated for each target child's interactions with peers and again for that child's interactions with the teacher (i.e., practicum student). These mean frequencies/target child were then compared for every behavioral category for retarded versus nonretarded target children using the Mann-Whitney U test.

These analyses revealed a significant difference between retarded and nonretarded target children on the mean frequencies of occurrence of only two of the behavioral categories. The nonretarded target children initiated more vocalizations in the proximity of peers than did the retarded children ($p < 0.03$, two-tailed test). Likewise, the nonretarded children engaged in simultaneous manipulation of different objects with peers more often than did the retarded children ($p < 0.005$, two-tailed test).

For all of the other categories, no significant differences were found between retarded and nonretarded target children on their mean frequencies of peer interactions initiated or received, or on simultaneous peer interactions. Similarly, the retarded and nonretarded target children showed no significant differences in their frequencies of interactions with the teacher on any of the categories of social behavior.

A similar series of statistical comparisons for male versus female target children (collapsed over the retarded-nonretarded groups) revealed only one significant sex difference: female target children initiated more approaches towards peers than did their male counterparts ($p < 0.04$, two-tailed test). No further significant differences between males and females were found for any of the categories of behavioral interaction with either peers or teacher.

PEER PREFERENCES

For each target child, frequencies of interaction with each of the peers were ranked within each of the observational categories (similar to the ranking described above for proximity preferences). Rank 1 was assigned to the peer with whom the target child had the greatest mean frequency of occurrence of the behavior in question, with ranks 2 and 3 being assigned, respectively, to the peers with intermediate and lowest mean frequencies on that behavior. As described above, the total number of retarded versus nonretarded children included in each rank was compared to that expected by chance alone for the retarded and again for the nonretarded target children.

Analyses of the ranked peer preferences within each category indicated that for the nonretarded target children, there was a significantly greater number of nonretarded than retarded peers within preference rank 1 for the following behavioral categories: approaches initiated, follows initiated, total behavior initiated, vocalizations received within the proximity of another peer, vocalizations received outside of the proximity of another peer, vocalizations initiated within peer proximity, manipulation of different objects simultaneously with a peer, and offers received from a peer (see summary, Table 3). Finally, within the category of simultaneous manipulation of different objects, significantly more retarded than nonretarded peers were included in preference rank 3 (designating the lowest mean frequency of interaction with the target) for the nonretarded target children.

The retarded target children showed no significant differences in frequencies of retarded versus nonretarded peers within any of the preference ranks for any of the behavioral categories listed in the appendix.

When rank preferences were analyzed for male versus female target children, males were found to initiate withdrawals from other males significantly more often then from females in rank 1 (see Table 4). For the mean frequency of total behavioral categories initiated by the males, females occurred in rank 3 (least "preferred") significantly more often than did male peers. The female target children showed no significant preferences for male versus female peers within any rank for any of the categories in the appendix.

Table 3. Summary of significant ''preferences'' by nonretarded target children for retarded (R) versus nonretarded peers (N)

Behavioral category		1 (highest mean frequency of interactions)		2	3 (lowest mean frequency of interactions)	
Total approaches initiated	N	11	$p < 0.002$			
	R	1				
Follows initiated	N	5	$p < 0.04$			
	R	1				
Total behaviors initiated	N	11	$p < 0.01$			
	R	3				
Vocalizatons received (within peer proximity)	N	11	$p < 0.01$			
	R	3				
Vocalizatons received (outside of peer proximity)	N	8	$p < 0.03$			
	R	2				
Vocalizations initiated (within peer proximity)	N	10	$p < 0.04$			
	R	4				
Manipulate different objects	N	9	$p < 0.04$		0	$p < 0.01$
	R	3			10	
Offers received	N	7	$p < 0.04$			
	R	2				

Table 4. Summary of significant ''preferences'' by *male* target children for male versus female peers

Behavioral category		1 (highest mean frequency of interactions)		2	3 (lowest mean frequency of interactions)	
Withdrawals initiated	M	7				
	F	0	$p < 0.05$			
Total behaviors initiated	M				1	
	F				5	$p < 0.04$

DISCUSSION

The data presented above reveal a consistent tendency for nonretarded target children to interact most frequently with other nonretarded children rather than with retarded peers. This "preference" of nonretarded children for similarly categorized peers was found for measures of physical proximity as well as for several categories of behavioral and vocal interactions. Retarded target children, on the other hand, displayed no consistent preferences for other retarded versus nonretarded peers for any of the observed dependent variables. These differential preferences of nonretarded versus retarded children for "similar" peers may be at least partially a function of the greater ability to discriminate by the nonretarded subjects (cf. House and Zeaman, 1958; Zeaman and House, 1963). That is, the nonretarded target children might be better able to discriminate between members of the two subpopulations than would the retarded children, and therefore show a distinct preference for members of their own subpopulation. Furthermore, like the "preferences" shown by rhesus monkeys for conspecifics raised in a manner similar to themselves (Pratt and Sackett, 1967), the preferences of nonretarded children for nonretarded peers may be to some extent due to their avoidance of the dissimilar (i.e., retarded) peers.

The similarity in the results from the measures of peer proximity and social interactions suggest that tentative rankings of peer preferences may be obtained by the mean-distance-between-peers method used in the present study. The obvious advantages of this technique are that the data are easily obtained and require little training on the part of the observer, with data reduction and analysis being relatively straightforward. Of course, this approach alone would leave a lot to be desired and might therefore be considered an initial abbreviated method for studying social preferences necessitating further detailed observations before firm conclusions could be made.

In general, the preference data from the present study tend to corroborate and extend the results of a number of recent sociometric studies indicating that nonretarded children "prefer" other nonretarded children over retarded children in a classroom setting (Meyerowitz, 1967; Goodman, Gottlieb, and Harrison, 1972; Iano, Ayers, Heller, McGettigan, and Walker, 1974) or day camp (Shellhaas, 1969), or as partners during a competitive game (Gottlieb and Davis, 1974). Whereas these earlier studies generally focused on self-reports by the subjects of their peer preferences, preference data in the present study are based upon overt behavioral interactions, and may therefore be more accurate indicants of cross group acceptability or rejection.

The "preferences" of the male target children for male rather than female peers within the two categories "withdrawals initiated" and "total behaviors" lend some support to the often cited tendency of children to interact primarily with like-sexed peers (cf. Hutt, 1972). It should be noted, however, that the frequency of preferences (i.e., number of categories for which a significant preference was displayed) based upon sex of peers was not nearly as great as those preferences based upon the retarded versus nonretarded dichotomy.

A series of especially interesting findings consisted of the similar measures of mean peer proximity as well as the rarity of gross differences in mean frequencies of the various behavioral categories for the retarded versus nonretarded subpopulations. Thus, except for two behavioral categories, the retarded children behaved similarly to their nonretarded peers, at least as measured by frequency of behavior per se. The greater frequency of vocalizations within peer proximity initiated by nonretarded versus retarded children could simply be a reflection of a greater verbal aptitude on the part of the former group. A more noteworthy difference between the two subpopulations consisted of the greater mean frequency of simultaneous manipulation of different objects shown by the nonretarded children. This latter category appears to resemble to some extent (and overlap with) the categories of "parallel play" and "group play" as defined by Smith and Connolly (1972) as follows:

Parallel play

> The child plays independently, but the behavior he chooses naturally brings him among other children. If playing with toys then these are like those which nearby children are using, but he plays with the toys as he sees fit. If play is without toys then he uses the same apparatus or his behavior is of a similar nature to that of nearby children. In either case he does not attempt to influence the behavior of nearby children and there is little or no interaction with them. He plays beside, rather than with, the other children.

Group play

> The child plays with other children, interacting with them in the nature of the behavior. Interactions here include conversation, borrowing or sharing toys, following or chasing one another, physical contact, and organized play involving different roles.

One of the functions of play suggested by Bruner (1972) is that of serving "as a vehicle for teaching the nature of a society's conventions, and it can also teach about the nature of convention per se" (p. 699). Thus, through social play the child can learn rules and techniques basic to functioning adequately in society. Given that the above reduced rate of simultaneous manipulation of different objects (a reflection of social play behaviors) in retarded children is a general phenomenon, such low rates of "play" may be causally linked to some extent to the reduced social skills displayed by retarded individuals. The low rate of social play-like behavior by retarded children may be somewhat a function of their inability to emit appropriate signals to another child or to interpret signals given by others. These are among the questions that need to be answered before normalization can begin with very young retarded children because play seems to be a primary tool with which children learn about their environment.

Like any approach to the study of behavioral phenomena, the methodology employed above is not free from a number of shortcomings. Accordingly, it may be informative to enumerate the following major limitations arising from the specific methods of collection and treatment of the data.

1. As is true for most observational-descriptive studies, the techniques used in the present study were quite tedious, requiring a protracted effort by a number of observers to obtain data on relatively few subjects.
2. By focusing on frequencies of isolated motor events, the data do not reflect the ongoing flow of behavior and may therefore overlook major differences between the subpopulations. Thus, although quite similar on mean frequencies of behavior, retarded and nonretarded children may differ on the sequences or duration of their patterns of social behavior. In any event, this study must be viewed as a preliminary

approach to the problem, which should now be followed by a more sophisticated series of studies employing stochastic models.

3. The behavioral categories employed do not represent an exhaustive catalog. Further studies are now being planned which will be more finely focused upon such aspects of social behavior as greetings and dominance-subordination, rather than the more global categories of social interactions as used above.
4. The proximity (interpersonal distance) data were not integrated with the descriptive data. In this regard, one would ideally like to describe the extent to which social interactions vary as a function of the distance between the interacting individuals.
5. Use of a mental age (MA) matching strategy imposes a major confound in the data presented above. As stated under "Methods," the mean age of the retarded children was approximately 10 months greater than that of the normally developing children. Therefore, it might on first reading be concluded that the normally developing children were actually showing age-mate preferences rather than preferences based upon the retarded-normally developing dimension. It is our contention, however, that the retarded-normally developing variable was a more salient factor than age in the peer preferences displayed by the normally developing children. Earlier data (McGrew, 1972) showing age-mate proximity preferences in groups of normally developing children were likely a function of behavioral similarities among the children of comparable age concomitant with behavioral differences between children of different ages. Thus, one could argue that, if anything, an MA match (as used in the present study) might be expected to include retarded children who are behaviorally *more* similar to the normally developing children than would be the case for chronological age (CA) matched groups; thereby reducing the degree of subpopulation preferences relative to those resulting from a CA match. That is, we would hypothesize an even *greater* preference by normally developing children for other normally developing children when grouped with CA matched retarded children.
6. Since the present study was conducted in an experimental school containing heterogeneous groupings of retarded and nonretarded children, the results may not be generalizable outside of this setting. However, this is an empirical question, the elucidation of which will require further systematic observational research. It may be that the interactions of young retarded and normally developing children may be relatively independent of contextual constraints. In any case, the present results should be useful to the normalization movement, a basic goal of which is the integration of retarded and nonretarded children in natural settings. It is assumed that such integration will lead to interactions resulting in positive behavioral change for the retarded children. Thus far, however, there have been few attempts to test the validity of these assertions (cf. Ray, 1974).

Finally, the specific methodology employed above has several inherent advantages (some of which have already been alluded to earlier) as well as limitations. On the positive side, several points should be added. a) The noninferential behavioral categories are relatively easy to describe and observe, which allows for a fairly high degree of reliability. b) Use of video tapes enables the observer to review social interaction sequences as often as is necessary to extract the data in question. The same tapes can also be quite useful in training observers as well as in checking inter and intraobserver reliability. c) Behavior in such an unstructured "naturalistic" setting is probably a more valid reflection of social preferences than are responses to the more commonly used sociometric techniques discussed above. d) The population under study is uniquely suited to studies of social interactions and preferences in retarded and nonretarded individuals. First, the children were young, and therefore probably relatively free of prejudices. Furthermore, they had functioned in this heterogeneous setting for several months before the study began. Therefore, the observations tapped already established social behavior patterns uncontaminated by an "unfamiliarity" effect. e) The observations were conducted in a "normalization" context, which is the type of practical setting to which such data should be applied.

ACKNOWLEDGMENTS

We would like to express our appreciation to Luther Ludwig and Dr. Joel S. Ray who assisted in the preliminary phases of this study; and to the staff, children, and parents of the Experimental School of the John F. Kennedy Center for Research on Education and Human Development.

REFERENCES

Baxter, J. C. 1970. Interpersonal spacing in natural settings. Sociometry 33:444–456.

Blurton-Jones, N. 1972a. Ethological Studies of Child Behaviour. Cambridge University Press, Cambridge.

Blurton-Jones, N. 1972b. Categories of child-child interaction. In: N. Blurton-Jones (ed.), Ethological Studies in Child Behaviour. Cambridge University Press, Cambridge.

Bricker, D. D., and Bricker, W. A. 1971. Toddler research and intervention project report: year I. IMRID Monogr. No. 20. George Peabody College.

Bruner, J. S. 1972. Nature and uses of immaturity. Am. Psychol. 27:687–708.

Crook, J. H. 1970. Social organization and the environment: aspects of contemporary social ethology. Animal Behav. 18:197–209.

Eibl-Eibesfeldt, I. 1975. Ethology: The Biology of Behavior, 2nd Ed. Holt, Rinehart & Winston, New York.

Esser, A. H. 1968. Dominance hierarchy and clinical course of psychiatrically hospitalized boys. Child Dev. 39:147–157.

Esser, A. H. 1970. Interactional hierarchy and power structure on a psychiatric ward. In: S. J. Hutt and C. Hutt (eds.), Behaviour Studies in Psychiatry. Pergamon Press Ltd., Oxford.

Goodman, H., Gottlieb, J., and Harrison, R. H. 1972. Social acceptance of EMRs integrated into a nongraded elementary school. Am. J. Ment. Defic. 76:412–417.

Gottlieb, J., and Davis, J. 1974. Social acceptance of EMR children during overt behavioral interactions. Am. J. Ment. Defic. 78:141–143.

Grant, E. C. 1968. An ethological description of non-verbal behaviour during interviews. Br. J. Med. Psychol. 41:177–184.

Hall, E. T. 1966. The Hidden Dimension. Doubleday & Co. Inc., New York.

Hediger, H. 1950. Wild Animals in Captivity. Butterworth & Co. Ltd., London.

House, B. J., and Zeaman, D. 1958. A comparison of discrimination learning in normal and mentally defective children. Child Dev. 29:411–416.

Hudson, P. T. W., McGrew, W. C., and McGrew, P. L. 1970. Attention structure in a group of preschool infants. Proceedings of the C. I. E. Architecture Conference, Kingston-on-Thames.

Hutt, C. 1972. Males and Females. Penguin Books Ltd., Harmondsworth, Middlesex.

Iano, R. P., Ayers, D., Heller, H., McGettigan, J. F., and Walker, V. S. 1974. Sociometric status of retarded children in an integrative program. Except. Child. 40(4):267–273.
King, M. G. 1966. Interpersonal relations in preschool children and average approach distance. J. Genet. Psychol. 109:109–116.
Leach, G. M. 1972. A comparison of the social behaviour of some normal and problem children. In: N. Blurton-Jones (ed.), Ethological Studies of child behavior. Cambridge University Press, Cambridge.
McGrew, W. C. 1972. An Ethological Study of Children's Behavior. Academic Press, New York.
McGrew, W. C. 1975. Interpersonal spacing of preschool children. In: J. S. Bruner and K. J. Connolly (eds.), The Development of Competence in Early Childhood. The Developmental Sciences Trust Study Group.
Meyerowitz, J. H. 1967. Peer groups and special classes. Ment. Retard. 5:23–26.
Paluck, R. J. 1971. Territoriality and Operant Conditioning of Institutionalized Severely Retarded Boys. Unpublished doctoral dissertation, Columbia University.
Paluck, R. J., and Esser, A. H. 1971a. Controlled experimental modification of aggressive behavior in territories of severely retarded boys. Am. J. Ment. Defic. 76:23–29.
Paluck, R. J., and Esser, A. H. 1971b. Territorial behavior as an indicator of changes in clinical behavioral condition of severely retarded boys. Am. J. Ment. Defic. 76:284–290.
Pratt, C. L., and Sackett, G. P. 1967. Selection of social partners as a function of peer contact during rearing. Science 155:1133–1135.
Ray, J. S. 1974. Behavior of Developmentally Delayed and Nondelayed Toddler-age Children: An Ethological Study. Unpublished doctoral dissertation, George Peabody College.
Shellhaas, M. D. 1969. Sociometric status of institutionalized retarded children and nonretarded community children. Am. J. Ment. Defic. 73:804–808.
Smith, P. K., and Connolly, K. 1972. Patterns of play and social interaction in pre-school children. In: N. Blurton-Jones (ed.), Ethological Studies of Child Behaviour. Cambridge University Press, Cambridge.
Sommer, R. 1969. Personal Space: The Behavioral Basis of Design. Prentice Hall Inc., Englewood Cliffs, N.J.
Tinbergen, E. A., and Tinbergen, N. 1972. Early childhood autism—An ethological approach. Z. Tierpsycholo. Beiheft 10:1–53.
Wilson, E. O. 1975. Sociobiology. Harvard University Press, Cambridge.
Wolfensburger, W. 1972. The Principle of Normalization in Human Services. National Institute of Mental Retardation, Toronto.
Zeaman, D., and House, B. J. 1963. The role of attention in retardate discrimination learning. In: N. R. Ellis (ed.), Handbook of Mental Deficiency. McGraw-Hill Book Company, New York.

APPENDIX

Social Behavior Categories and Definitions

Degree of concordance appears in parentheses before each category. Asterisks denote categories that had a frequency of occurrence of *less than three* over the nine reliability check sessions (see page 316 of the text).

Vocalization (''Within peer proximity'' = within 3 feet of a peer; ''Outside of peer proximity'' > 3 feet from the nearest peer.)

(0.83) Laugh ''Open-mouthed smile together with audible vocalization (rapid or staccato expulsions of breath).'' (Smith and Connolly, 1972)

Cry ''Repeated usually low-pitched vocalizations; 'waah,' 'aaah-hah.''' (Smith and Connolly, 1972)

(0.65) Shout "Either a single loud, monosyllabic noise—but without the high-pitched 'urgency' of a scream, or more usually, a sentence, spoken loudly and emphatically, e.g., a command 'Don't do that.'" (Leach, 1972)

**(1.00) Scream* "High-pitched wail, of piercing quality." (Leach, 1972)

(0.86) Vocalization Any utterance other than the ones defined above.

Actions

Body Oppose "The trunk is forcefully inclined into contact with another individual's trunk; the body is upright and the feet are spread wide (giving a more solid supporting base). It resembles pushing or shoving except that the arms do not exert force; instead they are usually held away from the body, to its side" (McGrew, 1972).

(1.00) Give "An object, held in the child's hand or hands, is held out for another person to grasp and then is released; or the object may be placed on the other person's lap" (Leach, 1972).

**(1.00) Offer* An object, held in the child's hand or hands, is held out but not released.

Hit at "Sharp movement of hand towards another child, almost always with arm bent and hand held above shoulder before sharp downward movement. Sometimes hand out at side. But no actual contact with other child." (Adapted from Blurton-Jones, 1972b.)

**(0.0) Hit and Beat* A forceful downward movement of flexed arm from above shoulder height. Plus any other form of hard blow to the object child with hand. (Adapted from Blurton-Jones, 1972b.)

**(0.50) Hit and Beat with Object* Child uses object rather than hand to hit and beat another child.

Holds Hands Grasping another's hand. (After McGrew, 1972.)

Hug The arms are moved horizontally forward from a wide spread position toward each other and around an individual thusly encircling him/her. The movement is usually directed toward another individual's trunk in a peer-peer interaction or toward an adult's upper leg, if both are standing. (Modified from McGrew, 1972.)

Pat "The flat hand is gently tapped once, or twice, or three times, on some part of the other person—usually on the upper part of the body" (Leach, 1972).

(1.00) Physical Contact Any nonaccidental physical contact with another child. Excluding contacts falling into the other behavioral categories. (Modified from Smith and Connolly, 1972.)

Kick The child flexes one leg and swings it forward, so that the foot makes an impact on a person—usually the leg. If the child is sitting, or raised off the ground, both legs may be kicking simultaneously. (Modified from Leach, 1972.)

Poke "The child extends the arm and one finger, making contact with the body of another person. A poke is not usually hard enough to hurt the recipient if done with the finger (unless e.g., the eye is poked). But the child may use a weapon instead of the finger; the stick (or whatever) is grasped in the child's hand and then directed at the body of the other person" (Leach, 1972).

**(1.00) Push* The child flexes the arm(s) and then extends it with the hand flat against the other person's body, in one continuous, rather violent movement; or, the hand is placed on the person's body with the arm slightly flexed, and the arm is then extended. (Adapted from Leach, 1972.)

Body Push "Trunk is forcefully pushed into contact with another person. This pattern looks like pushing except that the arms exert no force and are held away." (Ray, 1974)

Push with Object Child uses object rather than hands to push another child.

**(0.50) Receive* "Child extends arm and takes in its hand an object given by another, does not flex arm until other has released his grip (contrast take-tug-grab)" (Blurton-Jones, 1972b).

Pull The child grasps another person and tries to draw the person toward himself. For a hard pull, the child will press hard on the ground with his feet, with the knees slightly flexed, and, after the person is grasped, lean away. Pulling may be reciprocal. (Modified from Leach, 1972.)

Point The child extends his arm, and usually also extends one or more of the fingers, in a specific direction. This action may be accompanied by alternating glances at the object/person being pointed at and another person, who is usually also addressed: " 'Look at that,' or 'What's that?' " (modified from Leach, 1972).

**(0.0) Throw* The child has an object in his grasp; the arm is flexed and then abruptly extended, and the object is released landing within 4 feet of another child. (Modified from Leach, 1972.)

(1.00) Take-Tug-Grab "A combination (i.e., any one or more) of the following three: (1) *Taking* an object from someone's hands (or an object which they are obviously using) when they have not held it out towards the subject. (2) *Grab* is a faster version of (1) and often with resistance from the other. (3) *Tug* is holding and pulling object which another is also holding and does not immediately release" (Blurton-Jones, 1972b).

Wave The child raises a hand to about shoulder height, and moves it to and fro, while looking at a person. Small children may do a modified wave, which consists of the hand being raised, and then opened and closed toward the person. (Modified from Leach, 1972.)

Movement Patterns

Follow The child moves (e.g., walks, runs, crawls) toward a person who is moving away from him. (Modified from Leach, 1972.)

(0.92) Approach Movement of a child to a stationary position in proximity to other child(ren), meeting the following criteria. 1) the child approaches within arm's reach and comes to a complete stop, or 2) the child contacts a specified object (specified objects consisted of the following nonportable objects: stairs, stove, refrigerator, table, store, crib, fence) with which other child(ren) are already in contact.

(0.88) Withdraw Movement of a child from a stationary position in which the distance is increased as follows. 1) the child is no longer within arm's reach, or 2) the child is no longer in contact with the specified object with which other child(ren) are in contact.

(1.00) Manipulate Same Object Mutual contact or use of the same portable object.

(0.75) Manipulate Different Objects Simultaneous use of different portable objects by children within proximity (as defined in the definition of approach).

Coding Specifications

1. Categories that can be continuous events (e.g., manipulation of different objects) are coded only at the onset. For example, if A and B are manipulating objects, it is coded. When C approaches and also manipulates an object, it is coded as a new event, but if C leaves, as long as there isn't more than a 2 sec delay in the object manipulation of A and B, it is not coded again.
2. If a continuous category (e.g., vocalization) ceases for more than 2 sec, it is coded as a new event when it occurs again.
3. The category take-tug-grab is coded either with a +, indicating a child takes possession of an object, or −, indicating the other child maintains possession of an object.

OBSERVATIONAL STUDIES OF BEHAVIOR IN COMMUNITY SETTINGS

Introduction

Nancy M. Robinson

The material presented in this section deals with the life styles of mentally retarded people. The Edgerton and Langness chapter contrasts sharply with the work of Landesman-Dwyer et al. in approaches to describing the behavior of retarded persons in the community. The former deals primarily with general characteristics of largely non-quantitative anthropological methods. The latter describes in detail an exemplar of an actual quantitative observational investigation. Chapter 16 by Butler and Bjaanes also illustrates how a variety of observational techniques might be used along with traditional attitude and performance scales to compare behavior between alternative residences. The differences between the quantitative and nonquantitative approaches are by no means artificial.

The distinctive type of research employed by anthropologists focuses on the method of *participant-observation.* In a larger perspective, the method is described as *naturalistic, cross cultural,* and *mentalistic.* In studying mentally retarded people, the participant researcher should be prepared to deal descriptively and theoretically with ethnically different subcommunities. Thus, the observational study of mental retardation must deal with cross cultural communication even within a single society such as our own. The mentalistic orientation assumes that the participant observer will be especially effective at elucidating the beliefs and symbols of mentally retarded persons. This allows the researcher to assess validly the ways in which the culture affects retarded people *and* the nonretarded people in the community whom they contact. Underlying the method is the idea that by living with retarded people the researcher will identify the cognitive means by which retarded people cope with their everyday lives. Gathering such data requires attention to information revealed both deliberately and inadvertently by informants, and a willingness to analyze the basic belief systems of the researcher's own culture.

Discussion of the participant observer method reflected the commitment of most conference participants to empirical, quantitative, methodologically "tight" observational approaches. The major issue of reliability centered about the fact that the participant observer is a "sentient, thinking human being," who is usually the only individual to report observations and conclusions from an ethnographic study. This produces the danger that because of bias or selectivity the participant observer will find exactly what he looks for. Moreover, the sample may be unrepresentative of the cultural group under study, and therefore it may be possible to repeat the basic observations.

In reply, Edgerton and Langness confirm that the participant observer does indeed need self-awareness. However, observations that seem to be unsystematic or anecdotal are in fact the product of a long acquaintance with the study group. This yields the opportunity and obligation to test the consistency of both behavior and interpretations. Furthermore, Edgerton and Langness stress that it is rarely possible to employ more than one observer because of funding, and because there are few researchers trained both to observe and to fit equally well into a particular culture.

Currently, the anthropologist seems to be in a unique position in the field of mental retardation. Because few ethnographers have been interested in this area, the leading anthropologists have become highly visible as social critics. This dual role of researcher and politician multiplies the potential effects of the ''personal equation'' which underlies the participant-observer technique. As any scientist must be appropriately cautious in interpreting data, particularly in a politicized arena, so must the anthropologist who carries the burden of a reduced opportunity to cross validate findings.

Despite these limitations, a mentally retarded population provides unique and demanding opportunities for application of the participant-observer technique. The observer must learn how to make meaningful social contacts despite language deficits and other handicaps. This can lead to an intense involvement with and commitment to the subjects under study. The researcher may become the most important person in their lives, with the responsibilities of a teacher, a benefactor, and a protector-advocate for helping the subjects cope. The observer soon learns of the special burden placed on the retarded individual, who must be more than normal to gain general social acceptance because of the high standards of conduct applied by the nonretarded community. Any nonretarded individual who becomes involved in this ''normalization'' process—including the participant observer—has the opportunity to help make a readily observable difference. This aspect of the anthropological method seems to be a gratifying asset and a methodological hazard.

Landesman-Dwyer et al. summarize a study of detailed quantitative recordings, at 15-min intervals for 48 hr, of the physical and social environments and behavior of 400 persons in 20 group homes in the state of Washington. Discussion centers about the purposes for which such research might be employed. Among the applied goals are planning of residential unit size according to the kinds of activities and social relationships that are found to relate empirically to the size variable. For example, the study revealed that more dyadic relationships and specific friendships were found in homes containing 20 or more retarded residents than in smaller homes. Other applied issues involved the types of residents in the home (homogeneous versus heterogeneous backgrounds), comparisons of the type of care and environment provided by profit and nonprofit group home systems, and the effects of urban versus rural geographic location of the home.

A number of possibilities were discussed with respect to the usefulness of such data for more scientific, theoretical purposes. The test method was in fact derived from laboratory techniques employing digital electronic instruments to code behaviors as they occur in real time. Whereas the content codes of the behavior categories were designed specifically for the group home environment, the general types of categories were derived from an extensive body of data involving both human and nonhuman primate populations. The observers were trained to very high standards of reliability before any data were collected. Besides coding specific predefined behaviors, these observers also wrote extensive notes describing subtle aspects of the quality of behaviors that were observed and detailed information about the homes themselves. Such data seem acceptable for rigorous testing of specific hypotheses about behavior and its relationships to variations in social and nonsocial environmental variables.

During the discussion, hope was expressed that a scientifically meaningful bridge might be built among divergent approaches such as the participant-observer and quantitative observational methods. The detailed quantitative data need to be understood within the context of real life problems of retarded people such as those exposed through the participant-observer method. On the other hand, the reliability and generality of ethnographic reports must be tested and found to be acceptable. In all fairness to the conference discussions, it must be concluded that these are ideas whose time has not yet come.

chapter 14

Observing Mentally Retarded Persons in Community Settings: An Anthropological Perspective

Robert B. Edgerton and L. L. Langness

There has been little discussion of the use of observational techniques in the study of mentally retarded persons in the community. In an effort to initiate such discussion, we shall consider certain practical, theoretical, and ethical aspects of observing mentally retarded persons, in that context. Because we believe that any discussion of methods can have value only insofar as these methods are relevant to particular research problems in particular contexts, we begin with a discussion of mentally retarded persons outside of large institutional settings. We then review some examples of observational research in a variety of community settings and conclude with a general discussion of methodological issues. As ethnography, the stock-in-trade of anthropologists from the beginning, can easily be seen as human ethology, it will be necessary to comment at times on the nature of anthropological research itself. We conceive ethology to be the systematic observation of animals, including man, in the natural environment. However, when attempted with human beings, there are two crucial dimensions that become problematic; the problem of reactivity and the problem of emic versus etic perspectives. In attempting to deal with these dimensions, as all ethnographers must do, we see no particular advantage in the term human ethology.

THE MENTALLY RETARDED IN THE COMMUNITY

It is most important to realize that the innocuous catch phrase, "the mentally retarded in the community," actually refers to an extraordinarily great diversity of persons, settings, and situations. As most diagnoses of retardation are made in early school years by

The research on which this paper was based was supported in part by PHS Grant #HD04612 NICHD, the Mental Retardation Research Center, UCLA, and #HD05540-02, Patterns of Care and the Development of the Retarded.

employing IQ tests, and as such tests are known to discriminate against various ethnic and lower class populations (Mercer, 1973), there is an immediate question of cultural or subcultural diversity. This diversity was increased during the 1960's when large residential facilities for the mentally retarded began to shift their "patients" to smaller community-based residences. These persons joined the ethnic and lower class populations mentioned, as well as many other mentally retarded persons who, for one reason or another, had never been institutionalized. As a result, the contemporary situation throughout the United States is characterized by an almost staggering heterogeneity. For example, some so-called mentally retarded persons are probably not properly labeled in the first place. Others are of such relatively high IQ and adaptive skills that they cannot easily be distinguished from the so-called "normals" who live in the same apartment or neighborhood, and still others have such low IQ's, minimal adaptive skills, and multiple physical handicaps that they spend their lives confined to beds or wheelchairs in some form of nursing home.

Between these extremes are many mentally retarded persons—at various levels of IQ and adaptive skills—who live with their parents, in small residential facilities, or in foster-care homes. Many of these people are quite sequestered from the community in which they live, their activities being restricted to employment in a sheltered workshop, supervised visits to church, and occasional organized entertainment, such as bowling or picnics. For some, life in "the community" means only that their place of residence is located in some sort of residential area; for others it means a degree of participation in the prevailing patterns of living found in their neighborhoods, towns, or cities. Many of these mentally retarded persons are small children, some are adolescents, others are elderly. Some are married; some have regular jobs; some have disabling physical handicaps; some are physically sound; some have concerned parents; many do not. Given this diversity, it is obvious that many kinds of research problems are posed and many opportunities exist for observational research among the mentally retarded in the community. It is also obvious that the kinds of observational methods appropriate in one type of situation may be quite inappropriate in another.

OBSERVATIONAL RESEARCH IN RESTRICTED COMMUNITY SETTINGS

The use of systematic observation to study the behavior of mentally retarded patients in large state institutions is well established (e.g., MacAndrew and Edgerton, 1964; Luckey, 1966; Davis et al., 1969). This research has systematically used checklists, activity logs, and rating scales in an effort to obtain precise records of ongoing patient or patient-staff behavior (Hutt and Hutt, 1970). Much of this research has involved the use of behavior therapy in relation to stereotyped or otherwise undesirable behavior (e.g., Campbell, 1968; Wills, 1973). Some of this research is similar in kind to the ethological observations recently used in the study of normal children (Blurton-Jones, 1972; McGrew, 1972). These methods have also been transferred to certain kinds of community settings, especially those that are "restricted" by space, time, supervision, or institutional rules. Common "restricted" settings include residential facilities, half-way houses, sheltered workshops, schools, and to a lesser extent, single family homes.

A good example of the use of systematic observation in residential settings is provided by Bjaanes and Butler (1974), who compared two kinds of alternative community care facilities in terms of the behavior expressed by the residents of these places. Confining their sample to a certain geographical area, two "home care" facilities (each with a resident population of four to six) were selected from a larger sample of 18 such facilities as were two "board-and-care" facilities with resident populations of approximately 30 and 50. Using an activity checklist (e.g., watching television, playing cards, doing chores, talking to peers, etc.) the observers recorded behaviors in four residential settings. Observation periods were selected on a time-sampling basis. Employing what they call "activity analysis," the investigators then coded these behaviors into five dimensions or domains: 1) passing-natural ("passing" refers to an effort to conceal incompetence and past institutionalization), 2) independent-dependent, 3) spontaneous-planned-routine, 4) structured-unstructured, 5) obligatory-discretionary. Behaviors in the four residential settings were then compared and substantial behavioral differences were observed from setting to setting. For example, residents displayed greater independence in board-and-care facilities than in home-care settings.

Similar observational research has often been conducted in restricted school settings of various kinds (Brandt, 1972; Kelly, 1967). Examples of this approach are available in the work of Gallimore, Tharp, and Speidel (1975), and of Forness and Esveldt (1975). This type of research often employs a formal observational technique called point sampling, in which a checklist of possible behaviors is constructed and repeated observations are then made at various points in time (Brandt, 1972). A recent checklist of this type, for example, in a study of Indian verbal behavior in the classroom, involves categories such as: statement of fact or direction, asking a question of another, commanding another to act using language, calling attention to oneself using language, and so on (Guilmet and Langness, 1976). This technique allows for a great many observations in a short period of time (it takes approximately 1 min to complete one column of observations on five or six children) and is both objective and efficient.

Some observational work has also been attempted in restricted family settings (e.g., White and Watts, 1973). Much of this research has been concerned with the modification of a child's problem behaviors (e.g., Zeilberger, Sampen and Sloan, 1968; Eyberg and Johnson, 1974), but some of it has focused more generally on the interaction between parents and their developmentally disabled child (Kogan, Wimberger and Bobbitt, 1969; Kogan and Tyler, 1973). There has also been some concern with methodological issues such as observer reactivity (Johnson and Bolstad, 1975).

Although there has been relatively little use of systematic "ethological" observation in the study of mentally retarded persons in community settings, it is clear that such techniques could be usefully employed, especially in what have been termed restricted settings. Such techniques permit a maximum of precision in measurement of variables, of interrater reliability, and of replicability. Where these goals are paramount, systematic observational approaches will serve well. Needless to say, however, these approaches, like all others, have limitations.

As Lipinski and Nelson (1974) point out, and as our own research confirms, systematic observation can be highly reactive when it is used with higher IQ adolescents or adults. This reactivity may increase still more when such research is attempted in a public setting rather than a restricted or private one. Furthermore, as the ''psychological ecology'' of Barker (1968) has shown, extending ethological observation to multiple or public settings, or to the everyday routines of life, can be both inordinately difficult and expensive (Willems, 1967; Brandt, 1972). However, the most serious limitation of these formal ethological techniques has to do with their tendency to distort the meaning of human behavior or, in some cases, to lose sight of meaning altogether. Distortion of meaning may occur as a result of the sometimes arbitrary process of chopping continuous human behavior into discrete but arbitrary units or categories that can be reliably counted. When these units or categories are then combined into higher order concepts, as in the previously mentioned work of Bjaanes and Butler (1974), further distortion may occur. Egon Brunswik (1955) referred to this problem as the ''artificial tying and untying of variables.''

Beyond this kind of distortion, ethological methods typically call for the observer to stand outside of the phenomena, like a naturalist, recording sequences of behavior strictly in terms of the observer's understanding of them. This kind of radically objective observation cannot easily penetrate the world of meaning which guides the action of human beings. Indeed, it can lead to a reductio ad absurdum, as in Marvin Harris', *The Nature of Cultural Things* (1964). Such observation can tell what it is that people do—at least in certain settings where observations are feasible—but it cannot tell how their thoughts, beliefs, emotions, and values are related to what they do. Because we believe, with Max Weber and Clifford Geertz, that ''man is an animal suspended in webs of significance he himself has spun'' (Geertz, 1973, p. 5), this is an omission that simply cannot be allowed.

To illustrate the problem, consider a typical ward for psychiatric patients. It is quite possible, as many investigators have demonstrated, for an observer to study such a ward ethologically. The result might well be an informative set of records that would reveal hitherto unexpected patterns of behavior among patients and the ward staff. However, it is difficult to imagine how this observational approach could apprehend the world of symbols and meanings that patients and staff possess with the success, for example, of that accomplished by D. Rosenhan (1973) who had his colleagues simulate mental illness in order to be admitted to such wards and then record not only what they saw and did, but what it meant to them to be pseudopatients.

We would conclude that although ethological observation can produce valuable data in certain kinds of community settings, especially those called ''restricted,'' these methods also have significant limitations.

OBSERVING MILDLY RETARDED PERSONS IN MULTIPLE SETTINGS

We would now like to discuss the problems of doing observational research with mildly retarded persons in a variety of community settings. There are several reasons for focusing our discussion on the mildly retarded. First, the overwhelming majority (perhaps 85%) of all retarded persons are mildly retarded. Second, as the principle of normalization (Wolfensberger, 1972) becomes more and more entrenched, as we believe it will, these people will spend a greater and greater percentage of their time in restricted community settings. That is, they will live, work, and play more or less as do other people in their communities. These circumstances pose obvious problems for ethological observation. Mildly retarded people are often sensitive to being studied, and they alter their behavior when they believe they are being observed (Edgerton, 1967). Some are actively and seriously trying to pass as normal and therefore resist being seen as subjects for study at all. Many are closely watched and protected by caregivers or parents who attempt to control or shepherd their lives, just as they also attempt to restrict the activities of researchers. To complicate the problems of systematic observations further, many of these retarded persons have surprisingly active and varied lives in the community, moving in and out of many private and public settings in the course of an ordinary day. Several investigators who have attempted to study the lives of such persons in community settings have reported that these people have lives that are both changeable and complex (Edgerton, 1967; Mattinson, 1970; Henschel, 1972; Edgerton and Bercovici, 1976).

In over 15 years of attempting to study mildly retarded persons in a variety of community settings, we have settled upon certain research procedures that seem to be the most effective in allowing us to understand at least some aspects of their lives. These techniques involve observation, but of a different sort than is used by ethologists. Because the methods we employ may be used to complement ethological observation, we shall attempt to describe them.

Our approach is primarily a version of what is often called participant-observation. John Madge (1953, p. 131) has summarized the goals of this approach as follows: "The primary task of the participant-observer is to enter into the life of the community being studied. If this task is achieved, there will be two consequences: his subjects will learn to take him for granted and thus to behave almost as though he were not there, and he will learn to think almost as they think." This is an old approach in anthropology, going back at least as far as the field research of Franz Boas before the turn of the century. It has served anthropologists well as a means of achieving at least a partial comprehension of alien ways of life. Full participation in an alien world is probably never completely possible, but careful observation and as much participation as is appropriate has proven useful in the study of even the most exotic of peoples in dramatically different circumstances (Lofland, 1971; Schatzman and Strauss, 1973; Bogdan and Taylor, 1975; Honigmann, 1976). The essence of the method lies in the prolonged and unobtrusive presence of a sensitive and trained observer among the persons being studied.

In applying this approach to mentally retarded persons we have, along with many research assistants, lived with mentally retarded persons, accompanied them in their everyday activities, and joined them for special occasions such as weddings or birthdays. We have also taken them places they have needed to go, and helped them with problems in their lives. In some cases we have made lasting friendships; in others we have served as patrons or benefactors; in still others we have been merely tolerated and never really accepted.

In all that we do, we spend large amounts of time—months and years—and proceed cautiously, making it entirely clear that we are interested in the people we study as persons and not simply as objects of scientific scrutiny. This can be accomplished only if we offer such persons a meaningful quid pro quo. For many years before the current HEW human subjects guidelines were established, we have begun each research contact with a retarded person by explaining in detail exactly what our research entailed. But even beyond this effort to achieve ''informed consent,'' we explain to people what we can offer them—help with their emergencies (involving their health, financial affairs, writing, etc.)—and this kind of help is usually appreciated. Most important, however, is our sincere demonstration of concern, companionship, and a certain amount of fun, especially for people who are so lonely. To say that we ''offer'' these things is somewhat misleading. As we attempt to explain our research goals we do discuss these matters, but we suspect that the discussion itself has little impact on most people. They listen, but they also wait and see. It is how we subsequently behave that establishes or fails to establish rapport. We attempt to provide help, concern, and affection to all persons we study. At times we fail, but most of the time we create and maintain relationships that last for years. From all of this it should be clear that our approach does not allow for disguised or covert observation. Anthropologists have rarely, if ever, deceived people as did Rosenhan in the study mentioned above or as John Howard Griffin did when he dyed himself brown to write *Black Like Me* (1960). Nevertheless, it is true, as many have recognized (e.g., Webb et al., 1966), that full disclosure of one's research goals and practices in natural settings may lend people to conceal their feelings or to alter their behavior. That is precisely why participant-observation requires such long periods of time if it is to be effective.

Participant-observation exists in many versions, some of which stress observation whereas others emphasize the degree of participation achieved. Typically, however, the end product is a set of field notes recorded by a single participant-observer (Pelto, 1970; Lofland, 1971). Our approach produces such field notes, but it does not rely solely upon them. For one thing, we employ multiple participant-observers, several of whom attempt to achieve a research relationship with the same person, and all of whom carefully record their field notes independently of each other. Field notes include everything of relevance that the participant-observer has seen or heard as well as his own interpretive comments, queries or working hypotheses. These participant-observers also record their observations in narrative form (Brandt, 1972) for certain specified periods of time in the routine of each individual. These narratives, sometimes called anecdotal recording, attempt to provide a precise word description of everything observed in a specified time period. Narratives, ideally, contain no subjective or interpretive comments. Theoretically, they are exact reproductions of observed behavior. The use of video tape or other recording devices may improve accuracy, but a narrative, however recorded, can never be more than a reasonably complete and accurate facsimile of human behavior.

In the early stages of our research, notes are not taken at all, allowing interactions to occur as naturally as possible. Then, after returning to a private place, each participant-observer reconstructs the sequence of the interaction as well as possible through memory. After many months, it may not only be possible to take direct notes of certain occurrences, but we may also ask the people we study for permission to audio or video tape certain of their activities. We explain that we want a record of the things they do and that we cannot see or remember everything without the help of recording devices. With the trust established over months of acquaintanceship, we are usually given permission to make such records. Bystanders seem to feel that the use of portable video cameras is innocuous enough, since we have received no complaints from such people. It goes without saying that we do nothing to embarrass the retarded person, and when we video tape in public places, we are able to use the camera in such a way that no one becomes upset. For example, we do not focus the camera directly on any bystander, making clear that our interest lies elsewhere. It also appears that the chance to hear one's voice or see oneself on a television monitor is a powerful incentive for many retarded persons (just as it is for many "normals" as well). We do replay the tapes as a regular practice, asking those recorded to explain what they were doing in particular behavioral sequences. We ask them to tell us what they were thinking or feeling, and what they were attempting to accomplish. Sometimes we video tape these replay interviews as well. Whenever we use video tape we offer the retarded person a chance to see what we have filmed; we also tell them that if they do not like anything about the film, we will erase it. On only one occasion so far have we been asked to do so, but we are prepared to do so whenever such a request might occur.

Our version of participant-observation, together with video tape narrative recording, is intended to provide a corpus of material that will permit an adequate description and understanding of a retarded person's everyday life. If the approach succeeds, we are able to say what someone's typical day, week, or month is like, but we may not obtain equally detailed material concerning infrequent but significant occurrences or episodes in a person's life. To study these infrequently occurring incidents we also use a form of event analysis similar to the critical incident technique (Flanagan, 1954; Fivars, 1973). Several versions of the technique have been used in mental retardation research (e.g., Fleming, 1962; Steiner and Cochran, 1966; Domino, 1967; Goroff, 1967; Jacobs, Nichols, and Larsen, 1973). Our study of incidents borrows from these past usages but modifies them by incorporating a multiple perspective technique akin to that called "indefinite triangulation" (Cicourel, 1974). We concentrate on incidents that facilitate or hinder normalization. We are also sensitive to the significance of "unguarded moments" (Langness, 1970) in reflecting the attitudes and feelings of the retarded. Such moments multiply and become increasingly significant with the length of the fieldwork period.

We conceive of a normalization incident as an occurrence or practice that significantly affects a mentally retarded person's achievement of a "more nearly normal way of life" (Wolfensberger, 1972). This significant effect can be either positive or negative with regard to normalization. The effect may result from a single important occurrence (e.g., a parent or caregiver refuses to "allow" a young mentally retarded woman to marry) or it may result from a routine practice (e.g., a caregiver routinely speaks to another person about one of her retarded residents, while that resident is present, *as if* the resident were not present at all).

Our past experience has indicated that in order to sample the full range of significant occurrences and routine practices related to normalization, it is necessary to study two kinds of incidents; those brought to light by a retarded person or some other person connected to the community-care system, and those directly witnessed by one of our research staff. Although more normalization incidents have come to our attention through the former source, both sources are necessary to give us a truly balanced view of how retarded persons do, or do not, come to live more nearly normal lives.

Our methods for the study of a normalization incident have several standard features: 1) multiple points of view, 2) a longitudinal perspective, and 3) ecological context. *Multiple points of view* refers to our practice of eliciting and recording the accounts of all persons whose views or actions are relevant to the incident. Beginning with the persons most directly involved (e.g., a caregiver and her resident) we seek out all those persons whose beliefs, attitudes, or behaviors appear to be, or in principle *could* be, relevant. Thus, to continue this example, we might seek accounts from other residents, from the attending physician, the supervising social worker, a parent, or a close relative. These persons would very likely be relevant. But so might a neighbor, a repair man at the caregiver's facility, a former social worker or caregiver, a friend at a sheltered workshop, or even a casual bystander. Whether two persons are involved, or a dozen, we attempt to carefully elicit and record as many accounts of the occurrence or practice at issue as we possibly can. We also record all relevant observations of behavior (at the time or later) to provide potential comparison. These multiple accounts (along with relevant records and documents) are then assembled for subsequent analysis.

Longitudinal perspective is added by the fact that our years of prior work often give us a background of recorded observations that bear directly upon the incident. These observations are added to our record. Similarly, our maintenance of close contact with the retarded person involved (and often with other persons as well) permits us to add pertinent information as it becomes available throughout subsequent years.

By *ecological context* we refer to the fact that by pursuing an incident until no more relevant information is available, or until saturation is reached (Glazer and Strauss, 1967), we learn which "persons, places, and practices" of the community-care system are salient and which are not, and we begin to see which parts of the ecological system tend to facilitate normalization and which do not. We may also discover connections between and among persons that may make up an informal or latent part of the system we would not otherwise have uncovered. We have in mind here such factors as attitudes held by state or regional center officials (they are not, of course, necessarily what they are said to be), availability of funds for certain programs, parental myths or misinformation about reproduction or the care of children, the economic concerns of caregivers, caseloads of social workers, and the unrecognized culture that pervades and helps to make sense of the entire system.

In the analysis of these incidents, every person's account is valuable since it expresses meaningful beliefs, attitudes, and values. Even when subsequent observations or information calls into question the accuracy or wisdom of someone's views, those views are nonetheless an important part of the record and must be considered in any effort to learn about normalization. In the aggregate, these incidents highlight the kinds of beliefs, practical concerns, fears, economic pressures, prejudices, stereotypes, therapeutic goals, and commonsense knowledge that play a vital part in the process of normalization. Without these different accounts, this mass of detail, the concept of normalization most probably must remain simply the latest in a long line of catchy phrases that attract attention, but which inevitably lead nowhere.

One of the most central tenets of anthropology, seen most clearly in the technique of participant observation, is that a fieldworker must attempt to see the "natives'" world through their own eyes. This is known in anthropology as an emic perspective and it contrasts most significantly with the observer's etic (and, it is often claimed, more scientific) point of view (Langness, 1974). Perhaps this more than any other single thing (with the exception of the problem of reactivity) points up the difference between ethological and ethnographic investigations. It is with this goal in mind that we concern ourselves so determinedly with what the retarded themselves believe and say about their lives. In our effort to achieve an emic perspective, we also attempt to use the retarded person's own observations. For example, in addition to our interviewing and observations, we often furnish such persons with a super-8 movie camera and a supply of film and instruct them to take movies of whatever they think is "really important," interesting, or personal about their lives. Some of the resulting films turn out to be incomprehensible jumbles of disconnected images, but others are remarkably coherent and well photographed. As we do with video tapes of behavioral sequences, we show these films to the person who made them, using the film itself as the eliciting device for more information about the incidents on the film, as well as on the motives, goals, attitudes, emotions, and values of the film maker.

A final observational approach we employ has to do with studying the same person over time in multiple settings. After some period of participant-observation, we are able to characterize a person's competence in many of the various settings that make up his ordinary world. We know how competent he or she is with regard to routine aspects of housekeeping, personal grooming, using public transportation, working, preparing meals, and social interaction in recreational settings. We compare repertoires of behavior in different settings, searching for similarities or differences in competence. We may find, for example, that a person is terribly inept in tasks that call for fine muscle coordination or the use of money, but this same person may be highly competent in ordinary conversation with strangers in public places. We systematically observe and compare the retarded person's behavior in all the settings to which we have access.

We also introduce many persons to new settings where we can carefully observe their reactions to new tasks and circumstances. Although this is not exactly experimentation, it is in some respects similar. For example, we may take someone to a large medical center, to a restaurant, to the beach, to a bowling alley, or to a job training center. Observing the person's efforts to cope with these novel experiences helps us to understand not only their everyday routines of life, but their potential for an increasingly competent way of life. It gives valuable information in learning, problem-solving, and adaptive strategies, information that is simply not available through any amount of IQ testing, interviewing, or questionnaires. Observations of this sort, within a single subject research design, are not terribly difficult to carry out and are of inestimable value.

The kinds of participant-observational techniques we have discussed here have many limitations. First, they are expensive. Trained participant-observers must spend long periods of time—a year is minimal—in data collection. Most forms of systematic observation can be carried out in much shorter periods of time (Willems, 1967). A second problem involves data reductions. The data produced by participant-observation are fieldnotes, narrative protocols, video tapes, and the like. If these data are to be "reduced" to variables or categories for quantitative manipulation and analysis, another long period is necessary for coding. Still a third problem has to do with the replicability of such data. It is often asserted that such data cannot be replicated at all, since neither the research procedures nor the resulting observations have been fully operationalized. Such complaints are not entirely justified. No science is as objective as it would like to be; and it has also been argued that complex episodes of human behavior cannot in principle be replicated since each is an ad hoc, separate, and individual experience that can never be recaptured or repeated in precisely the same form (Louch, 1966; Harre and Secord, 1972). Whereas there is something to be said for this contention, it can also be said that it *is* possible to estimate the reliability of the data yielded by participant-observation (Honigman, 1976). Multiple observers can be employed and some observations can be repeated. The real difficulty lies primarily in the fact that such data remain enmeshed in a broad social, cultural, and personal context. They do not come neatly packaged into variables or units that can easily be manipulated.

This leads to the final limitation, namely, the danger that participant-observation will suffer from observer bias. It is undeniable that participant-observers develop loyalties and dislikes, that they become involved in the lives of the persons they study. For example, our observers often find that the retarded persons they study become dependent upon them. This results in the possibility that our very research presence reduces, or at other times actually enhances, the displayed competence of the persons we are studying. These problems can be mitigated by the use of several observers, by self-conscious alteration of the role taken by the participant-observer, and by the use of audio and video recording so that ''uninvolved'' observers may also analyze, and sometimes ''correct'' the fieldworkers' behavior. Devices and safeguards such as these may reduce the problems of subjectivity somewhat, but the basic problem remains. Such problems take us directly into fundamental questions about methodology in the social sciences. It is interesting to note that there has been greatly increased interest in self-consciousness in anthropology in recent years (Nash and Wintrob, 1972).

CONCLUSION

As a complement to ethological observation, we have briefly described a set of ethnographic research procedures built around the technique of participant-observation. This approach has its roots in natural history, yet as we have seen it differs in many ways from the kind of observation done by ethologists. It emphasizes time and context, it utilizes participation, and it searches for meaning by talking to people and attempting to see and understand the world as they do. As Margaret Mead (1976) has pointed out in her Presidential Address to the American Association for the Advancement of Science, no single research approach—whether positivistic or humanistic—can be expected fully to comprehend complex systems of human behavior. Progress will be made not by rejecting one method in favor of another, but by combining several complementary methods.

Unfortunately, the current climate of research in the social sciences seems more likely to achieve polarization than complementarity. Indeed, social scientists who prefer ''qualitative'' or ''naturalistic'' methods often scorn those who utilize quantitative or experimental approaches, and these latter scientists often reject the former with equal acerbity. Thus Harre and Secord (1972) have challenged the positivistic philosophy that has long dominated thinking in psychology. Phillips (1973) has done the same thing in sociology, as have Winch (1958) and Louch (1966) with regard to social sciences in general. In anthropology, Geertz has emphasized the humanistic or artistic aspects of ethnographic research, saying:

> Cultural analysis is intrinsically incomplete. And, worse than that, the more deeply it goes, the less complete it is. It is a strange science whose most telling assertions are its most tremulously based, in which to get somewhere with the matter at hand is to intensify the suspicion, both your own and that of others, that you are not getting it right (Geertz, 1973, p. 29).

The challenge to positivistic methods was well posed by Irwin Deutscher:

> There was a time earlier in this century when we had a choice to make, a choice on the one hand of undertaking neat, orderly studies of measurable phenomena. This alternative carried with it all of the gratifications of conforming to the prestigious methods of pursuing knowledge then in vogue, of having access to considerable sums of monies through the granting procedures of large foundations and governmental agencies, of a comfortable sense of satisfaction derived from dealing rigorously and precisely with small isolated problems which were cleanly defined, of moving for 30 years down one track in an increasingly rigorous, refined, and reliable manner, while simultaneously disposing of the problems of validity by the semantic trickery of operational definitions. On the other hand, we could have tackled the messy world as we knew it to exist, a world where the same people will make different utterances under different conditions and will behave differently in different situations and will say one thing while doing another. We could have tackled a world where control of relevant variables was impossible not only because we didn't know what they were, but because we didn't know how they interacted with each other. We could have accepted the conclusion of almost every variant of contemporary philosophy of science, that the notion of cause and effect (and therefore of stimulus and response or of independent and dependent variables) is untenable. We eschewed this formidable challenge. This was the hard way. We chose the easy way (Deutscher, 1966, p. 244).

In the 10 years since Deutscher's challenge, there has been an impressive outpouring of books that present qualitative methods (e.g., Webb, Campbell, Schwartz, and Sechrest, 1966; Garfinkel, 1967; Filstead, 1970; Lofland, 1971; Harre and Secord, 1972; Phillips, 1973; Speier, 1973; Schatzman and Strauss, 1973; Bogdan and Taylor, 1975). The result is a growing awareness of qualitative methods, but as yet there has been little evidence of widespread desire to combine qualitative methods with quantitative ones.

Our approach does not derive from this recent interest in qualitative methods but rather from the traditional turn-of-the-century anthropological use of participant-observation in ethnographic fieldwork. As practiced and espoused by the founders of anthropology, such as Franz Boas and Bronislaw Malinowski, participant-observation has never consisted of more than general principles to be carried out by any means appropriate to a given research situation. This "personal approach" has recently been eloquently defined by John Honigmann (1976) and others. The *ad lib* quality of the method has alienated many researchers who prefer the precision of tests, interviews, experiments, or systematic observation. That participant-observation has many weaknesses is obvious, but its strengths should not be overlooked or underestimated. Through its reliance on prolonged involvement in the lives of others, it offers, perhaps beyond any other method, a means of reducing reactivity and comprehending meaning. If one is seriously searching for complementary methods for the study of human behavior, these are important benefits. That the method is imprecise and sometimes even inexplicable need not result in its rejection. As C. Wright Mills (1959) insisted, quoting the opinion of the Nobel Laureate physicist Percy Bridgman, good method consists primarily of common sense and hard work.

Participant-observation can produce results that are complex and even contradictory, but these are qualities that often characterize human life. The method need not be "artistic" or arcane; as participant-observation has developed over the years, its "naturalistic" procedures have become increasingly specifiable and replicable (Denzin, 1971). As a result we offer this approach as a complement to more systematic or ethological kinds of observation in the study of mentally retarded persons in the community. Many of these people lead largely normal lives in various community settings, and to study them in community settings by means of ethological observation could produce valuable insights. But to go beyond the information that such observation can yield, we need a method that will yield more understanding of the cares, hopes, fantasies, and values of these people. In addition to watching retarded people, we need to talk with them and listen to them. We need an approach, that is, that includes emics as well as etics. As Edgerton (1967) and Bogdan and Taylor (1976) have insisted, there is much to be learned by treating the retarded as both the *subjects* and the *objects* of study.

REFERENCES

Barker, R. G. 1968. Ecological Psychology. Stanford University Press, Stanford.

Bjaanes, A. T., and Butler, E. W. 1974. Environmental variation in community care facilities for mentally retarded persons. Am. J. Ment. Defic. 78:429–439.

Blurton-Jones, N. (ed.). 1972. Ethological Studies of Child Behaviour. Cambridge University Press, London.

Bogdan, R., and Taylor, S. J. 1975. Introduction to Qualitative Research Methods. Riley, New York.

Bogdan, R., and Taylor, S. 1976. The judged, not the judges. An insider's view of mental retardation. Am. Psychol. 31:47–52.

Brandt, R. M. 1972. Studying Behavior in Natural Settings. Holt, Rinehart & Winston, New York.

Brunswik, E. 1955. Representative design and probabilistic theory in a functional psychology. Psychol. Rev. 62:193–217.

Campbell, C. M. 1968. Stereotyped and expressive movements in imbeciles. Am. J. Ment. Defic. 73:187–194.

Cicourel, A. J. 1974. Cognitive Sociology: Language and Meaning in Social Interaction. The Free Press, New York.

Davis, K. V., Sprague, R. L., and Werry, J. S. 1969. Stereotyped behavior and activity level in severe retardates: the effect of drugs. Am. J. Ment. Defic. 73:721–727.

Denzin, N. K. 1971. The logic of naturalistic inquiry. Soc. Forces 50:166–182.

Deutscher, I. 1966. Words and deeds: social science and social policy. Soc. Probl. 13:235–254.

Domino, G. 1967. The identification of behavioral aggression in the mentally retarded. Train. School Bull. 64:66–72.

Edgerton, R. B. 1967. The Cloak of Competence. University of California Press, Berkeley.

Edgerton, R. B., and Bercovici, S. M. 1976. The cloak of competence—years later. Am. J. Ment. Defic. 80:485–497.

Eyberg, S. M., and Johnson, S. M. 1974. Multiple assessment of behavior modification with families: effects of contingency contracting and order of treated problems. J. Consulting Clin. Psychol. 42:594–606.

Filstead, W., (ed.). 1970. Qualitative Methodology. Markham, Chicago.

Fivars, G., (ed.). 1973. The Critical Incident Technique: A Bibliography. American Institutes for Research, Palo Alto.

Flanagan, J. C. 1954. The critical incident technique. Psychol. Bull. 51:327–358.

Fleming, J. W. 1962. The critical incident technique as an aid to in-service training. Am. J. Ment. Defic. 67:41–52.

Forness, S. R., and Esveldt, K. C. 1975. Classroom observation of children with learning and behavior problems. J. Learn. Disabilities 8:49–52.

Gallimore, R., Tharp, R., and Speidel, G. 1975. The relationship of sibling caretaking and attentiveness to a peer tutor (Tech. Rep. #20). The Kamehameha Schools, Kamehameha Early Education Program, Honolulu.

Garfinkel, H. 1967. Studies in Ethonomethodology. Prentice-Hall Inc., Englewood Cliffs.

Geertz, C. 1973. The Interpretation of Cultures. Basic Books Inc., New York.

Glazer, B., and Strauss, A. 1967. The Discovery of Grounded Theory: Strategies for Qualitative Research. Aldine Publishing Company, Chicago.

Goroff, N. N. 1967. Research and community placement—an exploratory approach. Ment. Retard. 5:17–19.

Griffin, J. H. 1960. Black Like Me. Houghton Mifflin Company, Boston.

Guilmet, G., and Langness, L. L. 1976. The Non-Verbal Ethnic Child in the Classroom. Research proposal submitted to The National Science Foundation.

Harre, R., and Secord, P. F. 1972. The Explanation of Social Behaviour. Basil Blackwell & Mott Ltd., Oxford.

Harris, M. 1964. The Nature of Cultural Things. Random House, New York.

Henschel, A. M. 1972. The Forgotten Ones. University of Texas Press, Austin.

Honigmann, J. J. 1976. The personal approach in cultural anthropological research. Curr. Anthropol. 6 (No. 2).

Hutt, S. J., and Hutt, C. 1970. Direct Observation and Measurement of Behavior. Charles C Thomas Publisher, Springfield.

Jacobs, A. M., Nichols, D. G., and Larsen, J. K. 1973. Critical nursing behaviors in the care of the mentally retarded. Int. Nurs. Rev. 20:117–122.

Johnson, S. M., and Bolstad, O. D. 1975. Reactivity to home observation: a comparison of audio recorded behavior with observers present or absent. J. Appl. Behav. Anal. 8:181–185.

Kelly, J. G. 1967. Naturalistic observations and theory confirmation: an example. Hum. Dev. 10:212–222.

Kogan, K. L., Wimberger, H. C., and Bobbitt, R. A. 1969. Analysis of mother-child interaction in young mental retardates. Child Dev. 40:799–812.

Kogan, K. L., and Tyler, N. 1973. Mother-child interaction in young physically handicapped children. Am. J. Ment. Defic. 77:492–497.

Langness, L. L. 1970. Entree into the field: highlands New Guinea. In: R. Naroll and R. Cohen (eds.), A Handbook of Method in Cultural Anthropology, pp. 220–225. The Natural History Press, New York.

Langness, L. L. 1974. The Study of Culture. Chandler & Sharp Publishers Inc., San Francisco.

Lipinski, D., and Nelson, R. 1974. Problems in the use of naturalistic observation as a means of behavioral assessment. Behav. Ther. 5:341–351.

Lofland, J. 1971. Analyzing Social Settings: A Guide to Qualitative Observation and Analysis. Wadsworth Publishing Company Inc., Belmont, California.

Louch, A. R. 1966. Explanation and Human Action. Basil Blackwell & Mott Ltd., Oxford.

Luckey, R. E. 1966. Adult retardates responsiveness to recordings as a functioning of music therapist participation. Am. Soc. Ment. Defic. 71:109–111.

MacAndrew, C., and Edgerton, R. B. 1964. The everyday life of institutionalized 'idiots.' Hum. Organization 23:312–318.

Madge, J. 1953. The Tools of Social Science. Longmans, Green & Co., Inc., New York.

Mattison, J. 1970. Marriage and Mental Handicap. Gerald Duckworth & Co. Ltd., London.

Mead, M. 1976. Towards a human science. Science 191:903–909.

McGrew, W. C. 1972. An Ethological Study of Children's Behavior. Academic Press, New York.

Mercer, J. 1973. Labeling the Mentally Retarded: Clinical and Social System Perspectives on Mental Retardation. University of California Press, Berkeley.

Mills, C. W. 1959. The Sociological Imagination. Oxford University Press, London.

Nash, D., and Wintrob, R. 1972. The emergence of self-consciousness in ethnography. Curr. Anthropol. 13, No. 5:527–542.

Pelto, P. J. 1970. Anthropological Research: The Structure of Inquiry. Harper and Row, New York.

Phillips, D. L. 1973. Abandoning Method. Jossey-Bass, Inc., San Francisco.

Rosenhan, D. L. 1973. On being sane in insane places. Science 179:250–258.

Schatzman, L., and Strauss, A. 1973. Field Research: Strategies for a Natural Sociology. Prentice-Hall Inc., Englewood Cliffs.

Speier, M. 1973. How to Observe Face-to-Face Communication: A Sociological Introduction. Goodyear, Pacific Palisades, California.

Steiner, K. E., and Cochran, L. L. 1966. The simulated critical incident technique as an evaluation and teaching service. Am. J. Ment. Defic. 70:835–839.

Webb, E. J., Campbell, D. T., Schwartz, R. D., and Sechrest, L. 1966. Unobtrusive Measures: Nonreactive Research in the Social Sciences. Rand McNally & Company, Chicago.

White, B. L., and Watts, J. C. 1973. Experience and Environment: Major Influences on the Development of the Young Child, Vol. 1. Prentice-Hall Inc., Englewood Cliffs.

Willems, E. P. 1967. Toward an explicit rationale for naturalistic research methods. Hum. Dev. 10:138–154.

Wills, R. H. 1973. The Institutionalized Severely Retarded. A Study of Activities and Interaction. Charles C. Thomas Publisher, Springfield.

Winch, P. 1958. The Idea of a Social Science. Routledge & Kegan Paul Ltd., London.

Wolfensberger, W. 1972. Normalization. National Institute on Mental Retardation, Toronto.

Zeilberger, J., Sampan, S. E., and Sloane, H. W., Jr. 1968. Modification of a child's problem behaviors in the home with the mother as therapist. J. Appl. Behav. Anal. 1:47–53.

chapter 15

A Behavioral and Ecological Study of Group Homes

Sharon Landesman-Dwyer, Jody G. Stein, and Gene P. Sackett

The current emphasis in the field of mental retardation is to get the retarded out of institutions and into the normal mainstream. The appeal of humanitarian goals (such as the opportunity for a more normal lifestyle, the right to privacy and personal dignity, freedom from discrimination and segregation), coupled with devastating critiques of the institutional environment, have paved the way for dramatic changes in social policy. At the national, state, and local levels, high priority is assigned to rapid deinstitutionalization and to the development of alternative residential facilities for the retarded. Concomitantly, detailed standards and elaborate tools for evaluating community residences have evolved, dictating precisely which features of the environment are thought to be "optimal" or "desirable." Unfortunately, these standards reflect untested assumptions and beliefs and are not based on empirical evidence. In effect, the movement to small community-based facilities may be viewed as a large scale, poorly controlled human experiment, guided by the good intentions and economic considerations of politicians, planners, parents, and professionals. What is lacking is an objective assessment of the physical and social impact of the environment on the mentally retarded.

Many retrospective studies have attempted to describe important factors in the adjustment of previously institutionalized individuals to community placement (Edgerton, 1967; Eagle, 1968; Stephens, Peck, and Veldman, 1968; Hoffman, 1969; Song and Song, 1969; Rosen, Kivitz, Clark, and Floor, 1970; Skaarbrevik, 1971; Kraus, 1972; Rosen, Floor, and Baxter, 1972, 1974; Nihira and Nihira, 1975; Edgerton and Bercovici, 1976). These studies have found that many retarded adults can "succeed" in community living, whereas many others cannot adjust, and are at high risk for being returned to an institution. However, they are *equivocal* as to which client characteristics might best predict "success." To some degree, the discrepancies may be attributed to differences in a) outcome measures of what comprises "success," b) types of clients and their previous life experiences, c) characteristics of the community facilities and the supportive services available to the clients, d) geography, history, and politics unique to each study, and e) data collection methods. The majority of studies relied on information obtained from client records, questionnaires, interviews, and standardized tests or test-like situations. Seldom do the investigators discuss the reliability or validity of their data. Rosen, Floor, and Baxter (1972) twice tried unsuccessfully to replicate their earlier findings relating client characteristics (inferred from records, staff ratings, and test performance) to adaptation to community living (evaluated by client interviews), and concluded that "this research effort cast doubt upon the efficacy of an empirical shotgun approach to predicting complex criteria of community adjustment" (p. 112).

A different approach to studying the retarded in community settings is simply direct observation of what happens from day to day. The potential usefulness of this method has been advocated for many years (Butterfield, 1967; Dingman, 1968; Balla, Butterfield, and Zigler, 1973) but only a few studies have reported systematic observations in a variety of community settings (e.g., Bjaanes and Butler, 1974; Landesman-Dwyer, Stein, and Sackett, 1976).

Bjaanes and Butler (1974) compared the behavior of 10 individuals in two home care facilities with that of 54 individuals in two board-and-care facilities, all in southern California. They coded and described all activities observed in four 2 to 3-hr sessions per subject, based on whether the activities were independent or dependent; spontaneous, planned, or routine; structured or not; obligatory or discretionary; and "passing" (defined as "a deliberate attempt by the retarded person to conceal his incompetency and history of institutionalization" p. 431) or "natural." The frequency and proportion of time spent in each major activity category, as well as the characteristics of the behaviors, were analyzed for the four facilities. The tentative conclusions were that social competence and independence were greater in the two large board-and-care settings than in the two small homes. Furthermore, from the observed differences in these four facilities, Bjaanes and Butler suggested that proximity to the community, geographic factors, and the degree of caregiver involvement may be important influences on resident activities.

More general assessment of the relationship of the environment to the ongoing behavior of groups and of individuals derives from the work of ecological psychologists (notably, Barker, 1960, 1968), environmental psychologists (e.g., Proshansky, Ittelson, and Rivlin, 1970; Wohlwill, 1970; Craik, 1973) and human social ecologists (e.g., Moos and Insell, 1974). Ecological principles relating various physical, social, and psychological characteristics of the environment to behavior have been proposed and empirically validated to some extent (e.g., Barker, 1960; Proshansky, Ittelson, and Rivlin, 1970; Stokols, 1972; Wicker, McGrath, and Armstrong, 1972; Evans, 1973; Ittelson, Proshansky, Rivlin, and Winkel, 1974; Stokols, 1975; Stokols and Marrero, 1976). Many of the ecological constructs appear heuristic for analyzing group behavior of the retarded and their caregivers. For example, Barker (1960) developed a theory of "undermanning" in which greater stress supposedly is exerted on individuals when a setting is understaffed relative to the tasks to be accomplished. Another construct used to study human groups is "crowding," which is viewed as both a physical and psychological phenomenon affecting aggression, territoriality, and social behavior (e.g., Stokols, 1972, 1975). Extension of these general fields, with their emphasis on naturalistic and longitudinal observations, appears promising for investigating groups of retarded persons in community settings.

Similarly, architectural features have been implicated as important factors influencing activities and the "psychological welfare" of individuals. The burgeoning literature on environments for the developmentally disabled offers an abundance of theories and ideas (e.g., Dybwad, 1968; Gunzberg, 1968; Schwerdt, 1968; Norris, 1969; Dybwad, 1970; Nirje, 1970; Pederson, 1970; Gunzberg, 1973; Bedner, 1974). For example, Bedner's review of facilities in Denmark, Sweden, and Holland (1974) focused on 15 investigative issues related to the concept of ''normalization'' and considered which architectural components were designed with specific behavioral objectives in mind. Currently, much money is being allocated for design and construction of ''better'' group living arrangements ''for'' the retarded. However, as Dybwad (1970) cautions:

> Much of what has been said is still speculative and . . . [there is] the need for careful research in a controlled setting. Unfortunately, there have been practically no instances where in designing of new facilities a deliberate attempt is made to create parallel settings differing in important exterior and interior features of architectural design to permit ongoing comparative studies (p. 48).

In sum, the reasons for studying the movement to community-based treatment range widely from practical and political considerations to basic theoretical issues. The practical reasons are virtually synonymous with ''accountability.'' That is, to what extent does a program measurably achieve its stated objectives? The theoretical issues concern the effects of the environment on behavior and the nature of social organizations. However, since very little is known about the behavioral repertoire or naturally occurring ''culture'' of the retarded, theorizing about the effects of certain factors (e.g., size and heterogeneity of group, amount of space, etc.) is likely to be premature or overly simplified at this stage. Moreover, the degree to which principles about group behavior can be generalized across different populations—particularly for individuals with abnormally functioning nervous systems or with very divergent life histories—is not known. Thus, the present investigation of group homes in Washington State was undertaken to provide some basic descriptive data about the daily lives of retarded children and adults in a variety of community settings.

HISTORY OF GROUP HOMES IN WASHINGTON STATE

Washington State has been a national leader in establishing small community-based group homes licensed for the care of the mentally retarded. These group homes are privately owned and operated, serve six to twenty residents each, and are supervised by a local advisory board and by the state's Bureau of Developmental Disabilities (Department of Social and Health Services). There is no single philosophy or set of objectives common to all group homes other than the goal of improving the quality of life. Generally, the group home concept emphasizes integrating clients into the community and encouraging advancement in skills for independent living, working, and interpersonal relationships. However, the degree to which individuals achieve these goals in their day-to-day activities has not been evaluated systematically or objectively. In fact, surprisingly little is known about the residents in these group homes or about the characteristics of the facilities.

The goal of the present study was to objectively describe the group home program in Washington State in terms of the behavior of residents and staff and the group home resources. It began as a pilot application of an ethological-observational methodology for assessing group living situations. Evaluating the usefulness and validity of such behavioral data, in contrast to the more conventional and subjective information from interviews and questionnaires, is an important and integral aspect of this research.

The specific aims of this study included 1) systematically observing the daily activities of both residents and staff; 2) describing in detail the ecological features of Washington's group homes; and 3) determining whether there were significant relationships between the observed activities and the measurable characteristics of the group homes or of the residents. To our knowledge, this study is unique in several respects. First, the scope is broad. More than 400 individuals in 23 facilities were observed over approximately a 40-hr period. The residents represent a heterogeneous group, including children as well as adults, the severely and profoundly retarded as well as the mildly and moderately retarded, and noninstitutionalized as well as previously institutionalized individuals. Second, the scoring methodology permits analyses of the relationship of time, sequence, and environmental resources to the ongoing behavior of both individuals and groups of individuals. Moreover, a complete scoring of all social interactions within a facility provides an opportunity to study social interactions and friendship choice. Third, the behavioral observations can be compared with information obtained from client records and from interviews with staff; and fourth, the entire research effort was coordinated with state planners and group home operators, so that the findings and their potential interpretation could be part of the changing social service delivery system.

METHODS

Selection of Group Homes and Subjects

Twenty of Washington's 43 group homes were selected to represent as closely as possible the eight characteristics in Table 1: geography, neighborhood, size, age of residents, level of retardation, co-ed living arrangements, proprietorship, and type of building. In addition, three half-way houses were studied. All residents and staff in these 23 settings were invited to participate and informed consent was obtained from 406 persons, with only 13 not consenting to be observed.

The residents ranged from 9 to 62 years old, with 75% in the 16 to 36-year-old range. Seventy-seven percent of the residents had previously resided in state institutions for the mentally retarded. According to medical records, 10% of the residents were classified as borderline or not retarded, 28% as mildly retarded, 41% as moderately retarded, 17% as severely retarded, and 3% as profoundly retarded. Fifty-five percent of the residents were males and 45% were females. (For a more complete description of the resident population, see Landesman-Dwyer, Stein, and Sackett, 1976.)

Naturalistic Observations and Scoring Procedures

Naturalistic observations were conducted using the Home Observation Code (HOC) (see Landesman-Dwyer, Stein, and Sackett, 1976, for definitions and scoring procedures), which provides a systematic and objective means for describing individuals' actual be-

Table 1. Basic characteristics of group homes in Washington State

Characteristics	All group homes		Group homes in study	
	Number	%	Number	%
Geography				
Eastern Washington	14	32.6	6	30
Western Washington	29	67.4	14	70
Neighborhood				
Urban	25	58.1	10	50
Suburban	7	16.3	4	20
Rural	11	25.6	6	30
Size				
6–10 residents (small)	14	32.6	5	25
11–17 residents (medium)	10	23.2	6	30
18–20 residents (large)	19	44.2	9	45
Residents' age grouping				
Children only	13	30.2	7	35
Adults only	26	60.5	11	55
Children and adults	4	9.3	2	10
Living arrangements				
All males	5	11.6	3	15
All females	5	11.6	0	0
Males and females	33	76.8	17	85
Residents' level of retardation				
Mildly-moderately retarded	26	60.5	13	65
Moderately-severely retarded	13	30.2	5	25
Severely retarded, multiply handicapped	4	9.3	2	10
Proprietorship				
Nonprofit	19	44.2	8	40
Proprietary	24	55.8	12	60
Building				
New—private funds	7	16.3	5	25
New—federal funds	7	16.3	4	20
Existing building	29	67.4	11	55

haviors and their relationship to the environment. Each observation or code entry contained information pertaining to 10 separate behavioral or ecological variables:

1. Subject ID number
2. time of day
3. location of subject

4. major activities of subject (see Table 2)
5. physical-gestural communication (see Table 3)
6. verbal communication (see Table 3)
7. assistance needed or received
8. use of objects (see Table 4)
9. minor stereotypies
10. with whom major activity of subject occurred

Table 2. Listing of major activities in Home Observation Code

	Basic sleep and wake behaviors		Social activities
1	Sleep	40	Affection and courting
2	Inactive	41	Intimate contact
3	Attentive looking	42	Approving or rewarding
4	General movement	43	Receiving approval or rewards
5	Specific transition	44	Assisting
6	Specific waiting	45	Defending/protecting
9	Other (to be specified)	46	Being defended/protected/consoled
		47	Sharing resources
	Self-care activities	48	Teasing and joking
		50	Initiates social interaction, general
10	Bathing	51	Responds to social interaction, general
11	Grooming	52	Mutual general social interaction
12	Dressing	53	Disapproving or punishing
13	Toileting	54	Receiving disapproval or punishment
14	Eating	55	Competition or aggression
15	Health-related activities	56	Receiving competition or aggression
19	Other self-help behaviors (to be specified)	59	Other social interaction (to be specified)
			Work and group maintenance activities
	Play, recreation, fine motor skills		
		60	Cleaning
20	Unstructured activity	61	Organizing
21	Focused activity	62	Preparing and planning
22	Gross motor/recreational skills	63	Directing or supervising
23	Externally structured activity	64	Building/constructing
24	Specific handicraft/fine motor skills	69	Other group activities (to be specified)
25	Formal game or recreation		
29	Other activities (to be specified)		Unusual, asocial, or repetitive behavior
	Educational and formal training activities	70	Abnormal-unusual
		71	Repetitive body movement
		72	Withdrawal
30	Transmitting information	73	Mimicking or echolalic behavior
31	Reception/observation of information	74	Persistent following
32	Active participation		
33	Imitation/simple rote		Unobservable or not in home
34	Focused symbolic behavior		
35	Specific problem resolution	75	Could not find, should be in house
36	Lack of or negative response to learning situation	76	Left house—score purpose separately
		77	Unable to observe—other reason(s)
39	Other learning situation (to be specified)	78	Ill
		79	Other (to be specified)

Table 3. Additional characteristics of behaviors in Home Observation Code

Physical-gestural communication	Verbal communication	Assistance needed or received	Minor stereotypies
0 None	0 None	0 No assistance-	0 Absent
1 Directive	1 Directive	1 No assistance-inappropriate	1 Present
2 Informative	2 Informative	2 No assistance-undeterminable	(to be specified further when observed)
3 Expressive	3 Expressive-conversational	3 Assistance desirable	
4 Physical contact	4 Question	4 Verbal assistance given but not essential	
5 Listening	5 Answer	5 Verbal assistance given and needed	
6 Laughter; gleeful sounds	6 Singing	6 Physical assistance given and needed	
7 Cry or distress sounds	7 Not understood by observer	7 Verbal and physical assistance given and needed	
8 Sign language	8 Repetitive	8 Physical assistance given, but not essential	
9 Other (to be specified)	9 Other (to be specified)	9 Other (to be specified)	

On one weekday and on one weekend day, the observers spent the entire day recording the behavior of staff and residents in each group home. Observers started collecting data early in the morning (usually between 5:00 and 7:00 a.m.) and continued until late at night (usually between 10:00 p.m. and 2:00 a.m.). Each subject (if available) was observed at least once every 15 min, and all 10 variables listed above were coded numerically. Table 2 lists the original 62 major activity codes and Table 3 summarizes the codes for physical-gestural communication, verbal communication, and the dimension of assistance from others. A sample of four code entries during an hour for a single subject is provided in Table 5, along with an interpretation of the codes. For the entire study, approximately 16,000 hr of behavior were sampled. Whenever possible, the observers joined the residents who left the home, and often continued to describe ongoing activities. In addition, the observers kept detailed notes, organized by coding categories, about the level or quality of each resident's behavior.

Table 4. Listing of objects in Home Observation Code

Code	Object
00	No Object
	Furniture and plumbing
01	Couches, chairs, stools
02	Tables
03	Storage spaces, closets, dressers, drawers
04	Beds
05	Toilets
06	Lamps, lighting
07	Bathtub, shower
08	Sink
09	Other (to be specified)
	Structural features
10	Floors
11	Walls
12	Doors and doorways
13	Windows
14	Ceilings
19	Other (to be specified)
	Toys, games, recreational equipment, and related items
20	Sports equipment
21	Table games
22	Indoor larger game equipment
23	Common children's toys
24	Outside play equipment
25	Craft and art supplies and tools
26	Musical instruments
27	Electrical equipment for construction (to be specified)
28	Exercise equipment
29	Other (to be specified)
	Reading, writing, and office related materials
30	Books
31	Newspapers
32	Magazines
33	Writing materials
34	Business related papers
35	Calendars
36	Schedules
37	Workbooks-programmed, school/work related
38	Typewriter, calculator, adding machine
39	Other (to be specified)
	Communication/transmission devices
40	TV
41	Radio
42	Phonograph
43	Tape recorder
44	Telephone
45	Intercom or walkie-talkie
49	Other (to be specified)
	Common household items
50	Stove
51	Refrigerator-freezer
52	Dishwasher
53	Washer-dryer
54	Common kitchen utensils
55	Small kitchen electrical appliances
56	Tools and special manual instruments (scissors)
57	Vacuum cleaner and floor polisher
58	Broom, mop
60	Food
61	Plants-garden
62	Cleaning agents
69	Other (to be specified)
	Personal items
70	Clothing
71	Trinkets
72	Towels, sheets, blankets, pillows
73	Personal items—wallet, purse, daypack, comb
74	Body parts
75	Drugs, medicine
79	Other (to be specified)
	Vehicles, transportation objects
80	Bus
81	Car
82	Bike, scooter, tricycle
83	Wheelchair
84	Other (to be specified)
	Pets, people, and multiple objects
90	Pets
91	People
99	More than one object (to be specified)

Table 5. Sample observations for a subject during 1 hr

	ID number	Time (24 hr clock)	Location	Major activity	Physical-gestural communication	Verbal communication	Assistance	Use of objects	With whom	Minor stereotypy
1.	10	1800	61	60	0	0	0	54	0	0
2.	10	1815	44	14	0	3	0	60	12 and 19	1
3.	10	1830	44	52	6	0	0	0	19	0
4.	10	1845	49	21	0	6	0	40	15, 18, and 19	0

Interpretation of code entries above:

1. Subject 10, at 6:00 p.m., was in the kitchen, organizing the silverware.
2. Subject 10, at 6:15 p.m., was in the dining room, eating dinner, having a discussion with two other residents (12 and 19), and repetitively rocking.
3. Subject 10, at 6:30 p.m., was in the dining room, laughing, continuing her social interaction with resident 19.
4. Subject 10, at 6:45 p.m., was in the upstairs living room, watching TV, singing along with the show, with residents 15, 18, and 19.

Table 6. Categories of ecological features of group homes

- I. Gross features
  - A. Home and property
    1. Dimensions—external
    2. Natural features (trees, hills, gardens, water, etc.)
    3. Additional structures (garages, buildings, walkways, etc.)
    4. Internal dimensions of home (number and arrangement of rooms, doors, windows, storage areas, etc.)
  - B. Neighborhood
    1. Other homes and property
    2. Residents (number, ages, socioeconomic status, etc.)
    3. Institutions and schools
    4. Commercial areas
    5. Parks and community resources in neighborhood
    6. Public transportation
  - C. Community
    1. General facilities (educational, recreational, protective, etc.)
    2. Specific community programs available to public
    3. Programs available for retarded children and adults
    4. Individuals and groups directly connected with group home
    5. Health-related services
- II. Specific resources within the home
  - A. Furniture
  - B. Lighting
  - C. TV's, radios, phonographs, musical instruments
  - D. Recreation and play equipment
  - E. Books and magazines
  - F. Craft supplies and tools
  - G. Transportation
  - H. Food—quality, quantity, accessibility
  - I. Private areas (individually or group-assigned)
  - J. Other resources
- III. Staff

Ecological Description Methods

The observers visited the group homes before the two observational days to map the number, arrangement, and type of rooms and to obtain a complete inventory of all resources and objects within each home. The general format for recording and categorizing ecological characteristics is shown in Table 6.

Interview Format

The observers interviewed group home staff to find out how the staff perceived individual residents and their service needs. A semistructured format was used and staff responses were coded on standard forms. Originally, we planned to interview residents also. However, we abandoned this plan after a pilot study because intraresident reliability in response to the same questions was very low, and often extremely contradictory.

RESULTS

The results presented here will focus on the relationship of major activities to characteristics of the residents and of the facilities. Other components of this study are analyzed elsewhere (Landesman-Dwyer, Stein, and Sackett, 1976; Landesman-Dwyer and Berkson, 1976; Sackett and Landesman-Dwyer, 1977).

Major Activities of Residents

The original 62 codes for major activities were reduced to 21 categories for summary and analysis. Table 7 shows the mean proportion of time (frequency of occurrence of each activity divided by the total number of observations per subject) that residents were observed in each activity category. Overall, more than 75% of the residents' time (excluding night sleep periods) was spent in five behavior categories: unstructured activities ($\bar{X}$ = 23.0%, s.d. =14.0%), inactive behaviors ($\bar{X}$ = 17.7%, s.d. =11.7%), general social behaviors ($\bar{X}$ = 13.1%, s.d. =9.4%), household maintenance ($\bar{X}$ = 10.7%, s.d. =8.5%), and eating ($\bar{X}$ = 10.7%, s.d. =4.8%). The "unstructured activities" included television watching and a variety of spontaneous, nonspecific pastimes, such as simply sitting and relaxing, waiting, or gazing into space.

"Organized activities," including games, handicrafts, sports, and hobbies, comprised nearly 5% of the residents' activities in their homes ($\bar{X}$ = 4.5%, s.d. =6.7%). "Self-care," including dressing, bathing, grooming, and toileting, occupied 4% of the residents' observed behavior ($\bar{X}$ = 4.2%, s.d. =3.6%).

The single event of "leaving the house" occurred in nearly 3% of the observation periods ($\bar{X}$ = 2.7%, s.d. =1.6%). Although 98% of the residents regularly participated in school, work, or other training programs during the weekdays, the single event of leaving to attend these scheduled programs would account for *less* than 1% of the observations. Thus, the residents left their homes over six more times than necessary, and frequently did so independently. The reasons for leaving ranged from visiting friends in neighboring group homes to participating in community activities such as dances, bowling, swimming, talent shows, or shopping.

Academic activities ("reading, writing, and arithmetic") accounted for less than 2% of the observations ($\bar{X}$ = 1.9%, s.d. =4.5%). "Undesirable behavior" also occupied less than 2% of the observation time ($\bar{X}$ = 1.6%, s.d. =5.2%). Behavioral profiles revealed that some subjects spent a considerable proportion of time in one or both of these activities, whereas many others never were observed in academic activities or undesirable behavior.

Relationship of Daily Activities to Resident Characteristics

To determine whether specific characteristics of the residents related significantly to observed behaviors, multiple regression analyses (model 3, stepdown regression analysis, Overall and Spiegel, 1969) were performed for the major activity categories. The individual resident characteristics entering into the regression analyses were: 1) level of

Table 7. Means and standard deviations for major activity categories[a]

Major activity category (original codes)	Mean (%)	Standard deviation (%)
Sleep (1)—excluding night sleep period	1.16	3.20
Inactive behaviors (2–9)	17.73	11.74
Self-care (10–13, 15–19)	4.21	3.61
Eating (14)	10.71	4.80
Unstructured activities (20–21)	23.02	14.04
Organized activities (22–29)	4.46	6.68
Active learning (30, 32, 39)	0.45	1.76
Reading, writing, arithmetic (34)	1.85	4.53
Problem solving (35)	0.04	0.24
Observation-imitation (31, 33)	0.43	1.12
No learning response (36)	0.02	0.38
Affiliative behaviors (40–42, 44, 45, 47)	0.29	0.88
General social (48, 50, 52, 59)	13.11	9.43
Received general social (43, 46, 51)	0.70	1.35
Initiated negative social (53, 55)	0.13	0.59
Received negative social (54, 56)	0.25	0.92
Household maintenance (60–62, 64–69)	10.72	8.48
Supervising (63)	0.09	0.59
Undesirable behavior (70–74)	1.57	5.19
Leaving house (76)	2.74	1.56
Unobservable (75, 77–79)	9.03	6.80

[a]These means and standard deviations were calculated for 240 group home residents who were observed for a minimum of 26 time periods.

retardation[1] (mild, mild-moderate, moderate, severe-profound), 2) age group (child or adult), 3) sex, 4) time living in home (months in present facility), 5) parent involvement (frequent visits, or unknown relationship), and 6) presence of Down's syndrome. From these regression analyses, F ratios were calculated, the level of significance was determined, and for all effects significant at $p < 0.01$, the percent of variance attributable to that variable was considered. The findings are summarized in Table 8.

Of the 21 major activity categories, 11 showed statistically significant main effects. The resident characteristics that most frequently related to the proportion of time residents spent in certain activities were 1) level of retardation, 2) sex, and 3) age group. Significant higher order interactions appeared for 10 categories, reflecting the fact that observed differences in behavior frequently were related to several combined resident variables. For

[1]Level of retardation was ascertained from records, then confirmed by observers in accordance with behavioral definitions provided by the American Association on Mental Deficiency. A considerable number of clients who could not reliably be classified as mildly retarded or moderately retarded were assigned to an intermediate category referred to as mildly-moderately retarded. Since very few individuals were functioning at a profoundly retarded level, and there was no apparent distinction between some individuals classified as severely retarded and those labeled profoundly retarded, these categories were combined into a severely-profoundly retarded category.

Table 8. Major activity categories: summary of significant effects of residents' characteristics from multiple regression analyses[a]

Major activity category (Original codes)	F ratio	Degrees of freedom	Significance level
Inactive (2–9)			
Main effect: Level of retardation	6.91	3	$p < 0.001$
Self-care (10–13, 15–19)			
Main effect: sex	29.93	1	$p < 0.001$
Interaction effect: age × time in home	19.46	1	$p < 0.001$
Eating (14)			
Main effects: Age	15.66	1	$p < 0.001$
Parent involvement	7.49	2	$p < 0.001$
Interaction effect: Age × sex × level	3.92	3	$p < 0.01$
Unstructured activities (20–21)			
Main effect: Sex	9.56	1	$p < 0.01$
Interaction effect: Sex × level × time in home	4.75	3	$p < 0.01$
Organized activities (22–29)			
Main effect: Age	8.41	1	$p < 0.01$
Interaction effect: Sex × parent involvement	7.68	2	$p < 0.001$
Reading, writing, arithmetic (34)			
Main effect: Sex	6.66	1	$p < 0.01$
Problem solving (35)			
Interaction effects:			
Time in home × level of retardation	6.93	3	$p < 0.001$
Time in home × level × sex	4.73	3	$p < 0.01$
Observation-imitation (31, 33)			
Main effects: Level of retardation	3.83	3	$p < 0.01$
Parent involvement	5.04	2	$p < 0.01$
No learning response (36)			
Interaction effects: Level of retardation × sex	4.64	3	$p < 0.01$
Level × age × sex	8.82	3	$p < 0.001$
General social (48, 50, 52, 59)			
Main effects: Level of retardation	6.17	3	$p < 0.001$
Down's syndrome	10.83	1	$p < 0.001$
Interaction effect: age × sex × time in home	4.13	1	$p < 0.01$
Received negative social (54, 56)			
Interaction effect: Sex × parent involvement	4.57	2	$p < 0.01$
Household maintenance (60–62, 64–69)			
Main effect: Level of retardation	5.79	3	$p < 0.001$
Age	22.23	1	$p < 0.001$

(continued)

Table 8. (*continued*)

Major activity category (Original codes)	F ratio	Degrees of freedom	Significance level
Undesirable behavior (70–74)			
Main effect: level of retardation	12.74	3	$p < 0.001$
Interaction effects: Level × age	5.97	3	$p < 0.001$
Age × parent involvement	8.08	2	$p < 0.01$
Time in home × level × sex	6.67	3	$p < 0.01$
Leaving house (76)			
Main effect: Level of retardation	12.63	3	$p < 0.001$
Sex	9.12	1	$p < 0.01$
Interaction effect: Time in home × sex	7.60	1	$p < 0.01$

[a]Multiple regression analyses were completed independently for each of 21 major activity categories. The independent variables entering into these analyses were: level of retardation, age, sex, time in home, parent involvement, and Down's syndrome. Only main effects and interaction effects significant at the $p < 0.01$ level are reported here. Only residents with at least 26 observations entered into these regression analyses ($N = 240$). For a full discussion of the statistical techniques and rationale see Overall and Spiegel (1969).

the present purposes, since the resident characteristics were not truly independent in the sample studied, only significant main effects will be discussed.

As shown in Figure 1, there was a direct relationship between level of retardation and the percent of time residents spent in inactive behaviors, observation and imitation, general social activities, household maintenance, undesirable behaviors, and leaving the house. Mildly retarded residents spent a significantly smaller proportion of time in inactive behaviors ($\bar{X} = 14.7\%$, s.d. $=8.3\%$) than did severely-profoundly retarded individuals ($\bar{X} = 24.4\%$, s.d. $=15.7\%$). There were dramatic differences in the proportion of general social activity of mildly retarded persons ($\bar{X} = 15.4\%$, s.d. $=10.0\%$). and that of severely-profoundly retarded residents ($\bar{X} = 7.9\%$, s.d. $=5.7\%$). Similarly, the mildly retarded engaged in twice the proportion of household maintenance ($\bar{X} = 12.7\%$, s.d. $= 2.7\%$) and leaving the house ($\bar{X} = 5.0\%$, s.d. $=2.7\%$) than the severely-profoundly retarded did ($\bar{X} = 6.5\%$, s.d. $=7.2\%$ for household maintenance; and $\bar{X} = 2.1\%$, s.d. $= 1.8\%$ for leaving the house). Very little undesirable behavior was observed for either the mildly or mildly-moderately retarded (less than 0.5%). The moderately retarded had three times the proportion of these negative behaviors ($\bar{X} = 1.5\%$, s.d. $=5.1\%$) compared with the mildly retarded, and the severely-profoundly retarded had more than 10 times as much undesirable behavior ($\bar{X} = 5.1\%$, s.d. $=8.8\%$). Some of the severely-profoundly retarded spent as much as 14% or more of their time in the home behaving in an abnormal, annoying, or destructive manner. Concerning imitative and observational learning behavior, the mildly-moderately and moderately retarded residents spent a slightly greater proportion of time in these activities than either the mildly or severely-profoundly retarded individuals. However, the overall proportion of observed imitative behaviors was very low ($\bar{X} = 0.4\%$, s.d. $=1.1\%$).

Figure 2 shows the significant behavioral differences for males and females. Essentially, males spent a greater proportion of time in unstructured activities ($\bar{X} = 25.2\%$, s.d. $= 14.3\%$) than did females ($\bar{X} = 19.9\%$, s.d. $= 13.2\%$), and left the home more often ($\bar{X}$

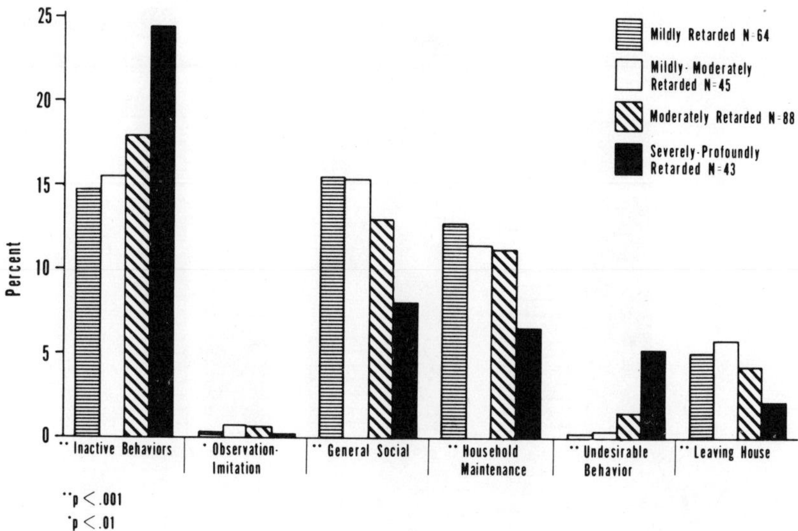

Figure 1. Relationship of level of retardation to proportion of time in major activities.

= 5.0%, s.d. =3.6%) than females did (X̄ = 3.7%, s.d. =2.4%). In contrast, females spent significantly more time in self-care activities and in academic activities of reading, writing, and arithmetic. In fact, females spent nearly twice the proportion of time in self-care activities (X̄ = 5.6%, s.d. = 3.8%) than males did (X̄ = 3.3%, s.d. = 3.2%). Similarly, females engaged in academic activities more than two times as much (X̄ = 2.7%, s.d. = 5.5%) as males (X̄ = 1.2%, s.d. =3.6%).

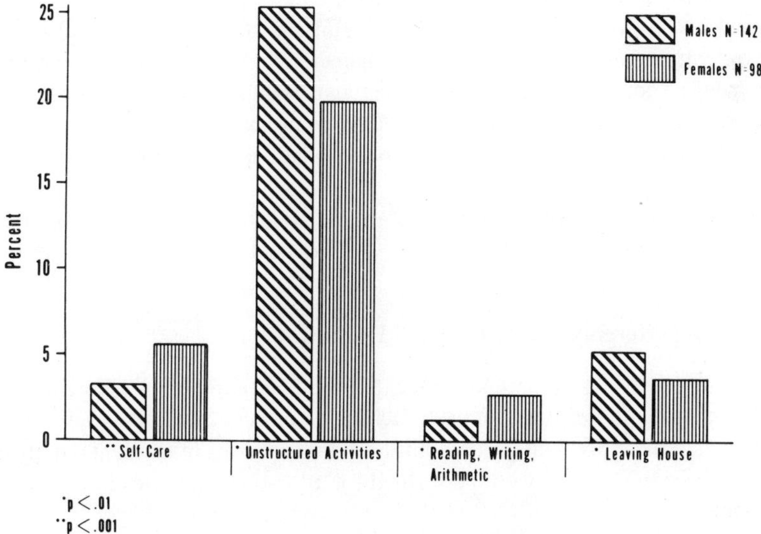

Figure 2. Sex differences in major activities of residents.

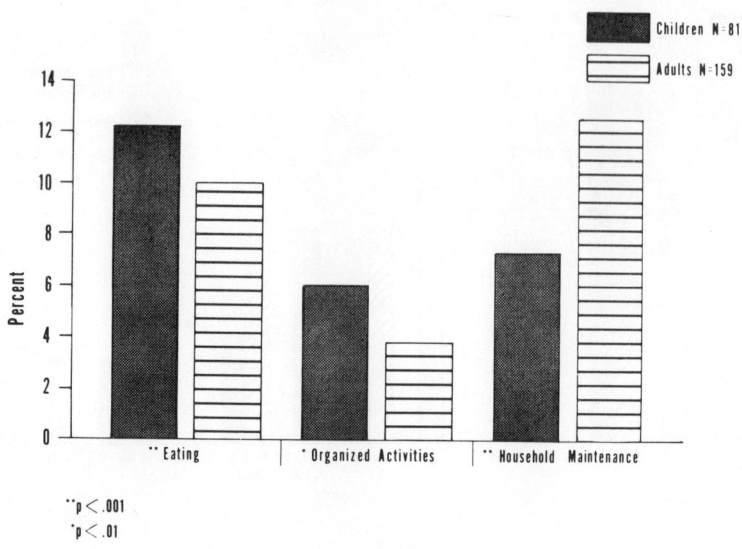

Figure 3. Relationship of age group to proportion of time in major activities.

Children and adults differed significantly in three major activity categories: eating, household maintenance, and participating in organized activities (Figure 3). Children spent a greater proportion of time in organized activities (children, $\bar{X}$ = 6.0%, s.d. = 6.9%; adults, $\bar{X}$ = 3.7%, s.d. =6.4%). They also spent 12.2% (s.d. = 5.3%) of their time eating and only 7.2% (s.d. = 7.4%) of their time in household maintenance, in contrast to adults who spent 10% (s.d. = 4.4%) of their time eating and 12.5% (s.d. = 8.5%) of their time in household maintenance.

Parent involvement with residents was significantly related to several major activity categories, often interacting with other characteristics of the residents. Preliminary analyses suggest that children whose parents visit frequently tend to be more dependent and to demonstrate more negative social behaviors or abnormal-unusual behaviors. However, the multitude of factors contributing to this relationship cannot be assessed in a study of this type.

Individuals with Down's syndrome (*N* = 53 residents) engaged in significantly less general social activity ($\bar{X}$ = 8.2%, s.d. =6.0%) than did other residents ($\bar{X}$ = 14.5%, s.d. = 9.8%).

Group Home Differences in Behavioral Profiles

A behavioral profile was computed for each of the 20 group homes, showing the average proportion of time the residents in each facility spent in various activities. To assess the degree to which the individual group homes differed in terms of residents' daily activities, multiple regression analyses were performed for all major categories in the Home Observation Code.

The data in Table 9 show that the distribution of residents' behavior differed considerably from home to home. For example, residents in Home 6 spent 33.8% of their time in low level inactive behaviors (the typical activity for this home), more than in any other home. They also had the least amount of general social activity (4.7%). Home 6 residents spent a fair proportion of time eating (14.3%) and moderate amounts of time in unstructured activities (17.7%) and undesirable behavior (3.6%), relative to other homes. In contrast, Home 7 residents spent the greatest percent of their time in general social activities (21.4%), and spent more time than any other group in academic activities (4.8%). Compared with other group homes, the residents of Home 7 spent a relatively small proportion of their day in inactive activities (13.2%) and moderate amounts in household maintenance (10.7%) and eating (12.8%). There was virtually no undesirable behavior observed in Home 7. Another home with a markedly different behavioral profile is Home 8, in which residents spent proportionately more time in three activities than residents of other homes: eating (22.2%), organized activities (15.4%), and active learning (2.8%). However, general social activities were fairly low (6.0%) in this home, as was household maintenance (2.4%). Also there was a moderate amount of undesirable behavior (3.3%) in Home 8.

To assess the significance of these home differences, multiple regression analyses for each major activity category were performed. The F values, significance levels, and percent of variance accounted for by the main effect of homes are reported in Table 10. For 13 of the 21 categories, the observed differences were statistically significant ($p < 0.01$). Thus, we undertook further analyses of the relationship between these 13 behaviors and known characteristics of the homes.

We have used several different approaches to analyze the relationship between home characteristics or variables and behavioral differences of residents in each home. This discussion concerns significant relationships that appeared during stepwise multiple regression analyses. A forward stepwise multiple regression was used because there was no a priori ordering of the independent variables, nor were the interaction effects considered to be particularly important at this stage. These findings are considered descriptive, rather than inferential. These methods have a number of limitations. Some of the independent variables are undoubtedly multidimensional and may actually be measuring the effects of other equally important factors (e.g., "size of home" may relate to wages paid to employees, the type of owner who chooses to set up a large versus a small home, the average age or educational level of employees, availability of resources per resident, etc.). Second, the findings are not appropriate for generalizing to a population at this point. In order to do this, it would be desirable to have more closely matched groups, a larger number of homes, a more complete description of the population being generalized to, and perhaps multiple measures over time to give some index of the stability of the group home profiles and their relationship to the home variables considered.

The eight major characteristics considered were:

1. Average level of retardation of residents
2. size of home (number of residents)
3. average age of residents
4. heterogeneity of residential backgrounds (i.e., number of different institutions or residential facilities from which residents came)
5. nature of proprietorship (state, single ownership, multiple ownership)

Table 9. Individual group home profiles for major activity categories[a]

Home	Percent of time spent by residents in each category										
	Sleep	Inactive behaviors	Self-care	Eating	Unstructured activities	Organized activities	Active learning	Academic activities	Problem solving	Observation and imitation	No learning response
H1	*0.9*	*11.8*	*1.8*	*12.7*	*25.9*	*0.0*	0.0	6.1	0.0	*0.0*	0.0
H2	*0.9*	*21.1*	*5.0*	*9.3*	*20.7*	*11.1*	1.0	0.1	0.0	*0.0*	0.0
H3	*0.9*	*7.5*	*2.2*	*11.6*	*19.6*	*13.7*	0.8	3.1	0.0	*0.8*	0.0
H4	*0.2*	*11.1*	*3.3*	*9.6*	*24.2*	*4.9*	0.0	3.5	0.0	*0.9*	0.0
H5	*5.9*	*17.8*	*7.4*	*11.7*	*14.5*	*5.2*	0.2	0.4	0.0	*1.4*	0.0
H6	*2.1*	*33.8*	*5.7*	*14.3*	*17.7*	*0.1*	0.0	0.4	0.0	*0.1*	0.0
H7	*0.0*	*13.2*	*4.3*	*12.8*	*21.6*	*2.5*	0.0	4.8	0.0	*1.0*	0.0
H8	*0.0*	*14.8*	*1.6*	*22.2*	*24.4*	*15.4*	2.8	1.5	0.0	*0.2*	0.0
H9	*0.9*	*20.5*	*6.3*	*7.7*	*19.9*	*2.6*	1.3	1.6	0.0	*0.0*	0.2
H10	*1.8*	*16.8*	*4.0*	*7.4*	*18.7*	*2.2*	0.8	1.8	0.0	*0.3*	0.0
H11	*0.4*	*21.9*	*6.8*	*13.9*	*19.3*	*3.5*	0.6	0.9	0.0	*1.4*	0.0
H12	*0.0*	*20.1*	*2.8*	*15.4*	*29.3*	*6.0*	0.0	0.4	0.0	*0.0*	0.0
H13	*1.0*	*23.8*	*4.2*	*6.5*	*34.6*	*3.1*	0.0	0.0	0.0	*0.0*	0.0
H14	*0.9*	*17.5*	*3.7*	*7.7*	*22.8*	*2.1*	0.0	2.4	0.0	*0.0*	0.0
H15	*0.4*	*12.1*	*5.7*	*10.8*	*32.1*	*0.8*	0.0	0.0	0.0	*0.0*	0.0
H16	*0.1*	*21.1*	*5.2*	*20.5*	*22.2*	*2.1*	1.6	1.0	0.0	*0.0*	0.0
H17	*0.0*	*14.0*	*3.8*	*20.3*	*26.2*	*9.8*	0.0	1.9	0.0	*0.3*	0.0
H18	*0.5*	*15.4*	*5.2*	*24.5*	*22.4*	*4.0*	0.1	0.7	0.0	*0.0*	0.0
H19	*0.1*	*14.2*	*1.5*	*9.0*	*24.6*	*3.8*	0.0	1.7	0.0	*0.0*	0.0
H20	*1.5*	*23.0*	*1.3*	*7.4*	*27.1*	*6.2*	0.1	1.5	0.0	*0.0*	0.0
Half-way houses											
HWH 1	*0.0*	*12.8*	*11.8*	*9.9*	*6.7*	*1.0*	*0.1*	1.2	0.0	*0.5*	0.0
HWH 2	*0.9*	*21.6*	*0.0*	*8.2*	*23.8*	*0.9*	*0.0*	0.2	0.0	*0.1*	0.0
HWH 3	*0.3*	*10.0*	*0.4*	*9.6*	*8.4*	*1.2*	*0.2*	5.3	0.0	*0.6*	0.0

Home	Affiliative behaviors	General social	Received general social	Initiated negative social	Received negative social	Household maintenance	Supervising	Undesirable behaviors	Unobservable
H1	0.5	*7.5*	0.9	0.0	*0.2*	*10.9*	0.0	*0.0*	*19.0*
H2	0.4	*6.1*	0.7	0.2	*2.0*	*5.2*	8.5	*8.5*	*7.0*
H3	0.0	*8.8*	0.9	0.2	*0.0*	*18.7*	0.2	*0.2*	*19.3*
H4	0.4	*15.2*	0.3	0.0	*0.1*	*13.0*	0.0	*0.0*	*11.5*
H5	0.1	*9.6*	1.1	0.2	*0.0*	*13.2*	1.4	*1.4*	*8.2*
H6	0.0	*4.7*	0.9	0.0	*0.0*	*6.4*	3.6	*3.6*	*8.8*
H7	0.0	*21.4*	0.6	0.0	*0.7*	*10.7*	0.0	*0.0*	*4.8*
H8	0.0	*6.0*	0.2	0.2	*0.2*	*2.4*	3.3	*3.3*	*3.3*
H9	0.9	*14.9*	0.3	0.0	*0.0*	*9.1*	2.0	*2.0*	*9.6*
H10	0.0	*13.9*	0.8	0.0	*0.3*	*22.1*	0.0	*0.0*	*7.5*
H11	0.2	*11.1*	0.8	0.2	*0.3*	*3.1*	0.5	*0.5*	*13.0*
H12	0.4	*7.8*	0.0	0.0	*0.0*	*4.3*	2.5	*2.5*	*9.6*
H13	0.0	*7.6*	1.1	0.1	*0.7*	*3.8*	9.6	*9.6*	*1.9*
H14	0.2	*17.7*	0.5	0.0	*0.0*	*12.5*	4.4	*4.4*	*6.1*
H15	0.0	*19.0*	1.5	0.0	*0.1*	*11.0*	0.0	*0.0*	*5.4*
H16	0.0	*10.3*	0.0	0.1	*0.0*	*13.2*	1.5	*1.5*	*9.6*
H17	0.2	*17.5*	0.3	0.6	*0.8*	*8.1*	1.1	*1.1*	*3.6*
H18	0.2	*10.0*	1.2	0.1	*0.5*	*7.6*	2.8	*2.8*	*11.5*
H19	0.2	*14.2*	0.8	0.1	*0.0*	*13.5*	0.0	*0.0*	*14.9*
H20	0.3	*13.0*	0.2	0.0	*0.0*	*6.7*	0.1	*0.1*	*10.5*
Half-way houses									
HWH 1	2.1	*17.1*	0.7	1.5	*1.3*	*10.5*	6.3	*6.3*	*24.7*
HWH 2	0.0	*8.1*	1.5	0.4	*0.0*	*9.8*	0.0	*0.0*	*22.9*
HWH 3	2.7	*15.6*	1.5	0.0	*0.4*	*10.8*	0.8	*0.8*	*30.4*

[a]The main effect of home was significant at $p < 0.01$ for all columns that are italicized.

Table 10. Results of multiple regression analyses for main effects of homes ($N = 23$)

Major activity category	F value	Significance level
Sleep	3.46	$p < 0.001$
Basic wake behaviors	3.33	$p < 0.001$
Self-care	5.39	$p < 0.001$
Eating	6.63	$p < 0.001$
Unstructured activities	2.26	$p < 0.001$
Organized activities	4.24	$p < 0.001$
Active learning	1.62	not significant
Reading, writing, arithmetic	1.37	not significant
Problem solving	0.66	not significant
Observation and imitation	3.07	$p < 0.001$
No learning response	0.64	not significant
Affiliative behaviors	1.05	not significant
General social	3.04	$p < 0.001$
Received general social	1.31	not significant
Initiated negative social	1.87	not significant
Received negative social	2.31	$p < 0.001$
Household maintenance	5.06	$p < 0.001$
Supervising	2.03	$p < 0.01$
Undesirable	2.01	$p < 0.01$
Leaving house	2.01	$p < 0.01$
Unobservable	9.29	$p < 0.001$

6. geographical location (eastern or western Washington)
7. neighborhood (urban or rural)
8. type of building (new or old)

Table 11 shows the intercorrelations for these eight variables. The two most highly correlated variables were home size and age of residents ($r = +0.64$). This reflects the fact that there were few children in the larger group homes of 18 to 20 residents.

For each group home characteristic, a forward stepwise multiple regression analysis was performed with the 13 major activity categories that differed significantly among homes (see Tables 9 and 10) as independent variables.[2] This approach tests the extent to which each group home characteristic can be predicted from the distribution of residents' activities. The findings are summarized in Table 12. The overall regressions for each of the eight home characteristics were significant at the $p < 0.001$ level. Furthermore, the residents' activities accounted for more than 20% of the variance among homes on five of the eight characteristics: 1) average level of retardation, 2) heterogeneity of residential backgrounds, 3) type of building, 4) size of home, and 5) nature of ownership.

Figure 4 shows the relationship of five major activities to the average level of retardation in a home. Essentially, these relationships reveal the same pattern found in the

[2]An alternative analysis of using home characteristics as the independent variables and each single behavior as the dependent variable was computed. All relationships between home characteristics and behaviors that were significant ($p < 0.01$) in these analyses were significant also when the behaviors were the independent variables.

Table 11. Intercorrelation matrix for group home characteristics

	Average level of retardation	Average age	Neighborhood	Ownership	Geographical location	Building	Size	Hetereogeneity of previous residence
Average level of retardation	1.00							
Average age	−0.36	1.00						
Neighborhood	−0.23	0.21	1.00					
Ownership	0.14	0.14	0.11	1.00				
Geographical location	−0.21	−0.13	0.40	0.25	1.00			
Building	−0.10	0.37	−0.28	0.39	−0.08	1.00		
Size	−0.37	0.64	0.13	−0.38	−0.09	0.27	1.00	
Heterogeneity of previous residences	0.22	−0.11	0.27	0.31	−0.09	−0.02	−0.31	1.00

Table 12. Effects of multiple regression analyses for group home characteristics

Home characteristics	Step	Behavior category	Percent of variance	F value
		Significant major activities		
Average level of retardation of residents	1	Leaving home	17.8	78.3[a]
	2	Unobservable	8.1	35.5[a]
	3	Household maintenance	6.4	28.0[a]
	4	Inactive	4.2	18.3[a]
	5	Undesirable	3.7	16.2[a]
Total percent of variance accounted for = 41.25%; F = 22.83, 8 df[a]				
Diversity of previous residences	1	Self-care	13.6	49.2[a]
	2	Social	4.9	17.6[a]
	3	Unobservable	3.2	11.7[a]
	4	Sleep	2.0	7.3[b]
Total percent of variance accounted for = 28.76%; F = 11.53, 9 df[a]				
Type of building	1	Imitation	7.9	28.2[a]
	2	Unobservable	7.4	26.6[a]
	3	Leaving home	3.6	3.1[a]
	5	Organized activities	2.7	9.7[b]
Total percent of variance accounted for = 28.16%; F = 12.62, 9 df[a]				
Size of home	1	Eating	9.9	34.1[a]
	2	Organized activities	3.3	11.2[a]
	3	Social	3.1	10.6[b]
	4	Unobservable	2.5	8.5[b]
Total percent of variance accounted for = 24.67%; F = 9.43, 9 df[a]				
Type of ownership	1	Inactive	7.5	24.3[a]
	2	Imitation	4.0	12.9[a]
	3	Eating	7.1	23.0[a]
Total percent of variance accounted for = 20.01; F = 9.26, df[a]				
Average age of residents	1	Unobservable	4.1	12.6[a]
	2	Household maintenance	3.7	11.5[a]
	3	Organized activities	2.4	7.4[b]
	4	Self-care	2.6	8.0[b]
Total percent of variance accounted for = 16.37%; F = 7.26, 7 df[a]				
Geographical location	1	Imitation	4.8	14.4[a]
	2	Unstructured activities	2.7	7.9[b]
	3	Leaving home	2.7	7.9[b]
Total percent of variance accounted for = 12.73%; F = 5.39, 7 df[a]				
Neighborhood	1	Leaving home	2.7	8.0[b]
	2	Organized activities	2.5	7.3[b]
Total percent of variance accounted for = 12.27%; F = 3.99, 9 df[a]				

[a] $p < 0.001$
[b] $p < 0.01$

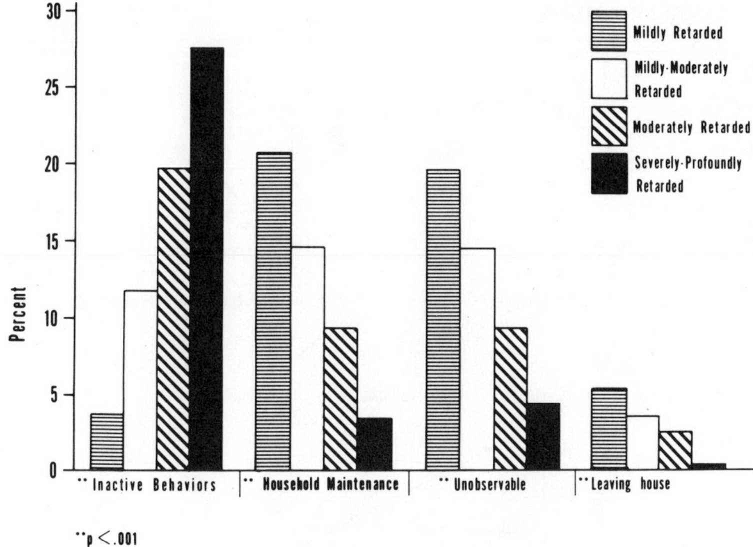

Figure 4. Average level of retardation in a home related to ongoing major activities.

analyses using individual subject characteristics (see Table 8 and Figure 1). Characteristically, homes with a collectively higher level of intelligence had residents who left the home more frequently, spent proportionately more time participating in household maintenance activities, and were "unobservable" for a greater percentage of the time they were at home (e.g., in bedrooms or in bathrooms with the doors closed). Also, residents in the higher level homes had a much lower proportion of inactive behaviors and less undesirable behavior than residents in homes with a lower average intelligence. Overall, the behavior of residents accounted for 41.25% of the variance in average level of retardation represented in a home.

Figure 5 depicts the significant relationship between heterogeneity of residential backgrounds and three major activities. In homes where residents all came from the same institution prior to current placement (heterogeneity = 1), there was a greater proportion of time spent in general social activity than in homes where the residents came from several different institutions or previous community placements. Similarly, in homes with greater *homogeneity* of residential backgrounds, the residents spent a smaller proportion of time in inactive behaviors or in self-care. Although there was a significant relationship of this variable to proportion of time residents were observed sleeping, there were extraneous factors that may have distorted the measurement of sleep (e.g., a few residents who worked night shifts slept during the day; or several residents who were ill slept more on 1 day). The residents' behavior accounted for 28.76% of the variance in number of different residential placements in a home.

Figure 6 compares three behaviors—imitation, unobservable behaviors, and leaving the home—for residents living in old versus new buildings. The most striking difference was that residents in older buildings left their homes *much* more frequently to go into the community than those living in new buildings specially designed as group homes ($\bar{X}$ =

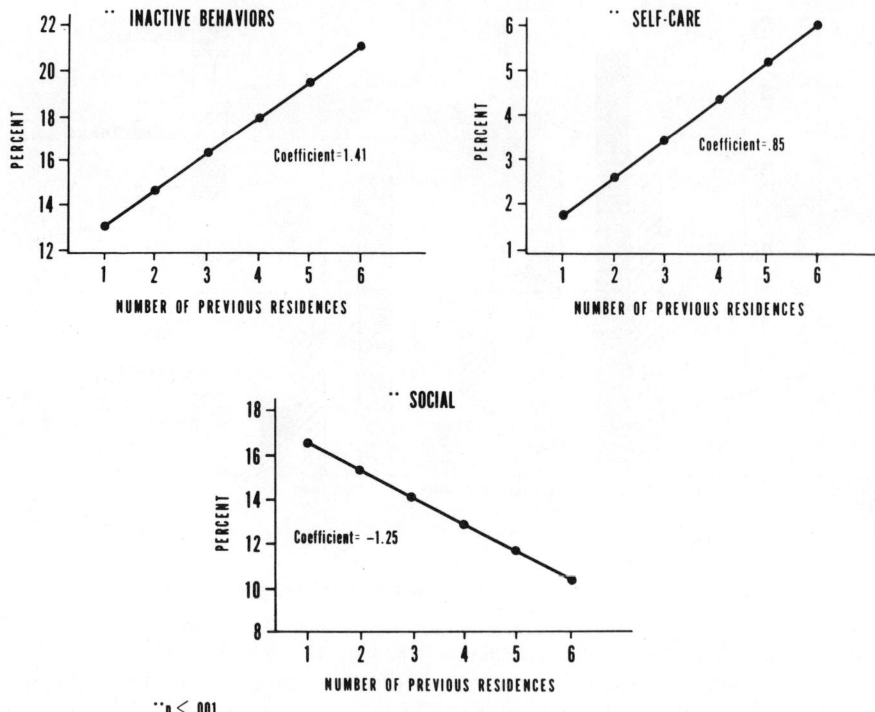

Figure 5. Heterogeneity of residents' backgrounds related to ongoing major activities.

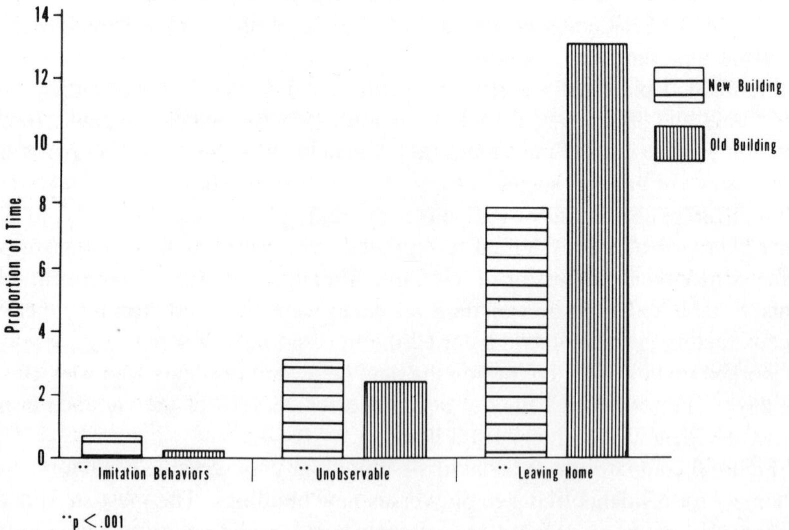

Figure 6. Type of building related to ongoing major activities.

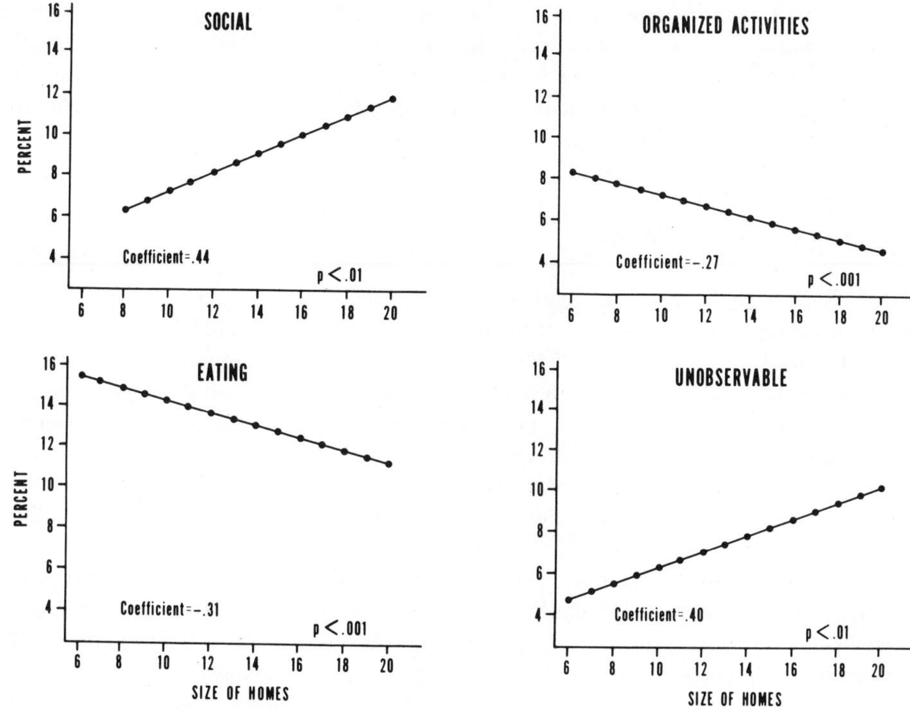

Figure 7. Resident behaviors related to group home size.

13.1%, s.d. =10.6% for old buildings; $\bar{X}$ = 7.9%, s.d. =6.6% for new buildings). The residents' behaviors accounted for 28.16% of the variance related to type of building.

The number of residents living in a home was predicted to some extent by the proportion of time residents spent in eating, organized, social, and unobservable behaviors. Figure 7 shows these activities as they related to the home size. Generally, the larger the home, the less the proportion of time residents spent eating or participating in organized activities, and the more they spent in social behaviors and in unobservable behaviors. Collectively, the residents' behaviors explained 24.6% of the variance in group home size.

There were several other significant findings. Homes that were part of a chain or multiple ownership had a significantly higher proportion of inactive behaviors than homes that were under single ownership ($\bar{X}$ = 22.9%, s.d. =13.9% for multiple ownership; $\bar{X}$ = 15.7%, s.d. =10.7% for single ownership). Homes with a younger average age of residents tended to have a greater percentage of organized activities and self-care, but significantly less household maintenance and unobservable activities. Again, these findings reflect the same relationships found for individual subject characteristics (see Figure 1). Concerning geographical location, homes in eastern Washington had residents who spent proportionately more time in imitative behaviors ($\bar{X}$ = 0.55%, s.d. =1.31% for eastern Washington; $\bar{X}$ = 0.34%, s.d. = 0.87% for western Washington) and in unstructured activities, primarily watching television ($\bar{X}$ = 25.25%, s.d. =15.73% for eastern

Washington; $\bar{X}$ = 20.37%, s.d. = 13.18% for western Washington). Moreover, homes in urban settings, relative to those in rural neighborhoods, had residents who less frequently left the home ($\bar{X}$ = 2.5%, s.d. =1.5% for urban; $\bar{X}$ = 3.0%, s.d. =1.6% for rural) and who spent less time in structured activities within the home ($\bar{X}$ = 3.28%, s.d. =5.36% for urban; $\bar{X}$ = 5.18%, s.d. =7.46% for rural).

DISCUSSION AND SUMMARY

The findings from this investigation may be interpreted at several levels. Basically, what we learned may be related to 1) confirmation of observational methodology as a feasible means for describing the behavior of the retarded people in community residential settings, 2(the usefulness and validity of descriptive behavioral data for program planning and evaluation, and 3) the potential for understanding some fundamental principles about the interaction of the environment and behavior.

The data provide a direct answer to our original question, "Can we conduct such a study on a large scale?" Within 4 months, for less than $30,000, we were able to collect and compile the observational data. Admittedly, we spent a full year in advance coordinating the research with state planners and group home operators, and have spent the past 9 months since the study analyzing the reams of data; and still are far from finished. Nonetheless, the successful completion of this observational study of more than 400 persons in 23 facilities is confirmation that such studies are feasible.

Concerning the usefulness of the behavioral data for program planning and assessment, the findings are being used by the state and the community to 1) develop new programs for residents who behaviorally appear able to move into a "less restrictive setting" and 2) consider more adequate evaluation of residential facilities in general. A series of workshops to interpret our findings and to consider their implications has been planned. However, the critical issue about the comparative *validity* of the data is not resolved. Comparisons have been made among data from more usual sources, such as staff, administrators, clients, ratings, and case records. Sizable discrepancies appeared for some residents between observed behavioral capabilities and these other information sources. Which of these views most closely approximates "truth" is not known. What is needed is a study that is: 1) *prospective*—looks at clients over time in at least two different settings; 2) *broadly comparative*—accounts for the natural variation that may occur within any generic set of services (e.g., compares several different institutional settings *and* an equal number of varied community residences); and 3) *partially experimental*—allows for some empirical manipulation of the environmental variables that appear critical in determining "success." Moreover, at the level of long term program planning, there are many other issues besides individual client progress that need to be considered in the deinstitutionalization movement, including the economic, social, and psychological impact on the community and family (Arnhoff, 1975).

The issue about test-retest reliability (i.e., stability of measurements) or how representative 2 days of observation are for describing individuals' daily patterns of activities is being analyzed. For three facilities, an entire replication was conducted 1 month after the initial set of observations. These results will be reported and discussed in another paper.

Similarly, random subsamples of the observations will be compared with the entire data set to determine whether *fewer* observations would have yielded the same findings.

The findings presented in this paper identify certain significant relationships between observed behaviors and characteristics of the residents and the homes. The most consistent findings, for both individual and home characteristics, related "level of retardation" and "age" to observed proportion of time in certain activities. The findings are not surprising. What is surprising is that only 2 days of fairly gross time sampling of behavior reliably detected these relationships. Also, these findings serve as a reminder that the retarded are a very heterogeneous group of individuals, whose progress should not be evaluated in simple-minded terms that fail to consider baseline differences and social preferences of individuals. All of the value judgments about who is leading a "normal" or "independent" life assume that specific behaviors or accomplishments are a true index of progress, and that behavioral accomplishments (e.g., having a job, taking a bus, shopping for groceries, being married, going to a clinic) lead to a happier, more fulfilled life for retarded people. Since we have few notions as to what produces successful adaptation or happiness in "normal" people, our professional advocacy for retarded people should protect them from premature programming of all of their activities to make them "seem" normal.

Some of the findings, although still considered tentative, suggest that many hypotheses held about the merit of small homes, family involvement, specially designed buildings, and heterogeneity of groupings may *not* be correct. In our sample of group homes, serving six to 20 residents (mostly mildly to moderately retarded young adults), we found that:

1. more positive social behaviors occurred in *larger* facilities;
2. families that visited more often tended to have children who were *less* independent;
3. specially designed new group homes were related to decreased community interaction; and
4. more homogeneous groupings of residents was associated with more positive social behavior.

Of course, cause and effect cannot be inferred from only one set of observations. However, the findings are sufficiently strong to suggest that *no* one environment will be optimal, or even appropriate, for all types of developmentally disabled people.

Another difficult problem for this type of research concerns the choice of control groups. At this stage, we need comparisons with several groups that are similar to the retarded population studied in group homes in size (such as large families or small communes), in functional abilities (such as elderly persons or very young children), in socially deviant behavior (such as juvenile delinquents or mentally ill persons), in transition stages in their lives (such as first year college students or recently married persons), or in diversity of backgrounds (such as families with natural and adopted children or foreign student groups). Observations of the daily behavior of such control groups will yield more meaningful comparisons for interpreting the patterns of activity in groups of retarded people, in terms of the "success" of the programs and the degree of "normalization" achieved. Furthermore, such comparisons will allow us to assess whether certain principles of daily social behavior are related systematically and generally to certain environmental variables.

ACKNOWLEDGMENTS

The scientific and humanistic value of this investigation ws greatly enhanced by the remarkable dedication of the observers who spent hours collecting the data, organizing and compiling the information, and asking questions about how to improve the daily lives of the developmentally disabled. No words can fully express our gratitude to Denise Boelens, Renate Coulsen, Christine Curtis, Maureen Miltenberger, and Debra Tombari.

Without the special efforts of Courtenay Bell, John Stern, Cameron Dightman, Bob Sharpley, and the Washington State Association of Group Homes to coordinate and review, in great detail, the proposed research, this study could not have been conducted with the thoroughness and success we experienced. Above all, the group home residents, staff, and administrators extended themselves warmly to us, and voluntarily gave us permission to enter their homes and their lives for a few days.

We thank each and every one who shared in this effort for their hard work, concern, ideas, and friendship.

REFERENCES

Arnhoff, F. N. 1975. Social consequences of policy toward mental illness. Science 188:1277–1281.

Balla, D. A., Butterfield, E. C., and Zigler, E. 1973. Effects of institutionalization on retarded children: a longitudinal cross-institutional investigation. Am. J. Ment. Defic. 77:654–669.

Barker, R. 1960. Ecology and motivation. Nebr. Symp. Motiv. 8:1–50.

Barker, R. 1968. Ecological Psychology: Concepts and Methods for Studying the Environment of Human Behavior. Stanford University Press, Stanford.

Bedner, M. J. 1974. Architecture for the Handicapped in Denmark, Sweden, and Holland: A Guide to Normalization. University of Michigan, Ann Arbor.

Bjaanes, A. T., and Butler, E. W. 1974. Environmental variation in community care facilities for mentally retarded persons. Am. J. Ment. Defic. 78 (4):429–439.

Butterfield, E. C. 1967. The role of environmental factors in the treatment of institutionalized mental retardates. In: A. A. Baumeister (ed.), Mental Retardation: Appraisal, Education, and Rehabilitation, pp. 120–137. Aldine Publishing Company, Chicago.

Craik, K. 1973. Environmental psychology. Annu. Rev. Psychol. 24:403–422.

Dingman, H. F. 1968. A plea for social research in mental retardation. Am. J. Ment. Retard. 73:2–4.

Dybwad, G. 1968. Planning facilities for severely and profoundly retarded adults. Hosp. Comm. Psychiatry 19 (2):392–395.

Dybwad, G. 1970. Architecture's role in revitalizing the field of mental retardation. J. Ment. Subnorm. 16 (1):45–48.

Eagle, E. 1968. Prognosis and outcome of community placement of institutionalized retardates. Am. J. Ment. Defic. 72:232–243.

Edgerton, R. B. 1967. The Cloak of Competence. University of California Press, Berkeley.

Edgerton, R. B., and Bercovici, S. M. 1976. The cloak of competence: years later. Am. J. Ment. Defic. 80 (5):485–497.

Evans, G. 1973. Personal space: research review and bibliography. Man-Environ. Systems 3:203–215.

Gunzberg, A. L. 1968. Architecture and mental subnormality: II. Sensory experiences in the architecture for the mentally subnormal child. J. Ment. Subnormal. 14 (1):57–58.

Gunzberg, H. C. 1973. The physical environment of the mentally handicapped: VII. "39 Steps" leading toward normalized living practices in living units for the mentally handicapped. Br. J. Ment. Subnormal. 19 (37):91–99.

Hoffman, J. L. 1969. An investigation of factors contributing to the successful and nonsuccessful adjustment of discharged retardates. Social and Rehabilitation Services, Department of Health, Education and Welfare, Washington, D.C.

Ittelson, W., Proshansky, H., Rivlin, L., and Winkel, G. 1974. An Introduction to Environmental Psychology. Holt, Rinehart & Winston, New York.
Kraus, J. 1972. Supervised living in the community and residential and employment stability of retarded male juveniles. Am. J. Ment. Defic. 77:283–290.
Landesman-Dwyer, S., and Berkson, G. 1976. Social interactions among group home residents. Paper presented at the American Academy on Mental Retardation, Chicago.
Landesman-Dwyer, S., Stein, J., and Sackett, G. P. 1976. Group homes for the developmentally disabled: a behavioral and ecological description. State of Washington, Department of Social and Health Services, Division of Planning and Research Report. Library of Congress #76-12318.
Moos, R., and Insel, P. 1974. Issues in Social Ecology. National Press Books, Palo Alto.
Nihara, L., and Nihara, K. 1975. Jeopardy in community placement. Am. J. Ment. Defic. 9 (5):538–544.
Nirje, B. 1970. Symposium on normalization: The normalization principle—Implications and comments. J. Ment. Subnormal. 16:62–70.
Norris, D. 1969. Architecture and mental subnormality: V. The environmental needs of the severely retarded. J. Ment. Subnormal. 15 (1):45–50.
Overall, J. E., and Spiegel, D. K. 1969. Concerning least squares analysis of experimental data. Psychol. Bull. 72 (5):311–322.
Pedersen, J. 1970. The physical environment of the mentally handicapped. I. Progress in building for the mentally handicapped. J. Ment. Subnormal. 16 (2):121–125.
Proshansky, H., Ittelson, W., and Rivlin, L. 1970. Freedom of choice and behavior in a physical setting. In: H. Proshansky, W. Ittelson, and L. Rivlin (eds.), Environmental Psychology: Man and His Physical Setting. Holt, Rinehart & Winston, New York.
Rosen, M., Floor, L., and Baxter, D. 1972. Prediction of community adjustment: a failure at cross-validation. Am. J. Ment. Defic. 77 (1):111–112.
Rosen, M., Floor, L., and Baxter, D. 1974. IQ, academic achievement, and community adjustment after discharge from the institution. Ment. Retard. 12 (2):51–53.
Rosen, M., Kivitz, M. S., Clark, G. R., and Floor, L. 1970. Prediction of post-institutional adjustment of mentally retarded adults. Am. J. Ment. Defic. 74:726–734.
Sackett, G. P., and Landesman-Dwyer, S. 1977. Toward an etholoty of mental retardation. In: P. Mittler (ed.), Research to Practice in Mental Retardation, pp. 27–37. Vol. II. Education and Training. University Park Press, Baltimore.
Schwerdt, J. 1968. Architecture and mental subnormality. IV. Therapeutic variety: a day-to-day basis of design for the subnormal. J. Ment. Subnormal. 15 (2):101–103.
Skaarbrevik, K. J. 1971. A follow-up study of educable mentally retarded in Norway. Am. J. Ment. Defic. 75:560–565.
Song, A. Y., and Song, R. M. 1969. Prediction of job efficiency of institutionalized retardates in the community. Am. J. Ment. Defic. 73:567–571.
Stephens, W. B., Peck, J. R., and Veldman, D. J. 1968. Personality and success profiles characteristic of young adult male retardates. Am. J. Ment. Defic. 73:405–413.
Stokols, D. 1972. A social-psychological model of human crowding phenomena. J. Am. Inst. Planners 38:72–83.
Stokols, D. 1975. Toward a psychological theory of alienation. Psychol. Rev. 82:26–44.
Stokols, D., and Marrero, D. G. 1976. The effects of an environmental intervention on racial polarization in a youth training school: a field-experimental investigation. Paper presented at the 7th Annual Meeting of the Environmental Design Research Association, Vancouver, B.C.
Tizard, J. 1972. Research into services for mentally handicapped: science policy issues. Br. J. Ment. Subnormal. 18 (1):6–17.
Wicker, A., McGrath, J., and Armstrong, G. 1972. Organization size and behavior setting capacity as determinants of member participation. Behav. Sci. 17:499–513.
Wohlwill, J. 1970. The emerging discipline of environmental psychology. Am. Psychol. 25:303–312.

chapter 16

Activities and the Use of Time by Retarded Persons in Community Care Facilities

Edgar W. Butler and Arne T. Bjaanes

Varying levels of competence have long been moral and social problems in our society. In the past, individuals who have fallen below some level of ability to cope with demands of the larger environment have generally been removed from it and placed in a special environment which completely isolated the individual from the demands of society, and, incidentally, "protected society from the individual." However, few will disagree that the historic total institution has failed to increase competence among its residents. Some research indicates that it may even have contributed to retrogression of some individuals (Lyle, 1959; Bennet and Rudolph, 1960; Dentler and Mackler, 1961; Stedman and Eichorn, 1964; Tizard, 1964; Woloshin, Tardi, and Tobin, 1966).

In more recent years, there has been a major change in philosophy regarding care of the retarded. The asylum notion has been increasingly abandoned with a concomitant increase in emphasis on community care in various alternative settings (O'Connor and Justice, 1973). These alternative settings are expected to break down the social and economic walls that isolate the retarded from meaningful experience and learning. They include board and care and home care facilities as well as special schools, special classes, sheltered employment, and recreation. The objective of community alternatives is that impaired individuals should have available all community resources to use to the extent of their needs and capacities. The current concept is perhaps best illustrated by the term "normalization" (Nirje, 1970). Each individual is to be treated in all possible respects as though he falls within the normal range, the premise being that only in a relatively typical

The observations and data used in this paper were made possible by NIMH Grant MH 08667 and Office of Developmental Disabilities Contract 542A1, State of California. This paper includes only a small portion of observations gathered to date. A revised version will include expanded analyses of observations in a stratified sample of therapeutic, maintaining, and custodial community care facilities.

community environment can normalization occur (Kugel and Wolfensberger, 1969).

In California, there is a definite trend for more community placement of the retarded. The Lanterman Mental Retardation Services Act of 1969 emphasized community services for the mentally retarded and placed much of the decision making upon Regional Centers for the Mentally Retarded. Under this act, state hospitals and other state institutions, as well as local community units, became more integrated into a total system of care. Furthermore, there is currently an increasing emphasis on developing other community programs aimed at enhancing social competence among mentally retarded persons. There has been expansion of efforts to habilitate and to give sheltered employment for the less severely mentally retarded and to provide some degree of habilitation for the more severely retarded.

So far, the trend in community care is neither nationally nor universally accepted. Perhaps this is reasonable inasmuch as community-based facilities—foster care homes and group homes—are developments whose values and achievements beyond reduced costs have not yet been objectively certified. Whether or not current concepts of habilitation and treatment in various alternative community settings will increase social competence requires much more objective research than has been carried out to date. These trends, involving alternative community settings for the placement of mental retardates, require systematic study and evaluation. Many decisions that have been made and policies that have emerged have been based on emotion, economy, or expedience (Farber, 1968). The essential ingredient of evidence is often missing. Given the trends indicated above, a number of community alternatives have emerged. There is a wide range of community care environments, physical plants, types of supervision, and methods of care. The central question is which type of environment, or which combination of the various elements that comprise the total environment, is successful in the normalization process. Merely removing an individual from a large institution and placing him in a small unit does not necessarily result in normalization. A variety of factors must be considered. The objective of this research is to provide data on which factors are most important in developing effective habilitative programs and guidelines on which to base policy decisions which, in turn, should help place the mentally retarded in optimum settings for enhancing their potential and opportunities for a "normal" and quality life.

There are essentially three basic assumptions underlying changes in policy related to the care of the mentally retarded: 1) historic total institutions, i.e., large state hospitals, have failed to increase the competence of their residents, and may in fact have been detrimental to the development of social skills; 2) an environment providing "normal social contact" and the potential for "normal social interaction" has a positive "normalizing" effect on the mentally retarded; 3) community care facilities provide a relatively "normal environment," and therefore have a "normalizing" effect on retarded people, i.e., an increase in competence ensues.

A number of questions arise regarding the general validity of the assumptions outlined above. As indicated earlier, there is little doubt about the validity of the first assumption. There is considerable evidence indicating that total institutionalization tends to have a detrimental effect on motor skills, communication skills, learning skills, and social competence in general (Farber, 1968). There is, on the other hand, a limited number of studies supporting the second assumption. Several "special programs" have shown that *if the environment is significantly different* from that of the larger total institution, normalization can occur, and social and intellectual competence can be increased (Baller, 1936; Skeels and Dye, 1939; McKay, 1942; Kennedy, 1948; Mundy, 1957; Edgerton, 1967).

The last assumption is the most problematic. Are most current community care facilities significantly different from the total institution and do they provide a relatively "normal" environment and thus have a "normalizing" effect on their residents? Obviously, the first problem is that this assumption takes for granted *uniformity* or *similarity* among various community care facilities. In fact, our observations indicate that there is a lack of uniformity and that a great deal of dissimilarity exists (Bjaanes and Butler, 1974; Butler, Bjaanes and Hofacre, 1975; Moore, Butler and Bjaanes, 1976; Butler and Bjaanes, 1977; Butler and Bjaanes, in preparation). Community care facilities range in size from three or four retarded persons up to 30 and more. There is considerable variation in the type and "quality of life" support afforded individuals in community care facilities. Furthermore, there are significant differences in the amount of social interaction, incentives for normalization, and in caregiver knowledge, attitudes, behavior, and experience. In addition, there are geographical differences, e.g., rural versus urban settings, and differences in physical plants, to mention but a few of the facets in which considerable variation exists. Generally, variations range from small family care units to facilities which are replicas of larger total institutions: "mini-institutions." In view of the dissimilarities and lack of uniformity, it is clear that systematic investigative activities on the use of time by retarded persons in alternative community care facilities is urgently needed.

An evaluation of the interrelationships between various factors in community care facilities affecting the success of placement is, by nature, a complex and difficult task (Butterfield (1967) summarizes major problems which must be taken into account). The ideal method of study would be experimental in which the investigator had both the ability and the authority to control and manipulate significant activities and use of time, as well as caregiver characteristics, placement, and specific environmental components. Although this is not feasible, and perhaps not ethical, a similar in vivo experiment is taking place in the "social experiment" of placing retarded individuals in community care facilities. Substantial numbers of retarded persons are currently being transferred from large state institutions to a variety of community care facilities. Thus, we have available different types of environments and a substantial population entering different types of environments, making possible a longitudinal study starting with initial exposure to a changed environment.

Given a variety of community care alternatives, it is possible, and necessary, to investigate the relationship between environment, activities, use of time, and social development. Our hypothesis is that different types of environments result in *different kinds of normalization and social competence outcomes.* The speculative literature provides support for this hypothesis; however, to date the effects of specific factors in the environment on social development have not been determined. Such information is essential to future planning, organization, and training required to optimize community care for the mentally retarded. Outcomes of community care are seen as being predicated upon three major groups of variables. These major groups are 1) preplacement factors, 2) community care facilities characteristics, and 3) type of care facility. A systematic assessment of *each*

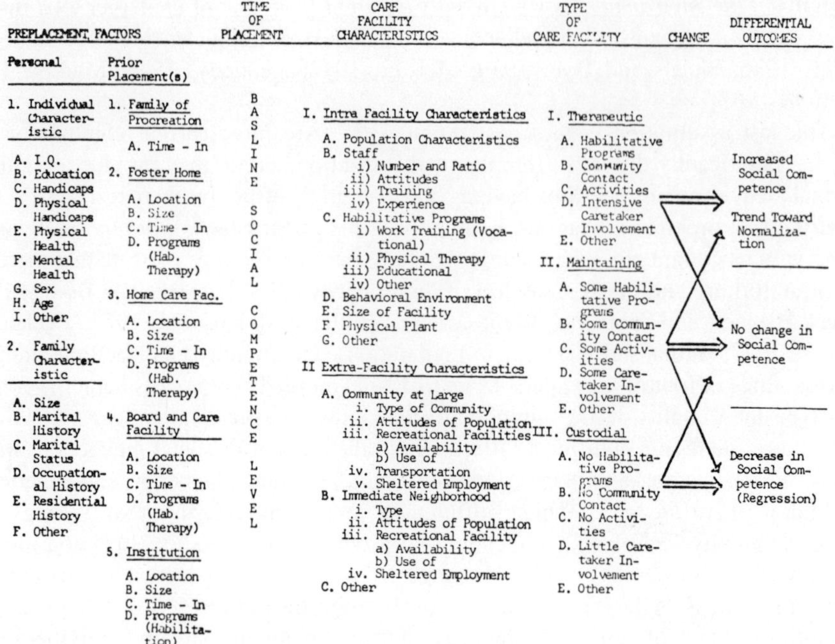

Figure 1. A model for the evaluation of alternative community care facilities.

of these major groups is essential to determine the relationship among environments and social competence outcomes.

Preplacement factors are those characteristics which the individual brings with him at the time of community care placement. Two categories of data are included under this heading shown in Figure 1. Individual characteristics include diagnosis, IQ, impairments, age, and family characteristics. Furthermore, preplacement information provides data on prior institutional or community care experience. In addition, level of social competence at the time of community care placement through such instruments as the Client Centered Evaluation Model (CCEM) provides baseline data against which competency levels over time can be examined by type of community care facilities. Assessment includes information about the facility as well as the characteristics of the surrounding neighborhood and community context.

Both individual changes and patterns of change in social competency in each facility are examined. At the individual level, the direction and magnitude of change in social competence relative to each individual's baseline social competence are determined. At the care facility level, *mean* changes and directions of change can be computed, and thus, patterns can be established that may be different from individual change. If individual changes are regressive for some individuals and progressive for others within the same facilities, whatever changes take place are primarily due to individual factors. On the other hand, if a facility shows a specific uniform pattern of change among its residents, factors in the environment of the facility are associated with this pattern and specific factor(s) related to these changes must be determined. Mean changes and direction of change provide a basis for comparing various facilities in terms of their effect on residents. A detailed analysis will provide information on which specific activities and use of time in the environment are related to successful outcome, i.e., an increase in social competence and achievement of normalization.

METHODS

The research model illustrated in Figure 1 assumes that there are preplacement factors—individual and family characteristics, prior placement history mediated by exposure to institutional and community based intervention programs—that lead to differentially successful social competency outcomes. The ''methods of procedure'' are devoted to evaluating this model.

Two interrelated research endeavors are necessary to evaluate this model: 1) observations in community care facilities, and 2) abstracted data from official records.

Sample

This research involves sampling 1) care facilities, 2) residents in each care facility, and 3) times of observation in each care facility.

Care Facilities A variety of community sources, including the Inland Counties Regional Center, the Riverside Mental Health Association, and the San Bernadino and Riverside Welfare Agencies, provided listings of community facilities with mentally retarded residents. A list of 171 care facilities was compiled of which 11 refused to participate. We completed interviews at 160 facilities in three counties: San Bernadino (85 facilities), Riverside (69 facilities), and Los Angeles (5 facilities); 53 facilities were located in rural areas, 91 in suburban areas, and 13 in urban locations.

Facilities ranged in population size from 1 to 95 residents, with the modal facility housing from three to six clients. The age range for the total population was as follows: 634 clients under age 18; 446 clients between 19 and 44 years of age; 116 clients between 45 and 64 years of age; and 24 clients over age 65.

Resident Sample The careprovider from each facility was interviewed. Using a schedule containing 260 questions, information was collected on the careprovider's education, experience, and attitudes; and the educational, social, recreational, and vocational programs within the facility. In addition, the interview asked about the utilization of community resources and other types of involvement with the community. The physical characteristics of the neighborhood and the facility itself were covered in the interview as well as by personal observation. In addition, observations of activities and time use, etc., were carried out on residents of facilities that were considered 1) therapeutic, 2) maintaining, or 3) custodial.

Time Samples Observations were conducted on random days of the week. Time sampling also included various times of the daily and weekly cycle and thus include a broad spectrum of activities and use of time. Observations provide data for control of variations in social space as well as in behavioral patterns.

Preplacement Factors

Preplacement factors deemed important in this research were explicated in Figure 1. Preplacement data were obtained primarily from available official records and community care placement forms. Protocols for the systematic gathering or preplacement data were designed with extensive input by practitioners, by research personnel at the Pacific State Hospital Research Group, the Developmental Disabilities Regional Planning Board, and the Client Centered Evaluation Model Research Group.[1]

Individual and Family Characteristics At the initiation of the project and for all new placements during the course of the research, we obtained prior history data for retardates in our sample. This included preplacement individual characteristic data such as diagnosis, IQ scores, educational experiences and attainment, ambulation and level of physical abilities and handicaps, mental health, and a variety of demographic characteristics such as age and sex. Similarly, family characteristics along the above indicated dimensions were obtained as well as size of family, birth order, marital history, occupational and educational history of parents, sibling data, IQ information, residential history, and so on.

Prior Placements In addition to individual and family procreation data, information about previous institutional and community care (e.g., foster homes, home care, board and care, etc.) was obtained. These data included the location, size, type of habilitation program, and so on.

Time of Placement: Social Competency

As a means of obtaining an objective measure of the level of competence of the mentally retarded, in preliminary pretesting (Knox, in preparation) we used items derived from a variety of scales measuring social competence: Nihara's Adaptive Behavior Scale (Nihara et al., 1969), and Doll's Vineland Social Maturity Scale (1965). In this project, the Vineland scale and either the Cain-Levine or the Nihara scale were administered to residents of various facilities. The first measures obtained were used as a *baseline* upon which to measure subsequent change. For those who were in a community care facility at the beginning of this project, a control for time in the facility can be made in subsequent data analyses; of course, for newly assigned residents, baseline data will coincide with their move to the community care facility.

Our major objective was to compare various *types* of care facilities and determine whether an increase in social competence took place across time. If normalization is taking place, we assume that it will be reflected in an increase in social competence and social skills; the baseline data measure allows such longitudinal *change analyses*.

Community Care Facility Characteristics

Preliminary observations indicate that there is considerable variation among care facilities in facility size, location, habilitative programs, and caregiver characteristics. Facilities

[1]Center for the Study of Community Perspectives, 3627A Canyon Crest Drive, Riverside, California. Client Centered Evaluation models are available upon request.

range in size from three residents up to a maximum of 95 residents. Locations of facilities vary from the proximity of the central business district of the city to isolated rural areas. Between these extremes are those facilities located in suburban and semirural areas. In some facilities there are well organized habilitative programs and extensive participation in sheltered workshops, and in others, neither exists (Butler, et al., 1975; Moore, et al., 1976). Some care facilities are operated by caregivers who have had both formal training and institutional experience in care of the retarded, and in others, the caregivers have not had training or experience with the retarded and have little knowledge about mental retardation.

Pretest observations indicate that the resident populations of facilities are relatively homogeneous in terms of initial characteristics. The IQ range is on the order of less than 30 points. Furthermore, all residents are ambulatory and remarkably uniform in terms of associated handicaps. On the other hand, in spite of these demographic similarities, there are considerable differences in behavioral patterns and social competence among residents of different care facilities. Initial demographic similarities are expected in that those first placed in alternative community care facilities represent the upper levels of social competence in state institutions.

A number of diverse factors seem to be significant to the normalization process. These include intrafacility factors such as the behavioral characteristics, physical plant layout and condition, and habilitative efforts. Also, extrafacility factors such as location, neighborhood characteristics, and available recreational facilities are important. However, these factors are significant only insofar as they are related to the retarded individual's life experience and placement outcome. Research, then, must be flexible and inclusive enough to take into account these variables, but at the same time be precise enough to discriminate those variables that are significant to positive outcomes.

Intrafacility Characteristics

Intrafacility characteristics were determined through the use of several forms specifically developed for that purpose.

1. Population characteristics were determined primarily from official records; however, observers also made note of population characteristics for cross checks with official data. Age, sex, number, length of time spent in the facility, ambulation, handicapped status, IQ, etc. are examples of important data obtained.
2. Residence profiles were developed for each community care facility, which summarized data concerning the physical setting in which the mental retardates are living. The systematically gathered data included the nature of the physical plant, e.g., size, number and size of rooms, living arrangements, and condition of the physical plant.
3. Caregiver profiles for each facility were collected through the use of questionnaires and in-depth interviews. In addition, data were obtained on the extent of knowledge about mental retardation and mental illness on the part of the caregiver and his staff. The behavior and activity patterns of the caregivers as they related to residents were observed concurrently with observations of the mental retardates in the facility. Primarily we are concerned with a) the caregiver's attitude toward the residents in terms of their retardation and their potential, and b) the caregiver's knowledge and

experience in mental retardation, the care of retarded individuals, and the development of programs, specific activities, and use of time in developing their social skills and competence. We hypothesized a systematic relationship between attitudes and background of caregivers and outcomes in terms of normalization and social competence.

4. The behavioral environment was examined in terms of the amount of time spent on different types of activities. This process established which types of activities constituted the major portion of the behavioral environment.

In view of these considerations, this research utilized the concept of *life space*. By life space is meant the physical, temporal, and social space utilized by an individual in the course of his life experience. For the purposes of this research, the concept is divided into the following specific components: a) temporal space, b) physical space, and c) social space; which has behavioral, attitudinal, and supportive components.

Temporal space is the time blocks allocated to different activities by the individual or by the caregiver or supervisor. *Physical space* is the physical plant and geographic area in which the retardate's activities take place. To discriminate between significant and nonsignificant environments, we have subdivided physical space into three categories: primary, secondary, and tertiary. *Primary physical space* is the geographic or physical area in which a major portion of the individual's activities take place. *Secondary physical space* is the geographic or physical areas into which the retardate frequently, but not routinely, moves. *Tertiary physical space* is the geographic or physical area that the retardate uses only once or on rare occasions. The most significant environment obviously is the primary physical space and, to some extent, secondary physical space.

By *social space* we mean the prevalent attitudes and range of social acts that take place within the temporal and physical space occupied by the retarded. Social acts include 1) acts initiated by and engaged in by retarded individuals directed toward others, either retarded or normal, 2) acts initiated by and engaged in by another person or persons, either retarded or normal, directed at the retarded individual, and 3) acts which occur between two or more other individuals in the presence of the retarded individual.

Social acts and physical movements become useful as analytic tools only when they have been classified into categories. Such categories have been developed for "normal" populations by Chapin, Brail, and others (Chapin, Butler, and Patten, in press). Our preliminary work indicates that these categories developed for normal populations have limited potential for use with retarded populations as a result of significant differences in behavior patterns. A set of behavioral categories for retarded populations was developed and modified on the basis of our exploratory work (available upon request). The currently used activity code has five major categories and some 80 subcategories within the major ones. These major categories were empirically developed on the basis of extensive observations in various community care facilities. Such a set of act categories is essential to activity analysis and the description of "typical" behavior systems prevailing within any given community care environment.

Social space may be divided into three components: 1) behavioral, 2) attitudinal, and 3) supportive. By the *behavioral component* is meant the behavioral systems or combinations of social acts which are predominant within a particular residence. It is within this framework that the individual retardate receives his cues and responds to perceived situa-

NAME ______ OBSERVATION
CASE ______ SCHEDULE ______
AGE ______ MEDICATION ______
TIME OF RELEASE ______ RESIDENCE ______
IQ ______
SEX ______
EMPLOYMENT

DATE ______
OBSERVER ______
OBSERVATION
PERIOD ______
CASE OBSERVATION ______

1=auto — private
2=bus
3=taxi
4=auto or bus inst.
5=walking

Page: ____

Time Start	Time End	Time Elapse	ACTIVITY DESCRIPTION	Number of Participants						Activity Code	Charact.	Sector code	Dist. from residence	Means of trans.	REMARKS
				Normal			Retarded								
				M	F	Total	M	F	Total						

Figure 2. Observational recording form.

OBSERVATION SCHEDULE

PAGE: ______

NAME ______ CASE# ______ DATE ______
SEX ______ EMPLOYMENT ______ OBSERVER ______
AGE ______ MEDICATION ______ OBSERVATION PERIOD ______
RELEASE DATE ______ RESIDENCE ______ CASE OBSERVATION # ______
IQ ______

ACT#	TIME	ACT CODE	ACTIVITY DESCRIPTION	1a	1b	2a	2b	3a	3b1	3b2	3c1	3c2	4a	4b	5a	5b

Figure 3. Observation schedule.

tions. It is clear that all acts, or units of behavior, are not equally frequent, nor are they equally significant. In this research we were interested in frequency of acts as well as in their significance to the retarded person. Behavior patterns were assessed by using participant observers. Observers classified observed behavior into activity categories and these were used to extract *modal behavior patterns,* i.e., behavior that is persistent, consistent, and frequent (a detailed description of the method is reported in Bjaanes and Butler, 1974). The observational recording form used in our study is shown in Figures 2 and 3. Furthermore, we developed a method which assesses the stimuli for the observed behavior. We examined activities in terms of whether they were generated by the retarded, the caregiver, or others in the environment.

By the *attitudinal component* is meant the attitudes of the caregiver or staff. We are particularly concerned with the attitudes of the staff and caregivers toward residents, type of care, discipline, and the process of "normalization." By the *supportive component* is meant the level of support and guidance provided for individuals in a care facility by the caregiver and staff, especially in terms of habilitation and "normalization." In addition, assessments were made of the "climate" of the setting. This assessment was concerned with the extent of supervised activities, frequency of absences, visits by relatives, resident participation in decision making, availability of medical care, and extent of medication used to control or depress the activity level of residents.

Data on the behavioral environment of the mental retardates were gathered through the use of a modified participant observation method involving the systematic recording of the following information: 1) when the activity took place, 2) a description of the activity, 3) who took part in the activity, i.e., number of retarded or number of normal individuals, 4) where it took place, 5) distance from the residence, and 6) means of transportation. Wide differences exist among community care facilities in time usage.

Further, each activity was coded as to the nature of the activity with the ultimate goal of systematically describing life styles of the mentally retarded in community settings. It is assumed that a variety of life styles are described and that these life styles are a result of the individual characteristics of mental retardates as well as the ''climate'' of a particular residential setting as affected by the caregiver and his staff, and of the opportunities present in the neighborhood sectors.

In addition, we assessed the extent to which the caregiver gave support in the sense of aiding individuals with personal care, finances, personal problems, and direction of activities. This assessment was made with rating scales, data being obtained through interviews of caregivers and by participant observation.

Extrafacility Characteristics

One of the expected outcomes of placing the retarded in community care facilities is that interaction with ''normal'' society will be enhanced and lead to normalization. Generally it is assumed that in facilities where there is a great deal of interaction with the surrounding community, there should be a greater amount of normalization.

Extrafacility characteristics are essentially concerned with the nature of the location and neighborhood of the board and care or family care facility. It is assumed that the immediate neighborhood is of crucial importance to the mentally retarded person. The retardates developing social skills and competence will be first tested in the immediate environment. Thus, we are concerned with the overall character of the street and neighborhood, dwelling types, type of businesses, deterioration and dilapidation present, presence of environmental hazards such as street traffic, ditches, and the like. The availability of outside recreational, commercial, and organizational facilities and activities is important in learning to deal with the community. In addition, the social class, age structure, and other demographic characteristics of the neighborhood are important to the mentally retarded person in his relationship to the larger society. Particular emphasis was placed in our research upon the neighborhood description in terms of location, condition, utilization (residential, business, rural, etc.),and potential for normalization related activities.

Also, the availability of transportation is seen as an important factor in normalization. An assessment was made of the availability of recreational facilities and of their use. In addition, we examined who used the available facilities, i.e., were they used exclusively by the retarded, or by the general population as well.

Thus, community opportunities for ''normal'' activities in the immediate environment were of particular interest since it was expected that only through expanded community activities would the mentally retarded become normalized.

Types of Community Care Facilities

Preliminary observations indicate that community care facilities can be categorized into three types: 1) custodial, 2) therapeutic, and 3) maintaining. *Custodial* residences are those in which little or nothing is done to achieve normalization, and in which a lack of organized and structured activities may lead to retrogression by facility residents. *Therapeutic* facilities are those in which there is an active, ongoing attempt at enhancing the normalization process. There is a constant effort through organized activities to increase social competence and skills of residents. In *maintaining* facilities, residents remain at more or less the same level of competence, i.e., little change takes place.

Preliminary determination of care facility type was made on the dimensions shown in Figure 4. Criteria were developed during the early phases of the project; they are somewhat rudimentary and are subject to refinement and modification when more extensive systematic data analyses are completed. Those care facilities that were identified as being custodial tended to have the patterns shown below, whereas therapeutic facilities were in direct contrast. These early findings suggest much closer analysis of factors that contribute to making a care facility either therapeutic, maintaining, or custodial; especially since they seem to be systematically related to the normalization process and development of social competence.

Specification of Outcomes

It can be safely assumed that measurable change can take place in levels of an individual's social competence and skill over time. Positive change may be seen as the acquisition of a larger vocabulary, social skills, and an increase in social competence. On the other hand, change may occur in the opposite direction, i.e., there is a decrease in vocabulary, social skills, and competence. It is assumed that different types of community care environments are associated with the development of different levels of skill and competence among their residents. At the initiation of the research project, baseline social competence data

	Care Facility Type		
Criterion	Therapeutic	Maintaining	Custodial
Habilitative Programs	+	+-	-
Community Interaction	+	+-	-
Recreational activities	+	+-	-
Sheltered workshop participation	+-	+-	-
Social Activities participation	+	+-	-
Resident participation in chores	+	+-	-
Active caretaker involvement in care	+	+-	-
Daily Activity routine	+	+-	-

Figure 4. Type of care facility.

were obtained for many individuals in our sample. Data on social competence is evaluated to determine 1) changes in social competence for each individual in the sample population, and 2) changes in social competence *patterns* in each care facility.

In this research, change in social competence is the primary dependent variable. As such, precision in measurement *and* analysis becomes of paramount concern. The research view changes from two points. One method of analysis uses raw scale score differences as a means of assessing change. Thus, if an individual at t_1 has a score of 40 on a social competency scale and at t_2 has a score of 55, a net gain of 15 will be recorded. Similarly, if in a care facility the following prevails:

	t_1 score	t_2 score	Difference	Change direction
Individual a	40	50	+10	+
Individual b	45	45	0	0
Individual c	50	60	+10	+
Individual d	55	60	+5	+
			+25	+3

then the mean net gain for this *facility* would be +6.25, i.e., a general increase of competence, and the overall pattern would be considered to be progressive with three persons recording positive change. Conversely, if the following pattern were to prevail:

	t_1 score	tb52 score	Difference	Change direction
Individual a	45	45	0	0
Individual b	50	40	−10	−
Individual c	40	35	−5	−
Individual d	60	55	−5	−
			−20	−3

then the facility would have a mean net loss of −5, and would be considered to have an overall retrogressive pattern, with three persons having negative changes.

In addition to these two polar types we would expect some care facilities to be static, i.e., there would be little or no change in social competency scores over time in terms of mean scores, in terms of deviation from the mean, and individuals. Another type would be one in which the mean scores changed relatively little but within which the deviation from the mean was extensive. This is the "mixed" type in which individual characteristics are of greater significance than facility characteristics. In those care facilities where the deviation from the mean is small, care facility characteristics are probably more significant. Deviation from mean change scores can thus be taken in part as an indicator of the relative importance of individual and care facility factors. On the basis of our early observations and tabulations, we expect deviations from the mean, in most cases, to be quite small, thus suggesting that such facilities are typical.

INTRAFACILITY ACTIVITIES

Clients living in a community care facility must utilize community opportunities to participate in outside normalizing activities. If not, the experience of the facility environment itself probably is not great enough to support the normalization process. Our data show that small facilities rarely utilize outside opportunities and that wide interaction with external settings is critically absent (Butler et al., 1975; Moore et al., 1976). Many small facilities are not providing the client with those activities considered necessary for individual development, and in effect are creating *socially isolated total institutions within the community*.

Care-provided interaction with clients *within* facilities varies with several important factors. Education of the caregiver influences both interaction and client opportunities more in a small facility than a large facility. Careprovider experience and attitudes were critical across family size. While experience has a negative effect on the amount of interaction, careprovider attitudes apparently create environmental support, or nonsupport of normalizing activities.

Careprovider attitudes were measured by a Therapeutic Orientation Scale measuring the careprovider's opinion of the capabilities of his/her particular clients and of the developmentally disabled in general. Confidence in client abilities and accomplishments, accompanied by specific means of achieving development, placed the careprovider in a "high" category; those seeing little or no potential for their clients' improvement were ranked lower.

Generally, a high therapeutic orientation was associated with both increased careprovider interaction and more outside activities for clients. However, previous careprovider experience negatively influences interaction with clients. The amount of time spent in related work experiences (e.g., nursing, technician, aide) and the length of time operating a facility has a dampening effect on interaction with clients.

Overall, the amount of *formal education* does not significantly affect the amount of careprovider interaction. This finding suggests that the Therapeutic Orientation Scale and previous experience are more important than formal education. However, these factors may all be related to size of facility, which has been shown to have an important impact on creating normalizing opportunities. In smaller family care homes, where the careprovider's influence may not be mediated by additional staff, the relative importance of education may be more evident. Careproviders with more formal education tend to interact more with clients in small facilities. The effect of education is apparent in utilization of outside activities for clients.

Perhaps of more interest is the extent to which specific types of behavior are participated in by clients within facilities. Table 1 illustrates such activity patterns in four community facilities by the five major coding categories referred to earlier.

Frequency of Specific Types of Behavior

Active leisure activities are those that involve playing games, doing craftwork, and dancing, and those that are goal-oriented. For this type of activity to occur, there must be considerable involvement on the part of the caregiver in terms of planning and supervi-

Table 1. Frequencies of observed acts falling in each activity category by percentage

Activity category	Board and care facility (%) I	Board and care facility (%) II	Home care facility (%) I	Home care facility (%) II
Active leisure	5.5	0.0	3.5	0.0
Passive leisure	12.5	37.1	15.7	3.6
Work and chores	6.9	0.0	14.0	1.2
Personal activity	18.0	9.7	28.1	6.0
Interaction	57.1	53.2	38.6	89.2
	100.0	100.0	100.0	100.0
Total of acts observed (*N*)	71	113	57	83

From Bjaanes and Butler, 1974.

sion. Table 1 shows that active leisure occurs rather infrequently, and not at all in one board and care and in one home care facility.

Passive leisure includes watching television, watching an activity take place, napping, staring into space, and nongoal-oriented behavior. This type of behavior requires little involvement on the part of the caregiver. The observed frequencies of passive leisure behavior were greater in all cases than were frequencies of active behavior. In contrast to the other care facilities, in one home care facility only 3.6% of all observed acts were of the passive leisure variety. Work and chores involve specific behavior such as cleaning, dusting, and cooking. This type of behavior was inconsistent between home care facilities and board and care facilities: in one board and care facility 6.9% of all observed activities were work and chores, whereas in the other board and care facility, no such behavior was observed.

Personal activities included grooming self, talking to self, talking to an inanimate object, and unintelligible mumbling. These activities were generally of an isolating type, not involving interaction with others. In terms of frequencies, there was a range from 6 to 28% in this kind of activity with no clear patterns of differences between the two types of community care facilities, although there was greater range within home care facilities. Interaction activities involved participation with others and included responses to suggestions, intelligible conversation, and physical show of affection. Of interest was the close similarity between the two board and care facilities, with a different of only 4%, as compared to the 51% between the two home care facilities.

In summary, activities participated in by retarded persons vary within as well as between board and care facilities and home care facilities. The greatest variation in facilities was in the proportion of behavioral acts that were socially interactive in nature. Slightly over half of the behavioral acts of retarded persons in both board and care facilities were interactive. However, in one home care facility, interactive behavior accounted for only 38.5% of the observed behavior, whereas in the other it accounted for 89.1%.

Percentage of Time Spent in Specific Types of Behavior

A different perspective on activities is shown in Figure 5 which presents the amount of time spent in each type of behavior, contrasted with frequency of occurrence. Here, instead of the number of acts as the unit of analysis, percentage of time spent in the activity is shown. The main effect is to reduce the apparent extent of social interaction and to increase the importance of other activity categories. Even so, Figure 4 and Table 1 give a rather similar picture of behavior taking place in a community care facility and, at the same time, illustrate rather large differences among facilities.

Overall, only 3% of time was spent in active leisure behavior, with only one care facility having a significant amount of time spent in such activities. Twenty-two percent of time was spent in passive leisure behavior, although there was considerable variation. Both home care facilities were similar and each had a relatively high amount of time spent in this type of behavior. Board and care facilities showed a greater variation, with one having an amount twice as large as the mean time spent in passive leisure behavior. Also, this facility was the one in which no active leisure behavior was observed.

The mean time spent on work and household chores was 8.0%. Both home care facilities showed some time being spent on this type of behavior, with one of the facilities having 22% of the time being spent on work and chores. In board and care facilities, work and chores took place in only one facility; however, the amount of time involved there was slightly greater than in one of the home care facilities.

Although there were significant differences among the four community care facilities in terms of the amount of time spent on personally oriented activities, there were no discernible patterns of difference between the board and care and the home care facilities, with variation within being as great as variation between. When passive leisure and personally oriented activity were combined, board and care facility II and home care facility I had a greater amount of time spent in behavior that tended to be isolated than did the other two care facilities. Social interactive behavior had a range of 55%, with the two board and care facilities being remarkably similar. There was, however, a significant difference between the two home care facilities. The amount of time spent on interactive behavior in one home care facility was almost twice the mean of 41%.

When comparing time usage for female and male populations, there were no significant differences in active and leisure activities. There was, however, a marked difference in work and chore behavior. In the home care facility with the female population, work and chores accounted for 22.5% of the time. In view of general patterns in society, perhaps this was to be expected. Although the amount of time spent by females in personally oriented behavior was relatively high, a greater amount of time was spent in this type of behavior by males in another facility, so there were no clear differences in this respect. There was a clear tendency for females to be less interactive and more socially isolated than males.

Characteristics of Activities

Two behavioral characteristics described earlier generally are individual characteristics: passing-natural and dependent-independent. The remaining are indicators of the care-

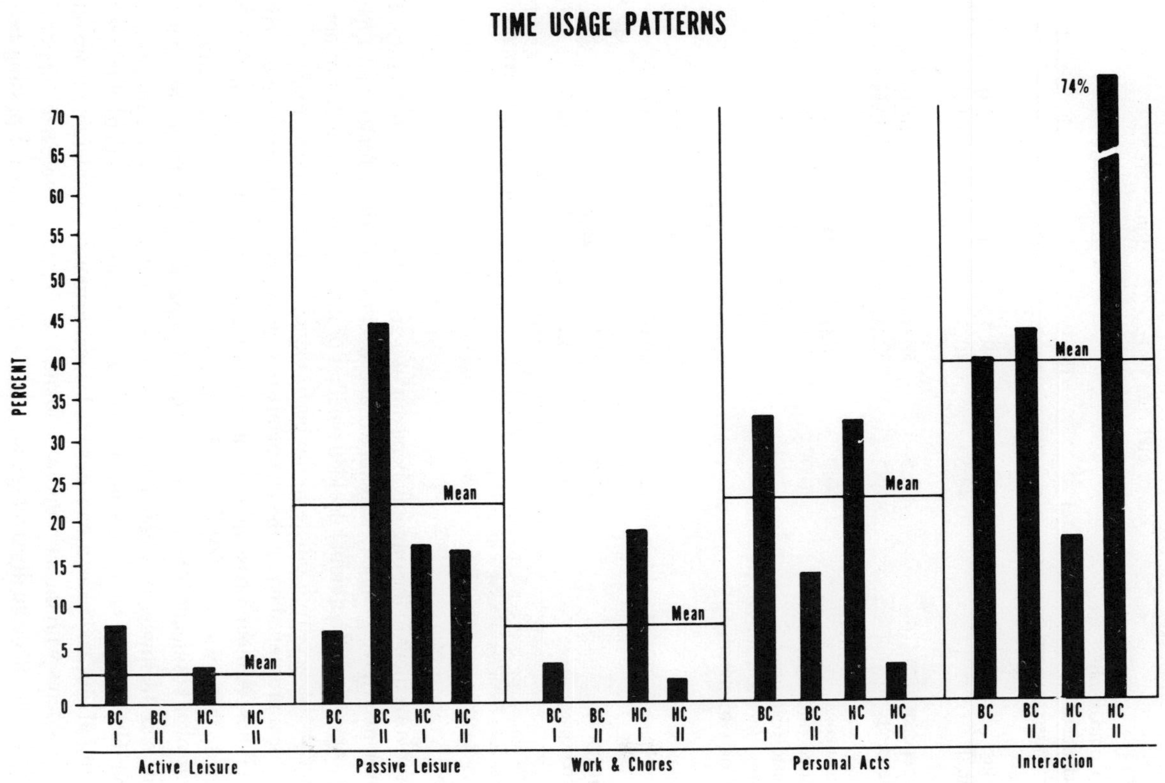

Figure 5. Time use patterns showing percentages of time spent in the different activity categories by the care facilities. BC, board and care facility; HC, home care facility.

Table 2. Characteristics of activities participated in by retarded persons in board and care and home care facilities

Comparison/ characteristics	Board and care (%)		Home care (%)			
	I	II	I	II	df	χ^2
One[a]					3	
Passing	51.5	59.5	43.0	39.0		
Natural	48.5	40.5	57.0	61.0		
Two					3	16.94[b]
Independent	83.5	68.0	59.5	65.0		
Dependent	16.5	32.0	40.5	35.0		
Three					9	37.39[b]
Spontaneous	90.0	98.0	74.0	94.5		
Planned (individual)	10.0	2.0	16.0	4.3		
Planned (caregiver)			10.0	1.2		
Routine (nonstructured)						
Routine (structured)						
Four					3	157.07[b]
Structured	8.0	1.0	38.0	85.0		
Unstructured	92.0	99.0	62.0	15.0		
Five					3	96.39[b]
Obligatory	15.0	27.8	28.0	85.5		
Discretionary	85.0	72.2	72.0	14.5		

[a]The chi square between care facilities was not significant but the chi square between board and care and home care facilities = 8.04 3 df, $p < 0.01$.
[b]$p < 0.001$.

giver's involvement in the ongoing behavior of a given community care facility. Thus, the caregiver may have planned, structured, and decided priorities for certain types of behavior, whereas the individual decided whether or not to pass and whether or not to accept cues and assistance from others in the performance of a given behavior.

Table 2 presents data on the characteristics of observed behavior in these community care facilities. Although passing-natural did not vary significantly when all facilities were compared, there was a significant difference between board and care and home care facilities, with residents of board and care facilities passing more frequently than residents of home care facilities. It is not clear at this point whether this was a function of size or location. However, it seems reasonable to assume that since both board and care facilities were centrally located in an urban area, and since there was considerably more interaction by their residents with the surrounding community, there was a greater "opportunity" to be accepted as intellectually average and thus a greater impetus for passing behavior.

Residents of board and care facilities tended to be somewhat less dependent, although one home care facility showed only a slightly smaller degree of such dependent behavior. This finding indicated that contact with the surrounding community reduced somewhat the need for cues and assistance from others. Perhaps this was related to the fact that only a minimal amount of observed behavior in board and care facilities was structured. It can be tentatively hypothesized that if the retarded person were presented with a structured situation (organized, planned, and prepared), he would be able to perform with a considerable degree of independence (guide himself in carrying out the game). Conversely, when posed with an unstructured situation, he would be more likely to depend on cues and assistance from others in the performance of the activity.

There were significant differences among care facilities in terms of the extent to which their activities were structured. As indicated earlier, only a small amount of the overall behavior in board and care facilities was structured, whereas in home care facilities, a substantial amount of the behavior was structured.

On the obligatory-discretionary characteristic, there was a significant difference among various care facilities. In one home care facility, virtually all activities were obligatory, whereas in one board and care facility virtually no activities were obligatory. There was a tendency for home care facility caregivers to structure a greater proportion of behavior as well as to require performance of the activity, thus making a considerable extent of behavior both structured and obligatory.

There was no significant difference between the frequencies of observed passing-dependent and independent behavior. There were some differences in frequencies of spontaneous and planned activities, with males tending to be more spontaneous than females. Activities in the home care facility with a male population were more structured and obligatory than in the facility for females.

CONCLUSIONS

To provide a normalizing environment, community care facilities must be activity-enriched with both internal programs and external contact and exchange. That is, the facility must be *therapeutic* as opposed to being a custodial or maintaining facility (Bjaanes and Butler, 1974). If normalization procedures are lacking, a deprived environment tends to develop which will effectively hinder the normalization process. Whereas this is obvious in large facilities, it is particularly critical in small care facilities which, by virtue of size, must include activities and external interaction to approximate a normal environment. Isolation in small care facilities results in a social setting populated only by developmentally disabled persons, thus restricting activities, the number of role models, and experiences necessary for normalization to occur. Some learning theory suggests that a wide range of behaviors are learned through the process of imitation. Furthermore, enriched environments provide increased stimuli for learning. If there are no normalizing activities available, the environment is deprived, the potential for normalization is negligible, and the facility is not fulfilling its intended function.

The results of this study, to date, clearly indicate several generalizations:

1. There are substantial differences in the utilization of community agencies, services, and programs by community care facilities, as well as variation in normalizing activities within facilities.

Generally, our data clearly indicate that, in our sample, interaction and exchange with the community is limited and intrafacility activities that could be considered as normalizing are restricted in most facilities. The size of the sample and the wide geographic dispersion indicate that this may be, in fact, a general characteristic of small care facilities as they are currently staffed and operated.

2. Variation in use of community agencies, services, and programs by community care facilities are associated with such factors as education and previous experience of the service providers, location of facility, size of facility, characteristics of the surrounding neighborhood, and extent of normalizing activities within facilities.
3. Larger facilities generally use agencies, services, and programs and have more internal normalizing activities; they thus appear to be closer to the objective of normalization and developing social competence than smaller facilities.

It has often been assumed, without carefully assessing the internal programs available and the extent of utilization of external community resources, that placing a developmentally disabled person in a community care facility is equivalent to providing a normalizing environment; however, *our data show otherwise*. This study so far shows quite clearly that if community care facilities are to provide normalizing environments, attention must be paid to the location, qualifications of service providers, and the nature and extent of internal programs and exchange with the community and utilization of community programs.

4. It cannot and should not be assumed that a community care facility is a priori a normalizing environment. That assumption is much too likely to result in a shift from larger total institutions to smaller, dispersed community based total institutions.

A custodial or maintaining facility that has few or no internal and external programs to facilitate the normalization process can be considered just as much a total institution as a large state institution. It must be recognized that for a facility to be considered as therapeutic and enhancing to normalization, internal and external programs must be planned, implemented, and evaluated.

REFERENCES

Baller, W. R. June 1936. A study of the present social status of a group of adults who, when they were in elementary schools, were classified as mentally deficient. Genet. Psychol. Monogr. 18.

Bennet, L., and Rudolph, L. 1960. Changes in direction of hostility related to incarceration and treatment. J. Clin. Psychol. 16(4):408–418.

Bjaanes, A. T., and Butler, E. W. 1974. Environmental variation in community care facilities for the mentally retarded. Am. J. Ment. Defic. 78:429–439.

Butler, E. W., and Bjaanes, A. T. 1977. A typology of community care facilities and differential normalization outcomes. In: P. Mittler (ed.), Proceedings of the 4th Congress of IASSMD. Vol. 1. Care and Intervention, pp. 337–347. University Park Press, Baltimore.

Butler, E. W., and Bjaanes, A. T. A model for the evaluation of alternative community care facilities. In preparation.

Butler, E. W., Bjaanes, A. T., and Hofacre, S. 1975. The normalization process and the utilization of community agencies, services, and programs by community care facilities. Preprint.

Butterfield, E. C. 1967. The role of environmental factors in the treatment of institutionalized mental retardates. In: A. A. Baumeister (ed.), Mental Retardation: Appraisal, Education and Rehabilitation. Aldine Publishing Company, Chicago.

Chapin, F. S., Jr., Butler, E. W., and Patten, F. C. Blackways in the Inner City. University of Illinois Press, Urbana, Illinois. In press.

Dentler, R. A., and Mackler, B. 1961. The socialization of institutional retarded children. J. Health Hum. Behav. 2(4):243–252.
Doll, E. A. 1965. Vineland Social Maturity Scale Manual of Direction. Condensed, Rev. Ed. Am. Guid. Serv., Inc., Minneapolis, Minnesota.
Edgerton, R. B. 1967. The Cloak of Competence. University of California Press, Berkeley.
Farber, B. 1968. Mental Retardation, Its Social Context and Social Consequences. Houghton Mifflin Company, Boston.
Kennedy, R. J. R. 1948. The Social Adjustment of Morons in a Connecticut City. Mansfield Sauthbury Training Schools, Social Service Dept., State Office Building.
Knox, L. Caretaker characteristics and variation in social competence. In preparation.
Kugel, R. B., and Wolfensberger, W. (eds.). 1969. Changing Patterns in Residential Services for the Retarded. President's Committee on Mental Retardation.
Lyle, J. G. 1959. The effect of an institutional environment upon the verbal development of institutional children: I. Verbal Intelligence. J. Ment. Defic. Res. 3:122–128, and 4:1013, 14–23.
McKay, B. E. 1942. A study of IQ changes in a group of girls paroled from a state school for mental defectives. Am. J. Ment. Defic. 46:496–500.
Moore, H., Butler, E. W., and Bjaanes, A. T. May 1976. Careprovider characteristics and utilization of community opportunities for mentally retarded clients.
Mundy, L. 1957. Environmental influence on intellectual function as measured by intelligence tests. Br. J. Med. Psychol. 30:194–201.
Nihara, K. R., Foster, M. S., and Leland, H. 1969. Adaptive Behavior Scales: Manual. Am. Assoc. Ment. Defic., Washington, D.C.
Nirje, B. 1970. Symposium on normalization: the normalization principle, implications and comments. Br. J. Ment. Subnormal. 62–70.
O'Connor, G., and Justice, R. S. 1973. National patterns in the development of community group homes for the mentally retarded. Paper presented at the 97th Annual Meeting of the American Association on Mental Deficiency.
Skeels, H. M., and Dye, H. A. 1939. A study of the effects of differential stimulation on mentally retarded children. Proc. Am. Assoc. Ment. Defic. 44:114–136.
Stedman, D. J., and Eichorn, D. 1964. A comparison of the growth and development of institutionalized and home reared mongoloids during infancy and early childhood. Am. J. Ment. Defic. 69:291–301.
Tizard, J. 1964. Community Services for the Mentally Retarded. Oxford University Press, New York.
Woloshin, A. A., Tardi, G., and Tobin, A. June 1966. The institutionalization of mentally retarded men through the use of a halfway house. J. Ment. Retard. 4(3):21.

Implications of Observational Methodology for Planning and Policy

chapter 17

Social Ecology and Ethology of Mental Retardation

Gershon Berkson

Formal study of the behavior of the mentally retarded began almost 200 years ago with Jean Itard's attempt to teach Victor the skills necessary for normal social living. He regarded the effort as a failure, but today we recognize his success: the demonstration of a theory-based method for dealing with a practical problem. The concept of sense training and the teaching devices he developed strongly influenced such apparently diverse areas as early childhood education and laboratory studies of the psychology of learning.

The next important step toward understanding occurred at the turn of the century with Alfred Binet's brilliant intuition that mentally deficient children not only have intellectual deficits but are slower than normal in their rate of behavioral development. The concept of mental *retardation* was born. Binet understood also that mental deficiency constitutes a failure in adaptation. He, like the American functionalists who took their inspiration from the theory of natural selection, regarded perception, learning, and cognition as central to adaptation. There were two major consequences of that view: a definition of mental deficiency that emphasized cognitive deficiencies was developed, and training programs to ameliorate cognitive deficits became the main goal of behavioral research.

In the last 70 years, diagnostic procedures have been developed in the laboratory and the clinic to help define the nature of cognitive deficits and to study how individuals differ in learning and thinking. Sophisticated learning theory has yielded spectacular improvements in performance, which have provided the basis for technologies to ameliorate behavioral deficits in practical situations.

ECOLOGICAL CONCEPT OF MENTAL DEFICIENCY

That is how things stood in the early 1960's. Then a revolution in thinking about mental deficiency occurred, which is now beginning to have important impact on mental retardation research. This revolution is best described by a discussion of change in definitions of mental retardation. Prior to 1960, low IQ was the main definer of mental retardation. The

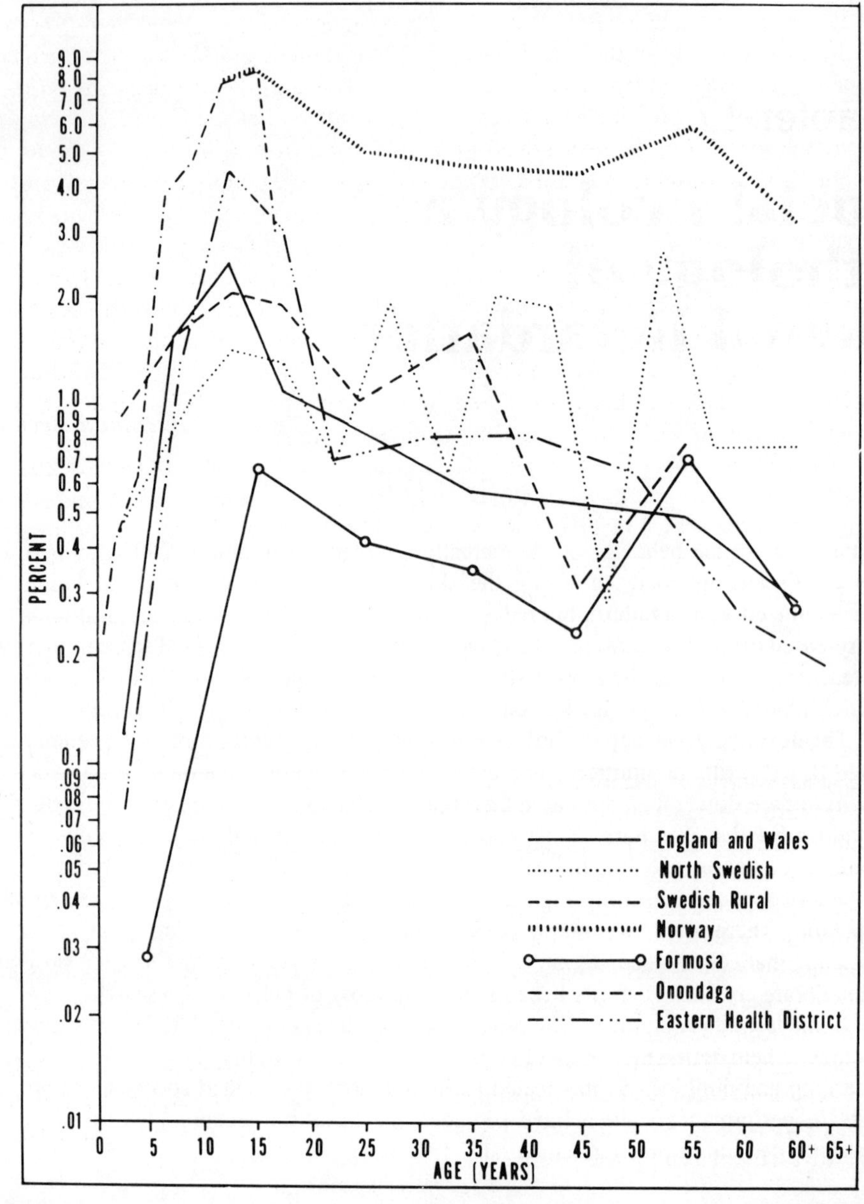

Figure 1. Results of seven community-wide surveys of mental retardation. Taken from Gruenberg (1964).

1960 definition of mental retardation introduced a new factor, social adaptation (Heber, 1961). This happened primarily because every survey of mental retardation had shown that prevalence of mental retardation changes with age. Prevalence rates increase from birth to about 12 years of age and decline thereafter (see Figure 1). This meant that a simple cognitive deficit or retardation notion predicting constant prevalence with age is not adequate. The variation in prevalence with age suggested that the degree of adaptation is a function not only of the individual's cognitive abilities but also of his environment (Gruenberg, 1964). For instance, junior high school makes greater demands on the intellect than does a preschool environment; the result is that more people are counted among the retarded in the later school years than early in development.

In combining failure of social adaptation with the more familiar criterion of low IQ, it was hoped that more valid criteria of adaptation could provide more precise bases for case management. To deal with this new concept, the American Association of Mental Deficiency developed the Adaptive Behavior Scales, which are widely used to define social adaptation. The scales are not completely successful as a defining characteristic of social adaptation because they continue to define mental deficiency primarily in terms only of the skills of the individual. This practice does not adequately follow the implications of the 1960 definition, which seemed to require a description of both the child's skills *and* the environment to which he is expected to adapt.

There are a number of reasons for this incomplete success. One is that those developing the scales were still caught in the ideology that retardation in development and a learning deficit are what mental retardation *is*. Although most clinical practice involves a description of both environments and behaviors, the classifiers had not yet begun to think ecologically. Another reason is that defining environments for taxonomic purposes is not so easily done. Imagine a fairly complete catalog of environmental factors that determine referral for mental retardation services. It would probably be tremendous. On the other hand, a start in this direction actually has been accomplished in the 1973 classification, which lists certain environmental demographic variables (e.g., family income) as a supplement for describing the characteristics of cases; this classification may aid in more precise assessment of adaptive behavior.

Perhaps the most important argument against using environments as definers of mental deficiency is the possible detrimental consequences for the delivery of services. Ecological concepts would involve a complication of planning by government and private services that would need ways of thinking that are not yet adequately worked out. This complication could result in inappropriate reduction of services. For instance, the development of early assessment programs and day care will probably result initially in an *increase* in the prevalence of mental retardation (before a reduction consequent on early training programs). It could be erroneously concluded that day care and early assessment ''cause'' mental deficiency, and there might ensue an inappropriate tendency to reduce such programs. Ecological thinking should therefore be used to describe cases more adequately, with an effort to explore ways of making the concepts clear, practical, and supportive of services for the retarded.

ECOLOGICAL RESEARCH STRATEGIES

How can this be done? Fortunately, we are not working in an intellectual vacuum. Ecological psychology, the community movement, service system sociology, and even ethology have been growing forces influencing the behavioral sciences during the last 20 years. Our conference, Application of Observational-Ethological Methods to the Study of Mental Retardation, is a reflection of these movements. The first of this series of conferences considered mental retardation services from the perspective of social scientists (Begab and Richardson, 1975). The last few days have had a different purpose. We have been exploring methods of studying ecological factors by a variety of behavioral observation techniques.

Most of us are psychologists interested in studying development and its disorders. Some of us have been describing behavior in natural settings for years, but most of us are experimental psychologists who are turning from the study of cognitive and social processes in relatively simple laboratory situations to the observation of complex events in homes, schools, service agencies, and the community at large.

The naturalistic orientations of ecological psychology, anthropology, and ethology have guided our discussions. They express the faith that studies in natural habitats can provide us with more valid answers than was possible when we worked only in the laboratory. They emphasize the ecological notion that descriptions of the environment as well as of the behavior of individuals in them constitute the phenomena to be studied, and they direct us toward the use of multivariate and interactional methods of design.

A central issue was the scope of the question that should be asked. Opinions varied. Some felt that the best approach was to describe as fully as possible every significant event in the child's life through combined description of details in his environment and of his behavior. In this approach the investigator is a recorder of events as they happen, and the organization of the events emerges naturally in the data analysis phase of the research.

Others believed that a more focused strategy is necessary. Defining major phenomena of interest, developing hypotheses about how they work, and choosing appropriate measures were seen as not only more intellectually satisfying and scientifically useful but also more economic of effort, time, and money. Furthermore, this more active strategy was seen as more likely to provide the scientific basis for social change than would a passive recording of events.

The apparent conflict in these positions was resolved by the agreement that two elements are necessary for understanding significant events. It is necessary to analyze causes, perhaps first through analyses of sequences of natural events, but ultimately, it is hoped, by gaining control of the phenomena through manipulation of antecedent events. To establish significance, the events in question must be shown to be important for adaptation in everyday life.

Whether the process is done consciously or not, by a single person or by many individuals working on a problem, each investigation ideally involves four major processes. The first is a qualitative description of major events occurring in natural environments. The approach involves seeing the situation from as many perspectives as possible. Sampling adequately across subjects and situations, use of informants, and participant observation are all features of this qualitative phase.

Qualitative description permits one to identify major important behaviors and environmental variables. However, it lacks quantitative precision and is ambiguous with regard to causal relationships. The second step is a specification of the frequency, duration, and order in which natural events occur. This involves a selection of behavioral events and characteristics of the environment to be recorded, followed by disciplined observation procedures with demonstrated observer and event reliability.

From this second process emerges the possibility of a third step, causal analysis. Finding different distributions of events in different situations allows one to think about the possible environmental factors determining these differences. Predictability among events through patterns of association in time permits one to imagine that the events are connected by a unifying process. The results of these interaction analyses undoubtedly provide more important descriptions of events than do the raw frequency and duration data derived in the second process. They are also important in the development of units of description for further study.

The fourth process cannot be called the most important because it depends on the quality of accomplishment in the previous three. However, it is the culminating stage that ensures true understanding and verifies the significance of the research. In this process, a change agent manipulates one or a group of events and measures the consequence of that manipulation. (The term ''change agent'' is used rather than ''experimenter'' because this stage is not only done in the laboratory, but also occurs frequently in natural settings when, for instance, new training procedures or other institutional arrangements are imposed.) Here again, disciplined, multivariate, multisituational observational methods of the kinds used in the third process are appropriate—and perhaps necessary—if one wishes to obtain a sophisticated understanding of the manifestations of causal events.

These four processes are the components of a full analysis. Of course, they ordinarily occur simultaneously with feedback between them. Proceeding through them requires ''common sense and hard work'' and also a long term commitment to the solution of what inevitably is a complex problem. Constant revision of hypotheses and categories of observation, without loss of the sense of the central issue of the research, is necessary for full success. In this area of investigation, the single isolated study has little place.

Given the basic strategy, we asked what types of data are useful and how events are to be classified. The answer was both simple and complex. On the one hand, the data taken are dictated by the questions asked and by the stage of the research. On the other hand, most people agreed that no behavioral taxonomy could ever be a complete description of all behaviors, nor could it be totally free of bias since it inevitably must reflect the categories used in approaching the problem. Purely physicalistic behavior units similar to those used in animal research were seen as appropriate at the initial stages of some research and at all stages for some populations (e.g., very young children and the profoundly retarded). However, as thinking about a problem proceeds, and relationships among behaviors and between behaviors and antecedent and consequent events become clear, these relationships can define the categories. More abstract and more heuristic categories can emerge as a result. For these more complex phenomena, the sequences of units themselves become the units of behavioral analysis. Varieties of tool use, semantic categories in language, and behavioral reflections of complex processes such as cognitive executive functions and animism are all examples that bring description out of the level used by ethologists in animal studies. This conference has demonstrated that complex environmental events such as parent attitudes, demographic indices of social organization, and cultural and historical variables are all necessary for full understanding. However, there is strong feeling that these complex sources of data need to be used with full consideration given to their degree of demonstrated reliability and validity, lest the promise of significance inherent in these abstract processes be denied by lack of attention to adequate procedure.

APPLICATIONS OF ECOLOGICAL METHODS TO MENTAL RETARDATION

Up to this point, I have tried to distill the sense of the conference with regard to the discussion of method. It remains now to relate the research described to the problems of research with the mentally retarded and to ask how this research might promote the quality of their lives.

Very little multivariate observational research has been done with the mentally retarded. A recent review (Berkson and Landesman-Dwyer, 1977) of 20 years of research with the severely and profoundly retarded (with whom one might expect much observational research) cited over 500 empirical studies, but less than 5% of the studies could be described as observational and few of those were more than pilot efforts. Most research with the retarded employs standardized tests, rating scales, or measurement of one response in a single highly controlled environment. Examples are the many comparisons of intellectual level or etiological category, surveys of attendant attitudes, and some form of task analysis and skill teaching paradigm. Missing is any direct observational account of the interaction of situations, individuals, and behaviors in a description of environment-behavior interactions.

The power of the latter approach in providing basic information about environments and the people in them was clearly demonstrated in the studies presented at this conference. Interaction analyses were shown to be more powerful descriptors than simple frequency counts. They are probably also more sensitive than rating scales and standardized tests. They could certainly be employed, not only in descriptions of environments, but also in evaluations of the effects of drugs, skill training techniques, and early assessment and intervention programs. Although still exploratory, their use in analyzing small group relationships in which the retarded are involved appears very promising. The methods have been demonstrated in family interactions, peer groups, and staff-client interactions, but the related literature is limited primarily to the pioneering efforts of the participants in this conference.

Beyond its use in applied psychology and small group social behavior, direct observation can be most useful in studies germane to the planning and administration of service systems for the retarded. Moving large numbers of the retarded from rural institutions to urban communities provides an opportunity to study the consequences of involuntary resettlement on the adaptation of intellectually limited persons. Furthermore, essentially comparable groups of the retarded living in environments of many sizes and types of social organization permit a look at the effects of size and organizational factors on long term affiliative relationships. Whether teachers and other staff function as parent surrogates, how they fulfill their training roles, and how they serve as agents of society in relating to deviant populations are questions whose answers would reveal the nature of the relationship between normal and deviant individuals in complex societies.

Under what conditions a disabled child is either a cohesive or a disruptive force in families and other groups is an old question that requires much more work because of the contradictory literature. How skill training adds or detracts from adaptation is a question that has produced many assertions, but these opinions have thus far had little empirical basis.

These are global questions that probably have no simple answers. Unfortunately, answers to these and to many other questions of practical significance are assumed without empirical support by academics, professionals, citizen advocates, and program administrators. Using assumptions rather than demonstrated principles to form the character of services leads to faddishness and shoddy programming that is expensive and undoubtedly the cause of much human suffering.

Given the will, alternatives would not be very difficult to develop. Direct observation is a growing possibility for monitoring service quality and providing an information input for program planners. These data sources probably would be no more expensive than those currently being developed so rapidly to manage fiscal resources. They are not now being widely developed because efficient and valid methods of direct observation in practical contexts have hardly been demonstrated.

This conference has shown that the basis for such a technology exists. What is missing are the questions. That is probably because there are not many people interested in asking them, although the conference has demonstrated that there are some. Perhaps our gathering here will help to stimulate more. Maybe those questioners will be people who, like Jean Itard, can see significant theoretical issues in practical problems and see also that the only way to solve those problems is to understand them.

REFERENCES

Begab, M., and Richardson, S. 1975. The mentally retarded and society. University Park Press, Baltimore.

Berkson, G., and Landesman-Dwyer, S. 1977. Behavioral research on severe and profound mental retardation (1955–1974). Am. J. Ment. Defic. 81:428–454.

Grossman, H. 1973. Manual on terminology and classification in mental retardation. Am. Assoc. Ment. Defic., Washington, D.C.

Gruenberg, E. M. 1964. Epidemiology. In: H. A. Stevens and R. Heber, (eds.), Mental Retardation, pp. 259–306. University of Chicago Press, Chicago.

Heber, R. 1961. A Manual on terminology and classification in mental retardation. Am. J. Ment. Defic. Monogr. Suppl. 2nd Ed.

Index